anatomy of
YOGA FOR BEGINNERS

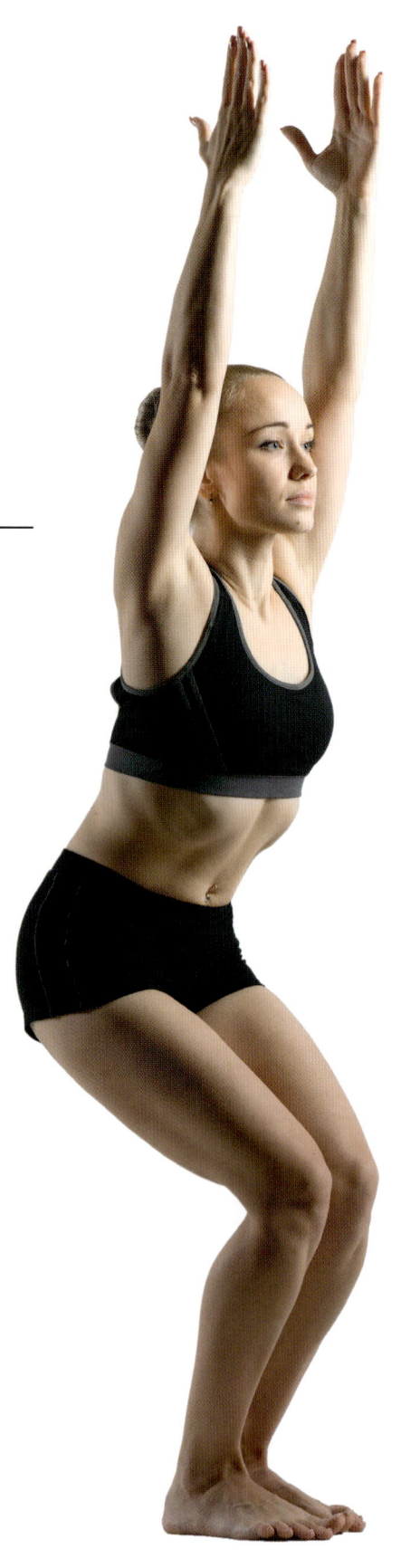

anatomy of
YOGA FOR BEGINNERS

Lisa Purcell

General Disclaimer

The contents of this book are intended to provide useful information to the general public. All materials, including texts, graphics, and images, are for informational purposes only and are not a substitute for medical diagnosis, advice, or treatment for specific medical conditions. All readers should seek expert medical care and consult their own physicians before commencing any exercise program or for any general or specific health issues. The author and publishers do not recommend or endorse specific treatments, procedures, advice, or other information found in this book and specifically disclaim all responsibility for any and all liability, loss, or risk, personal or otherwise, which is incurred as a consequence, directly or indirectly, of the use or application of any of the material in this publication.

Created by: Moseley Road Inc.
Editorial Director: Lisa Purcell
Art Director: Lisa Purcell , Adam Moore
Edited by: Finn Moore
Production by: Adam Moore

All rights reserved. No part of this publication may be reproduced, stored in a retrieval system, or transmitted, in any form or by any means, electronic, mechanical, photocopying, recording, or otherwise, without the prior permission of the copyright holder.

ISBN: 978-1-62669-178-0

Printed in China

CONTENTS

THE BASICS OF YOGA 8
    Yoga for the Mind & Body 19
    The Yoga Class 12
    Yoga at Home 14
    Yoga Tools 16
    The Language of Yoga 18
    Yoga Breathing 22
    Hand Gestures 28
    Full-Body Anatomy 30

STANDING POSES 34
    Mountain Pose (Tadasana) 36
    Prayer Pose (Pranamasana) 38
    Upward Salute (Urdhva Hastasana)) 40
    Awkward Pose (Utkatasana) 41
    Twisting Chair (Parivrtta Utkatasana) 42
    Tree Pose (Vrksasana) 44
    Garland Pose (Malasana) 46
    Eagle Pose (Garudasana) 48
    Triangle Pose (Trikonasana) 50
    Extended Side Angle Pose (Utthita Parsvakonasana) 52
    Low Lunge Pose (Anjaneyasana) 54
    High Lunge 56
    Warrior Pose I (Virabhadrasana I) 58
    Warrior Pose II (Virabhadrasana II) 60
    Warrior Pose III (Virabhadrasana III) 62

FORWARD BENDS & BACKBENDS 64
    Standing Toe Touch 66
    Standing Half Forward Bend (Ardha Uttanasana) 67
    Head-to-Knee Forward Bend (Janu Sirsasana) 68

Seated Forward Bend (Paschimottanasana) 70
Wide-Legged Forward Bend (Prasarita Padottanasana) 72
Extended Puppy Pose (Uttana Shishosana) 74
Cat Pose to Cow Pose (Marjaryasana to Bitilasana) 76
Upward-Facing Dog Pose (Urdhva Mukha Svanasana) 78
Cobra Pose (Bhujangasana) 80
Bow Pose (Dhanurasana) 82
Bridge Pose (Setu Bandhasana) 84
Camel Pose (Utrasana) 86
Reverse Tabletop Pose (Ardha Purvottanasana) 88
Fish Pose (Matsyasana) 90
Half-Frog Pose (Ardha Bhekasana) 92

SEATED POSES & TWISTS 94

Easy Pose (Sukhasana) 96
Staff Pose (Dandasana) 98
Bound Angle Pose (Baddha Konasana) 100
Bound Angle Pose with Forward Bend (Baddha Konasana Uttanasana) 101
Fire Log Pose (Agnistambhasana) 102
Cow-Face Pose (Gomukhasana) 104
Half Lotus Pose (Ardha Padmasana) 105
Full Lotus Pose (Padmasana) 106
Boat Pose (Paripurna Navasana) 108
Bharadvaja's Twist (Bharadvajasana I) 110
Marichi's Pose (Marichyasana) 112
Half Lord Of The Fishes (Ardha Matsyendrasana) 114
Reclining Twist 116

ARM SUPPORTS & INVERSIONS 118

Upward Plank Pose (Purvottanasana) 120

CONTENTS continued

    Plank Pose 122
    Four-Limbed Staff Pose (Chaturanga Dandasana) 123
    Side Plank Pose (Vasisthasana) 124
    Locust Pose (Salabhasana) 126
    Upward-Facing Bow Pose (Urdhva Dhanurasana) 128
    Supported Shoulderstand (Salamba Sarvangasana) 130

RESTORATIVE POSES 132
    Child's Pose Pose (Balasana) 134
    Downward-Facing Dog Pose (Adho Mukha Svanasana) 135
    Knee-to-Chest Pose (Apanasana) 136
    Corpse Pose (Savasana) 138
    Hero Pose (Virasana) 139

YOGA FLOWS 140
    Putting it all together 142
    Sun Salutation A 144
    Novice Flow 146
    Extended Novice Flow 148
    Spinal Flow 152
    Balanced Flow 154

Muscle Glossary 156
Index of Pose Names 158
Credits & Acknowledgments 160

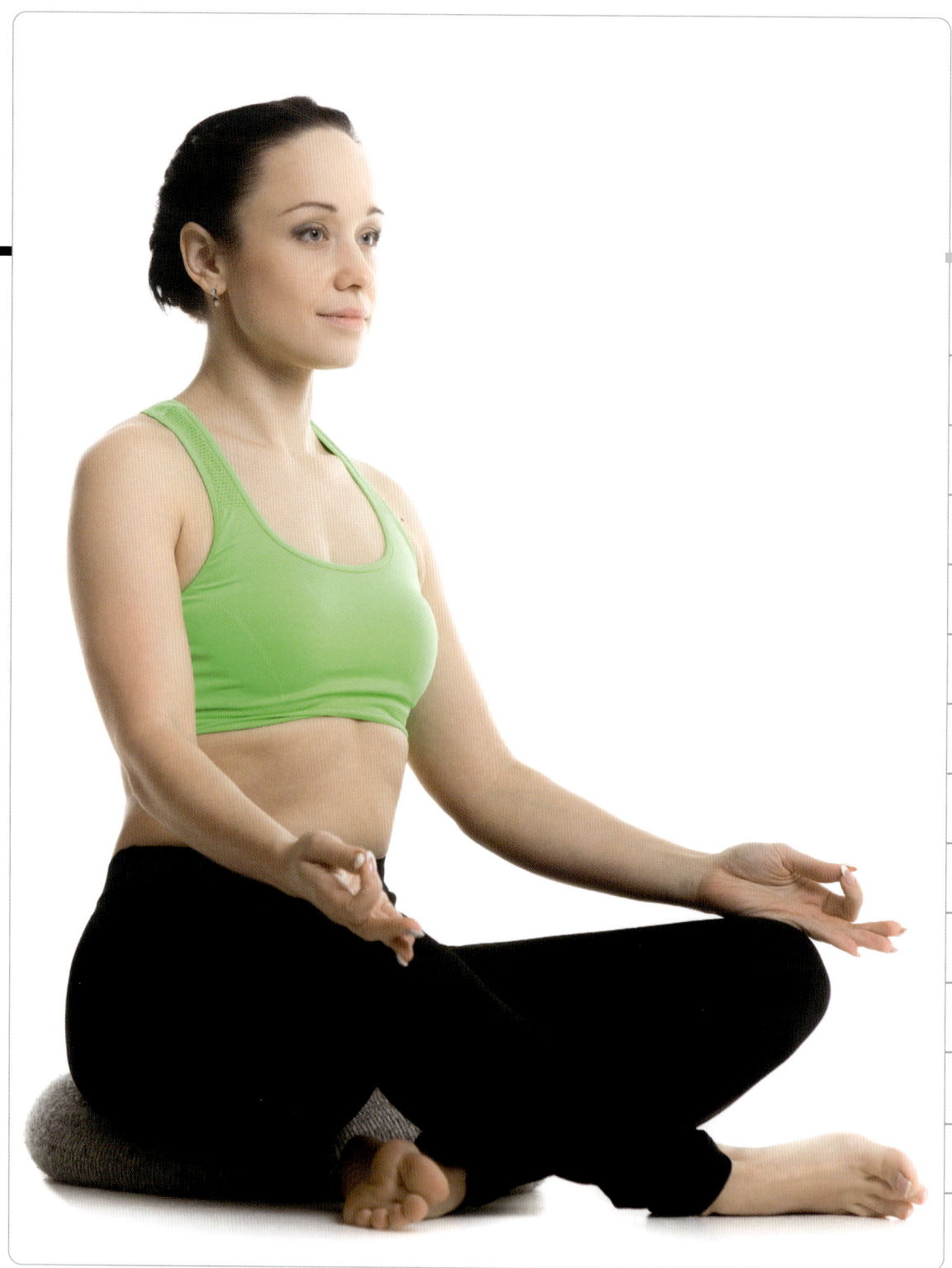

THE BASICS OF YOGA

With an ancient lineage that traces back thousands of year to India, the practice of yoga involves our entire beings—our bodies, our minds, and our spirits. By combining breathing techniques and a series of poses, students of yoga refresh all three. This venerable system is today one of the most popular ways of both getting physically fit and gaining mental clarity in today's stressful world.

Yoga for Beginners is your introduction to this practice, taking you first through the basics, such as where to practice, common yoga tools and lingo, hand gestures, and the all-important breathing techniques. Later chapters feature a range of poses common to many yoga disciplines that are suitable for a novice practitioner. Photos and anatomical illustrations guide you through the poses, with the muscles strengthened or stretched in each pose highlighted. There are also handy tips to help you achieve and hold each pose and that note each pose's focus to better allow you to target certain areas of your body, along with a section that helps you pull them altogether in flowing sequences.

YOGA FOR THE MIND & BODY

YOGA BASICS

Undertaking a yoga regimen can be transformative. The decision to include this practice in your daily life not only disciplines your body, it also helps you discipline your mind and rejuvenates your spirit.

Yoga is certainly a physical practice—even the easiest poses demand mental focus and muscle control. This self-control can help you in all aspects of life. Yoga transcends the physicality of the poses, aligning bodily control with control of the spirit and mind. In yoga, we are looking to calm the erratic fluctuations of the mind.

EXIST IN THE PRESENT

Too often we tend to focus our thoughts on the past and the future—even while our bodies are firmly grounded in the present. We have to concentrate to keep our thoughts in the present moment. Yoga teaches us that skill, so that we are more fully present on a daily basis.

BEGIN YOUR JOURNEY

This book contains a well-balanced selection of beginner poses that build strength and flexibility, while improving your concentration and willpower. As you come to master these poses, you will learn to control your body with your mind, and with that ability, you can begin to understand that, as in life, with time and patience you can overcome many obstacles. As you practice a pose, you will often feel as if your mind wants to give up before your body really needs to come out of a pose. If you listen to your body, you will learn to distinguish between pain and discomfort. Actual pain from an injury certainly signals that you should come out of a pose, but if what you feel is just discomfort, try breathing through it. While practicing a pose, you will, at times, feel intense sensations in certain muscles—this is normal while holding a yoga pose. Here then, you need to learn to ignore what your mind is telling you. Move beyond thinking, "I can't hold this any longer." Believe that your body is strong enough to hold the posture just a bit longer. By holding a pose even a few extra breaths, you will begin to build inner strength. You are stronger than you ever imagined.

SAVOR THE MOMENT

We live in a world of instant gratification, but that gratification is too often shallow amusement. By practicing yoga—working on the poses even when they become a bit uncomfortable—you will build patience. You will find that you can take a step back, pause, and breathe. Turn off your phone for an hour, and roll out your mat; the results will be worth it. When you finish your practice, you will have the

YOGA FOR THE MIND & BODY • THE BASICS OF YOGA

satisfaction of knowing that there is more than instant gratification; you will understand that you can take an hour to ignore your to-do lists and shut out other distracting thoughts, making an important decision to focus on your breath and the alignment of your body. The lessons learned on the yoga mat will translate into your daily life; you will come to realize that no challenging situation lasts forever—just as every yoga posture eventually ends. Yoga teaches you how to be completely present in every moment of your life, whether it is a good time or a bad one. Worrying about the future or dwelling on the past only elevates stress levels. Often the stress you feel is just triggered by the thoughts in your head—the moment you are actually in may not actually be all that stressful. With your yoga practice you will see that by changing how you think about things you can change your outlook. So give yourself an extra moment to pause, and take a deep breath.

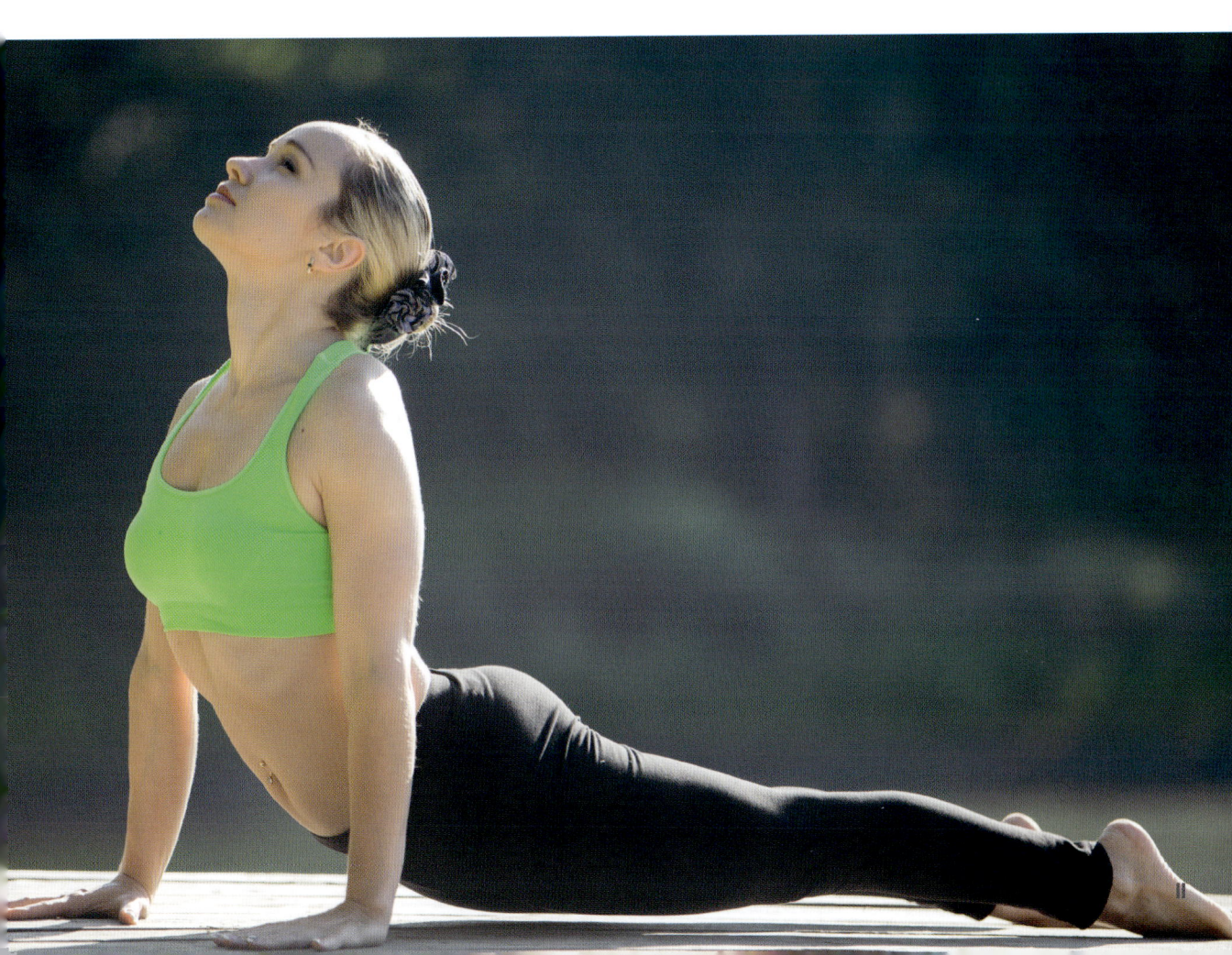

THE YOGA CLASS

Many of us begin our yoga journey by signing up for a class at a local yoga studio or gym. Yoga classes, however, are unlike other fitness classes. Here are some of the things you can expect as an uninitiated student.

Wherever it is held, a typical yoga class will call for students to spread out in organized rows positioned at least an arm's-length apart. Start by unrolling your mat so that the edges curl down toward the floor. Remove your shoes and socks—yoga is traditionally performed barefoot, which allows you to engage the toes, heels, and muscles of your feet. A typical gym or health club class often primarily focuses on the physical aspects of yoga, but those held in a dedicated yoga studio will likely emphasize all three aspects of yoga: body, mind, and spirit. To begin, the teacher might go over breathing methods—the pranayamas—lead a call-and-response chanting session, introduce you to the basics of meditation, or read a passage from an inspiring text. How much of this supplementation is included in a class depends on which yoga discipline your teacher practices. Before you enroll in a class, have a chat with the teacher so that you can decide whether you want a class that is strictly physical or one that incorporates a more spiritual approach. Whichever approach you decide upon, always remember that in yoga, it is the student who determines the extent of any pose, not the teacher.

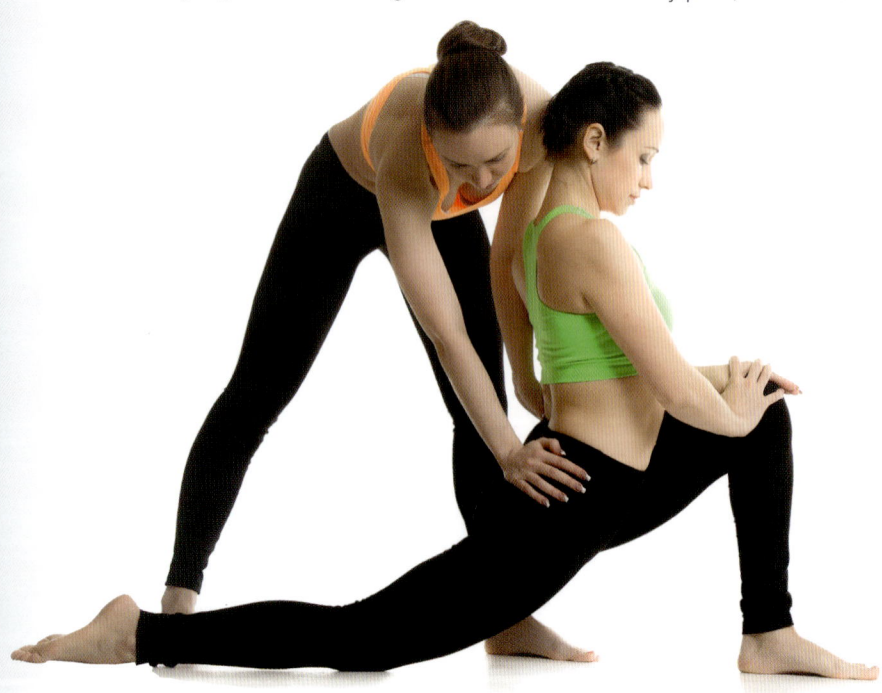

THE YOGA CLASS • THE BASICS OF YOGA

THE FLOW OF A CLASS

Classes are held both indoors and outside (many parks sponsor outdoor yoga classes in the warm months. Whatever your venue, before you begin, If this is your first yoga class, inform the teacher if you have any specific health issues or if you are pregnant or recovering from an injury or surgery, for instance. A beginner class starts with some warm-up poses, and then moves on to more challenging positions. Ease yourself into the discipline, and, at any point, you can modify a pose to suit your own comfort level, or you can ask the teacher for a less-difficult variation. If you need to rest, assume Child's Pose—knees bent, torso folded down, your chin on the floor, and your arms relaxed out in front of you or along your sides—to rejuvenate before joining in once more.

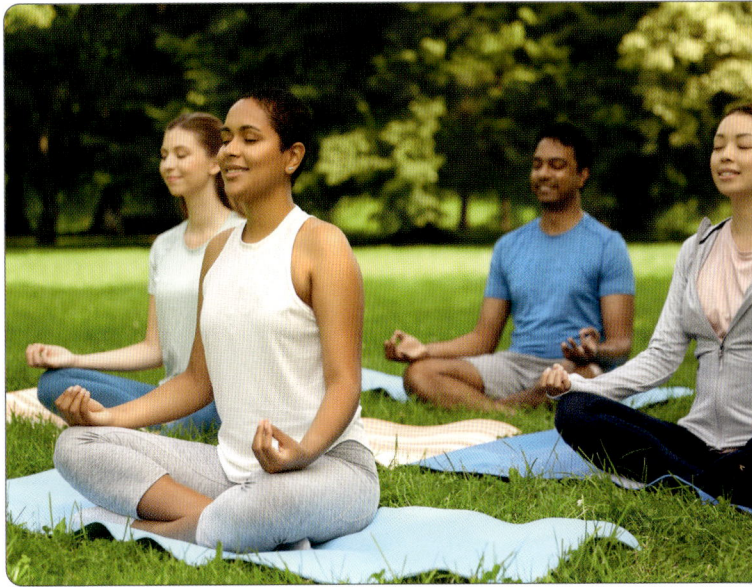

At the end of a session, you will rest for several minutes in Corpse Pose, lying flat on your back, with your arms and legs slightly outspread. After the physical effort of a session, you will likely experience a heightened awareness of your body as the outer world recedes. Don't hurry to rise from Corpse Pose—the change can be jarring. Once refreshed, rise up slowly, and, once you are upright again, thank your instructor, and gather up your supplies to leave your space as pristine as it was when you began.

YOGA IS A PRACTICE

We all have our own natural levels of strength and natural flexibility. Too often, people look at yoga poses and feel they are just not flexible enough to attain them. Yet, this is why we call yoga a "practice"—we can work on our bodies to improve ourselves. Each of us has a tendency toward either being more flexible or having tighter muscles, and in yoga we're trying to find that balance between our strength and our flexibility. Remember that your body and mind are constantly changing and evolving—every time you come to your mat you will feel differently than you did the last time.

This mutability is what keeps the yoga practice interesting. You will find that even as you perform the same poses time and time again, each time you will find something new to work on. As you master the beginner poses, you will be ready to take on the greater challenges. Yet, an advanced practitioner is not necessarily someone who can easily come into the most challenging poses; being advanced is having the body awareness and control to work the subtleties of each pose.

YOGA AT HOME

YOGA BASICS

Yoga is particularly suited to at-home practice, and it can afford you a sense of refreshment and renewal as you begin your day or a sense of peace and calm as you end it.

For home practice, all you really need is a mat, although beginners will find that a yoga block and a strap will help them attain the more challenging poses. Wear a comfortable clothing that allows a full range of movement, and leave off the socks. Practicing in bare feet will help you ground your hands and feet into the floor.

You can choose to practice poses you've already learned, or follow along with this book or an online tutorial.

A SPACE TO PRACTICE

To get the most out of your yoga regimen, dedicate a particular area within your home as your yoga space, where you practice on a regular schedule. For many, the greatest challenge to at-home practice is learning to shut out all of the potential distractions: your phone, computer, television, family members, and pets can all interfere with your concentration. If you live in a large house or apartment, you may have the luxury of transforming an entire room into a private yoga studio. The great thing about yoga, though, is that you don't need a lot of space—just the length of a yoga mat. Those in smaller spaces can still create a peaceful sanctuary in an area large enough to fully stretch and lunge freely, without obstructions. A movable screen, just as a folding Shoji screen, can lend you privacy, as will curtains or drapery that you can easily open and close.

SET THE MOOD

To keep your focus on your yoga practice, you need to create an oasis in which you can block out those distractions. Designate a room or area where you will always practice. If possible, the space should be free of clutter. Store your yoga mat and other gear within this space for easy access, and don't forget the atmosphere-setting extras. Calming colors, air-purifying houseplants, pretty stones or other natural objects, some mood lighting, and pleasing scents will encourage fruitful practice. A captivating image that you can meditate on or a flickering candle for your eyes to lock onto while you hold that pose just a few breaths longer can add to your yoga experience.

STICK TO A PLAN

Make a schedule for yourself, setting aside perhaps 30 minutes at the same time every day, five days a week for your yoga practice. When traveling, you can pack your mat in your suitcase, and then roll it out wherever you are.

YOGA AT HOME • THE BASICS OF YOGA

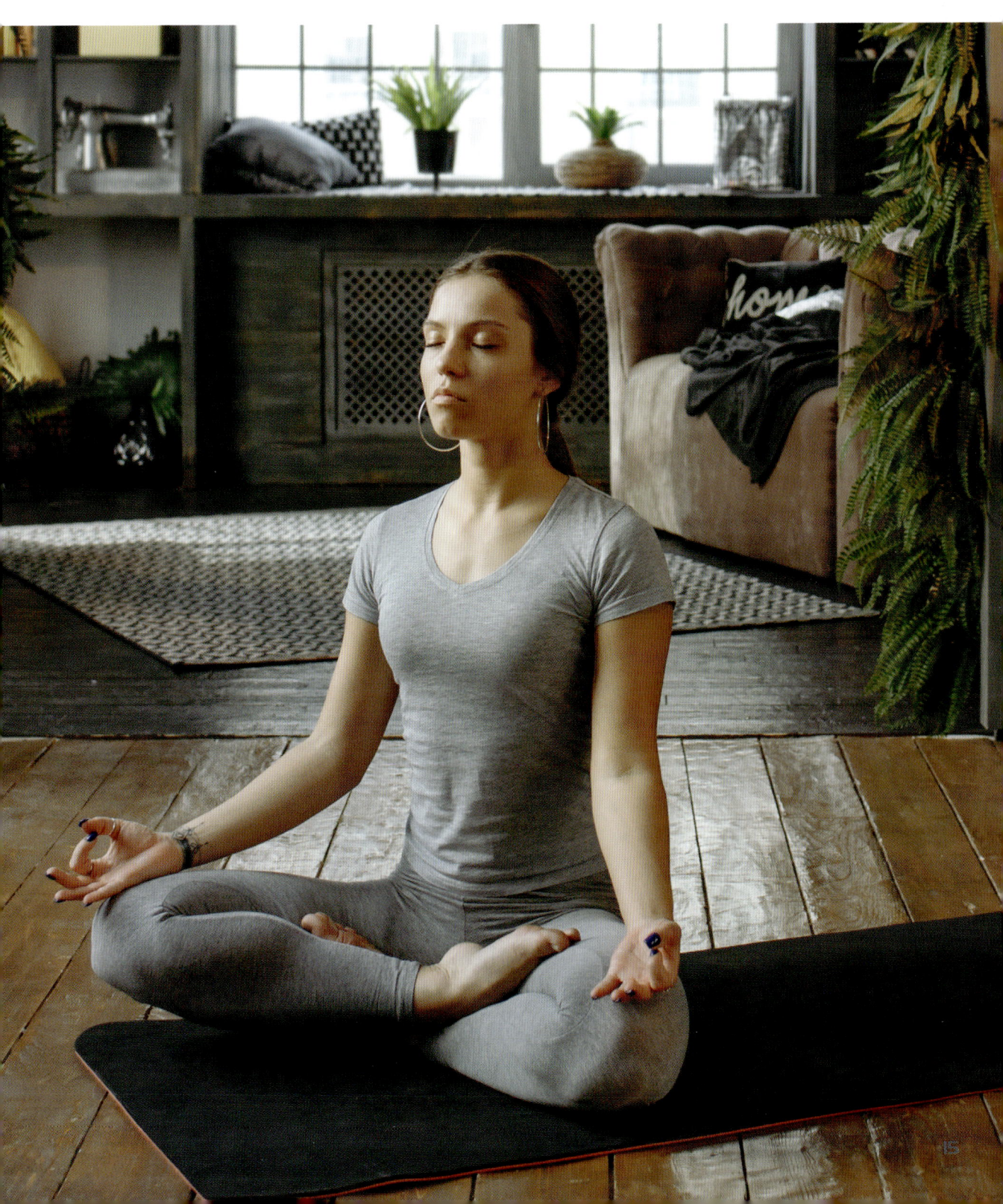

YOGA TOOLS

One of the great things about practicing yoga is that, unlike many other fitness disciplines, it calls for very little specialized sports equipment beyond a suitable mat.

You can work with just a mat, but there are several tools and other items that can enhance your yoga practice.

CLOTHING

Yoga clothing is simply any pieces that makes you feel comfortable and that allows you to move freely. Although there are many high-end choices these days, none of it is truly necessary—you don't need to splurge at the sporting goods store. Wear something relatively stretchy or flowing that is not confining. A comfy T-shirt and yoga pants are fine, as are a tank top and gym shorts. Jeans are usually out—they tend to be too stiff to accommodate bending and twisting movements. And don't worry about expensive footgear; yoga is traditionally performed barefoot.

THE MAT

To begin your practice you will need a yoga mat. The yoga mat is different than a Pilates mat or a padded gym mat. Buy a mat specifically designed for yoga. You can buy an inexpensive yoga mat for less than $20, but it might be worthwhile to invest a bit more than that—a good mat can make a difference in how you assume and hold poses. A good mat will be thin, sturdy, and slightly tacky to the touch, so that you have the traction to grip the floor with your hands and feet. It is true that you might be able to use a studio mat free of charge or for a small fee, but you will probably want your own for sanitary reasons—some people sweat a lot during yoga sessions. Plus, mats are quite light and easy to carry to and from class.

PROPS

For beginners especially, there are several helpful items. If a yoga pose is too difficult to complete, or if you find a position too painful to maintain, these aids can be employed to ease you into a pose. Some of these props are also used in restorative yoga to remove stress from your body.

- Blocks can help you achieve poses, deepen your stretches, and ensure correct alignment while holding a pose. At home, you can substitute a thick book for a block.

- Folded blankets can elevate your buttocks in poses in which your hips and thighs are opened.

- Webbing straps can help you reach down to your feet or raise your legs, as well as facilitate holds behind

YOGA TOOLS • THE BASICS OF YOGA

DEEPEN YOUR POSES

Your yoga props and equipment are tools that will help you deepen your poses. Never fear that using a yoga block or a strap "makes you a beginner," or that you're not correctly doing the pose if you use them. If they help you achieve better form, then they have done their job. In Triangle Pose, for example, the point of the pose is not to reach your palms to the floor; the point is to elongate the spine, finding length throughout your torso. If your hand is on the floor but the side of the body is crunched up and you can barely breathe, then you're not doing yoga—you are merely contorting your body. Instead, use your block to your advantage, and create the space you need to deepen the breath.

your back if you are knotted up or recovering from an injury. Straps also align your posture and help maintain the structure of a pose. A long towel can be used in place of a strap.

- Bolsters are like firm body pillows; you can use one during restorative yoga to foster relaxation, soften posture, and open your body.

Other useful props to consider include a meditation pillow, a yoga wedge, a neck pillow, yoga knee pads, a Swiss ball, toe spreaders, and yoga gloves.

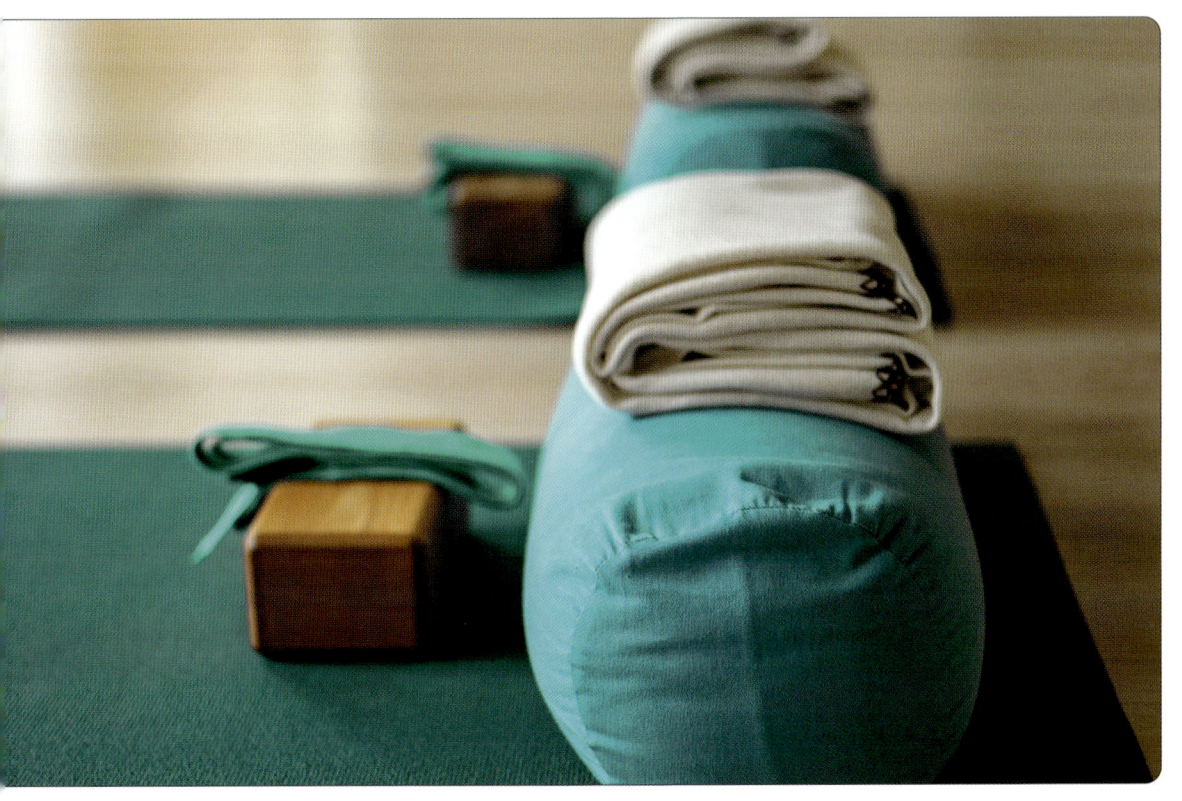

YOGA BASICS

THE LANGUAGE OF YOGA

Novice yoga students often find themselves a bit lost in their earliest classes when their teachers seem to speak a foreign language. It is foreign, Sanskrit, a language of the ancient Indians who formulated the discipline.

Asana: a "seat," or a physical posture of yoga.

Ashram: a hermitage; a monastic community or a religious retreat, especially in India and Southeast Asia.

Ashtanga: the eight-limbed yogic path, which includes:

1. **Yama** (restraints, moral disciplines or moral vows)
2. **Niyama** (positive duties or observances);
3. **Asana** (posture)
4. **Pranayama** (breathing techniques)
5. **Pratyahara** (sense withdrawal)
6. **Dharana** (focused concentration)
7. **Dhyana** (meditative absorption)
8. **Samadhi** (bliss or enlightenment)

Ayurveda: the ancient Indian science of health.

Bakti: devotion, as in Bakti yoga.

Bandha: internal muscular "locks" that, when engaged, support the toning and lifting of strategic areas of the body. The three major bandhas of Hatha yoga are:

- **Mula Bandha**: the pelvic floor muscles
- **Uddiyana Bandha**: the abdominals up to the diaphragm
- **Jalandhara Bandha**: the throat

Chakra: meaning a "wheel"; one of seven energy centers in your body located between the top of your head and the base of your spine.

- **Crown chakra (Sahasrara)**: the very top of your head
- **Third eye chakra (Ajna)**: the forehead, between your eyebrows
- **Throat chakra (Vishuddha)**: the throat area
- **Heart chakra (Anahata)**: the center of your chest
- **Solar plexus chakra (Manipura)**: the upper abdomen
- **Sacral chakra (Svadhisthana)**: the lower abdomen
- **Root chakra (Muladhara)**: the base of your spine

Core: the core is often thought of as the abdominal muscles, but it's more accurate to think of it as an apple core, running from the top of your head to the inner arches of your feet.

THE LANGUAGE OF YOGA • THE BASICS OF YOGA

Sahasrara
Crown Chakra

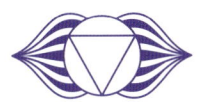
Ajna
Third-eye Chakra

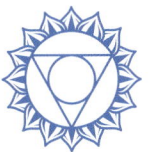
Vishuddha
Throat Chakra

Anahata
Heart Chakra

Manipura
Solar Plexus Chakra

Svadhishthana
Sacral Chakra

Muladhara
Root Chakra

THE LANGUAGE OF YOGA continued

Dosha: a physical body type; in Ayurvedic medicine there are three doshas: *pitta* ("fire"), *vata* ("wind"), and kapha ("earth").

Drishti: focal point of gazing during meditation or yoga practice—and quite useful during balancing poses.

Guru: teacher or master; one who illumines the darkness.

Hatha yoga: from *ha* ("sun") and *tha* ("moon"), hatha yoga seeks to unify opposites—body and mind—and describes any of the physical practices of yoga.

Kirtan: a gathering that includes chanting, music, and meditation.

Mantra: sounds, syllables, words, or groups of words repeated to create a positive transformation; a sacred thought or a prayer.

Meditation: the focusing and calming of the mind, often through breath work, to reach a deeper level of consciousness.

Mudra: a "seal," or hand gesture, that influences the energies of the body or mood. Most often the hands and fingers are held in a mudra to aid concentration, focus, and connection to yourself. The most common mudras are Anjali (palms pressed together at the heart) and Gyan (forefinger and thumb forming a circle, the other three fingers stretching away).

Nadi: the energy channels through which *prana*, or life force, flows. Pranayama uses the breath to direct and expand the flow of *prana* in the nadis.

Namaste: Sanskrit word commonly spoken at the end of a yoga class. One thoughtful interpretation: "I honor that place in you where the whole universe resides; and when I am in that place in me and you are in that place in you, there is only one of us."

Om: a mantra usually chanted at the beginning and end of a class. It is said to be the origin of all sounds and the seed of creation; often referred to as the "universal sound of consciousness."

Patanjali: an ancient sage who is said to have compiled the Yoga-sutras, a guide on how to live in order to advance along a spiritual path toward enlightenment.

Prana: life energy, or life force.

Pranayama: breath awareness used to facilitate inner stillness and awareness.

Props: tools such as mats, blocks, blankets, and straps used to extend your

THE LANGUAGE OF YOGA • THE BASICS OF YOGA

LEARN THE LINGO

The discipline of yoga has its roots in the centuries-old Indian Vedas, a large body of religious texts, and many of the words describing the poses and body positioning are in Sanskrit, the language of ancient India. As a yoga student you will quickly become familiar with words such as *asana*, *pranayama*, and *mudra*. When pronounced correctly, these words create distinct inhalations and exhalations that are similar to those employed in meditative mantras.

range of motion or facilitate achieving a pose.

Samadhi: a state of complete enlightenment.

Savasana, or **Corpse Pose**: the ultimate relaxation pose, typically at the end of yoga class.

Shakti: female energy.

Shanti: "peace," a word often chanted three times in class.

Shiva: a Hindu deity; male energy.

Surya Namaskar, or **Sun Salutations**: a sequence of dynamic asanas often used to warm up the body at the beginning of a yoga class.

Swami: a "master," or Hindu ascetic or religious leader, especially a senior member of a religious order.

Tantra: the yoga of union between mind and body.

Ujjay: a pranayama in which the lungs are fully expanded and the chest is puffed out; especially associated with the vinyasa style.

Upanishads: texts of a religious and philosophical nature, written in India between 800 and 500 BCE.

Vinyasa: movement linked with breath; postures are strung together to create a short flow or a long flow.

Yang yoga: a style that is rhythmic, repetitive, and energetic and is great for building strength and fitness.

Yin yoga: a series of long-held, passive floor poses that target the fascia, or connective tissue, in the body. A combination of yin and yang keeps students balanced and healthy.

Yoga: from the Sanskrit *yug*, meaning "yoke" or "union"; yoga is an ancient discipline in which physical postures, breath practice, meditation, and philosophical study are used as tools for achieving liberation.

Yogi/yogini: a male/female practitioner of yoga.

YOGA BASICS

YOGA BREATHING

Breathing is essential to life, although it's not something we need to think about in order to do. Yet, to truly benefit from your yoga practice, you must first learn to breathe properly. It is your breath that will guide you through your practice.

Pranayama, or the science of yoga breathing, is the first principle on which anyone beginning a yoga practice should concentrate. To fully benefit from your practice, you must first learn to breathe properly.

PRANAYAMA

In Sanskrit, *prana* means "life-force energy," and *ayama* means "to control or extend." Together, they form the word *pranayama*, which means "extension of the life force," or "breath control." Yoga calls for us to pay close attention to the process of breathing in and out, which we usually take for granted. *Apana* refers to the elimination of breath—the alternate action of *prana*. While you intake the breath of life, you must also eliminate the toxins within the depths of your respiratory system. Practicing pranayama means to control your internal pranic energy. See below to learn the pranayama technique.

As your progress through your yoga practice, you can learn how to alter the movement of prana. You can start breath control by familiarizing yourself with, and practicing, the other

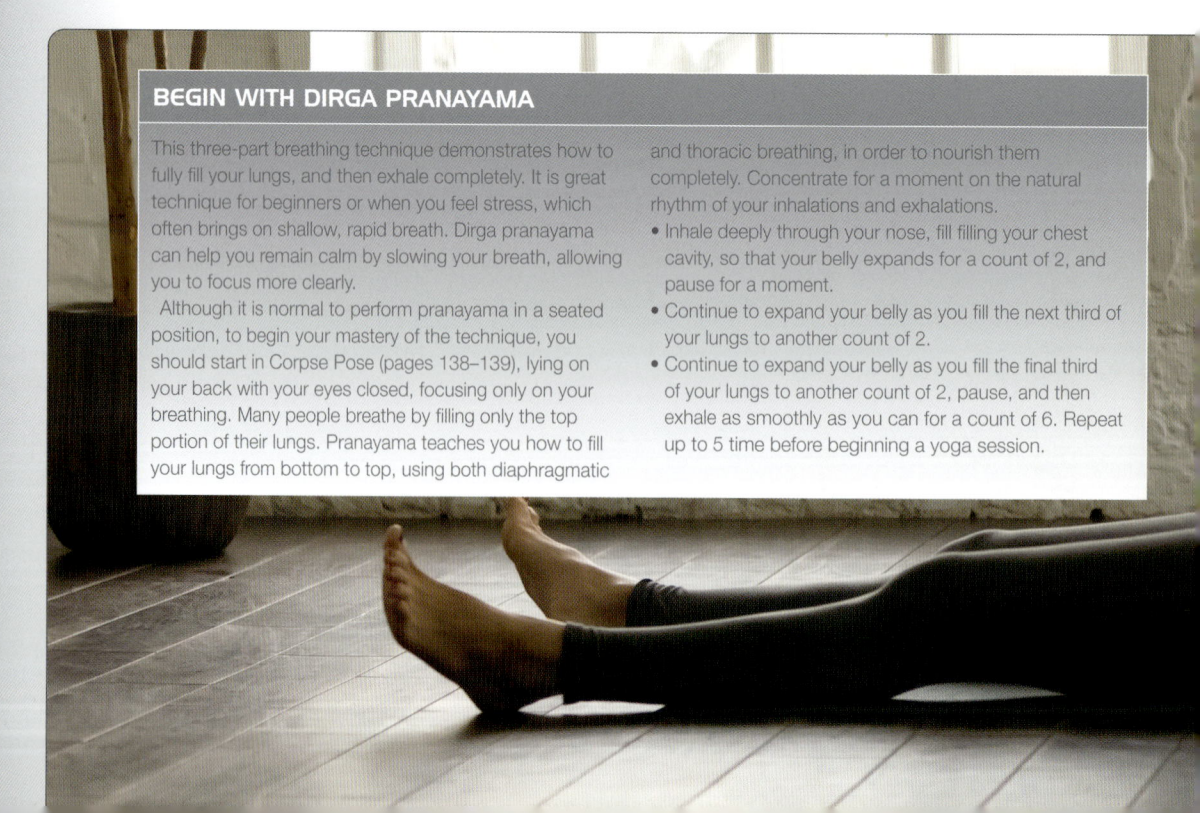

BEGIN WITH DIRGA PRANAYAMA

This three-part breathing technique demonstrates how to fully fill your lungs, and then exhale completely. It is great technique for beginners or when you feel stress, which often brings on shallow, rapid breath. Dirga pranayama can help you remain calm by slowing your breath, allowing you to focus more clearly.

Although it is normal to perform pranayama in a seated position, to begin your mastery of the technique, you should start in Corpse Pose (pages 138–139), lying on your back with your eyes closed, focusing only on your breathing. Many people breathe by filling only the top portion of their lungs. Pranayama teaches you how to fill your lungs from bottom to top, using both diaphragmatic and thoracic breathing, in order to nourish them completely. Concentrate for a moment on the natural rhythm of your inhalations and exhalations.

- Inhale deeply through your nose, fill filling your chest cavity, so that your belly expands for a count of 2, and pause for a moment.
- Continue to expand your belly as you fill the next third of your lungs to another count of 2.
- Continue to expand your belly as you fill the final third of your lungs to another count of 2, pause, and then exhale as smoothly as you can for a count of 6. Repeat up to 5 time before beginning a yoga session.

YOGA BREATHING • THE BASICS OF YOGA

exercises below. They will enable you to draw oxygen deep into your lungs, encourage a connection between your body and mind, and leave you feeling rejuvenated and refreshed.

BEGINNING YOUR BREATHING PRACTICE

Draw in even breaths as you concentrate on filling every portion of your lungs with oxygen. Begin at the bottom, expanding your diaphragm to inflate your abdomen; then raise your rib cage as oxygen floods the middle of your lungs. Finally, allow the top of your lungs to fill as your chest expands. Make sure both sides of your chest rise simultaneously.

Now you should be ready to practice pranayama in an upright, seated position. Once you are comfortable —perhaps with your legs folded, and shins crossed—place one hand flat on your chest and the other on your abdominal muscles. This will help you monitor your breath as it enters your body. Close your eyes, lift up from your spine, draw your chin in slightly toward your chest, and listen to your breath as your abdomen and rib cage expand and contract. Concentrate on the pathways the oxygen travels, the rhythm of your breathing, and the texture of the sound.

The following pages outline further examples of both rejuvenating and relaxing exercises, all of them aimed at replenishing fresh oxygen to your lungs and connecting your mind with your body.

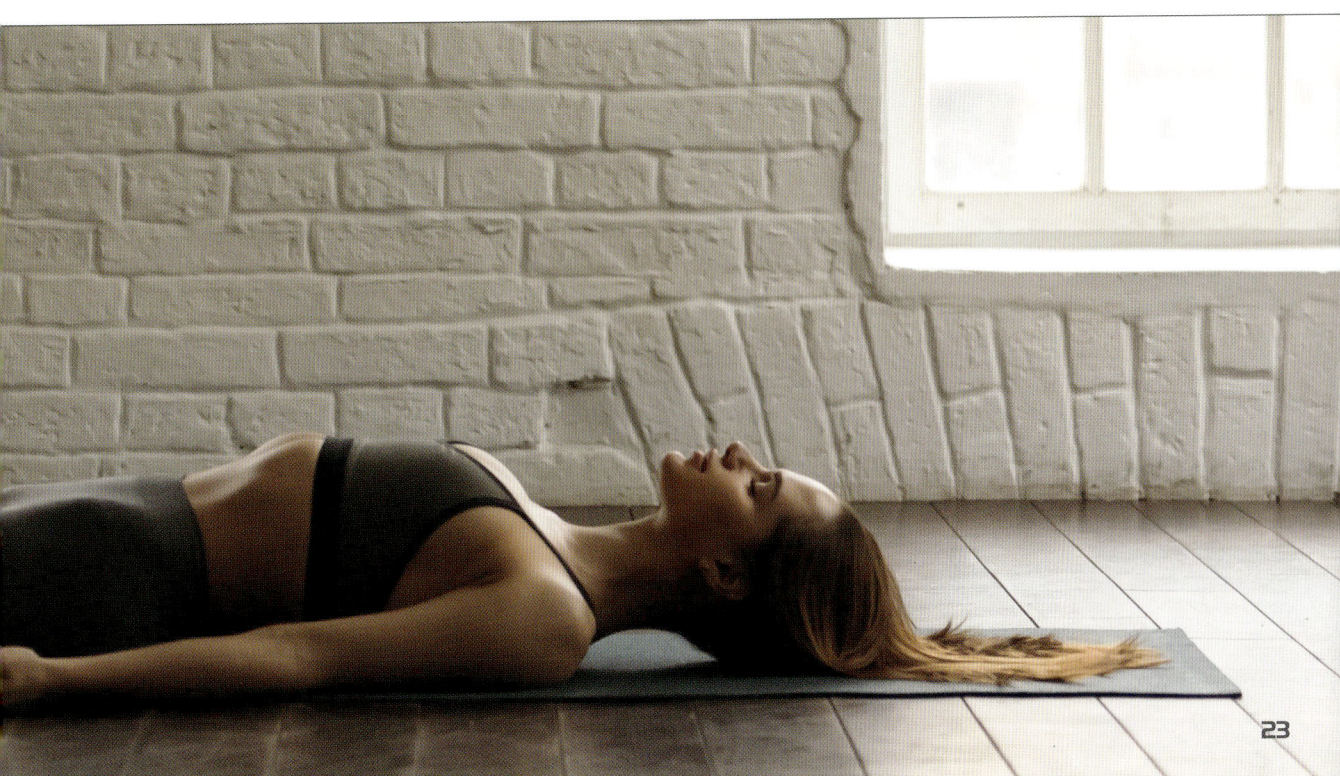

YOGA BREATHING continued

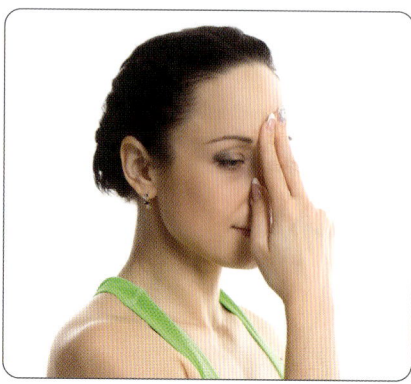

To stimulate Ajna chakra, place your index and middle fingers on forehead. The Ajna chakra is known as the chakra of the mind. This space between your eyebrows is said to be where the nadis energy channels through your nostrils and meets with the central nadi. This is a very powerful hand position in pranayama practice.

SAMAVRITTI, or THE SAME BREATH

If there are irregularities to your breathing, focus on transitioning into a slower and more even breath pattern. To achieve samavrtti, meaning "the same action," inhale for four counts, and then exhale for four counts. Repeat until you are doing it almost instinctively without the counting. This breathing technique calms the mind and creates a sense of balance and stability.

UJJAYI, or OCEAN BREATH

Also known as the Victorious Breath, the name "ocean breath" refers to the surflike sound that air makes as it passes through the narrow epiglottal passage in your throat. Maintaining an even rhythm, constrict the epiglottis, and keep your mouth closed as you listen for the hiss at the back of your throat. Ujjayi breathing tones your internal organs, raises your internal temperature, improves concentration, and calms your mind.

KUMBHAKA, or THE RETAINED BREATH

To practice this technique, begin with ujjayi or samavritti breathing, and after four breaths, hold your breath for four to eight counts. Exhale, allowing your exhalation to last longer than your inhalation. Initially, your retention, or kumbhaka, will be shorter than your other breaths. Eventually, reduce the number of breaths in between kumbhaka breaths and increase the number of counts in your inhale, exhale, and. Build up to an exhalation that is twice as long as your inhalation, and a kumbhaka breath three times as long. This breathing method strengthens the diaphragm, restores vitality, and purifies the respiratory system. Studies indicate it may even improve cerebral circulation.

KAPALABHATI, or THE SHINING SKULL

Kapal means "skull," and *bhati* means "shining"; together the two words mean "shining skull." This is a breathing technique that will cleanse your sinuses. In Kapalabhati, you control your breath

YOGA BREATHING • THE BASICS OF YOGA

by sharply exhaling while pumping your abdominal muscles in and out. The inhalation is passive, while the exhalation is forceful and sharp. The sharp and rapid exhales will help your lungs to clear any waste from your air passageways, purifying the respiratory system. This method also strengthens the diaphragm and revives energy. To practice Kapalabhati, follow these steps.

1. Sit up tall in a comfortable position, either in Easy Pose (see page 96) or Hero Pose (see page 139).

2. Close your eyes and your mouth, and relax your abdominal muscles.

3. Keeping your mouth closed, breathe only through your nose. Inhale once normally, and then exhale normally.

4. Inhale halfway, and begin to exhale sharply out of your nose in short, quick breaths while contracting your abdominal muscles. Continue doing this on each exhale. Think of drawing your stomach in and up as you pump and breathe diaphragmatically. Allow your inhale to be passive so that you are only focusing on the exhale.

5. When you are finished with your cycle, exhale all of your breath. As a begnner, start with two rounds of 10 cycles and work up to four rounds of 20 cycles.

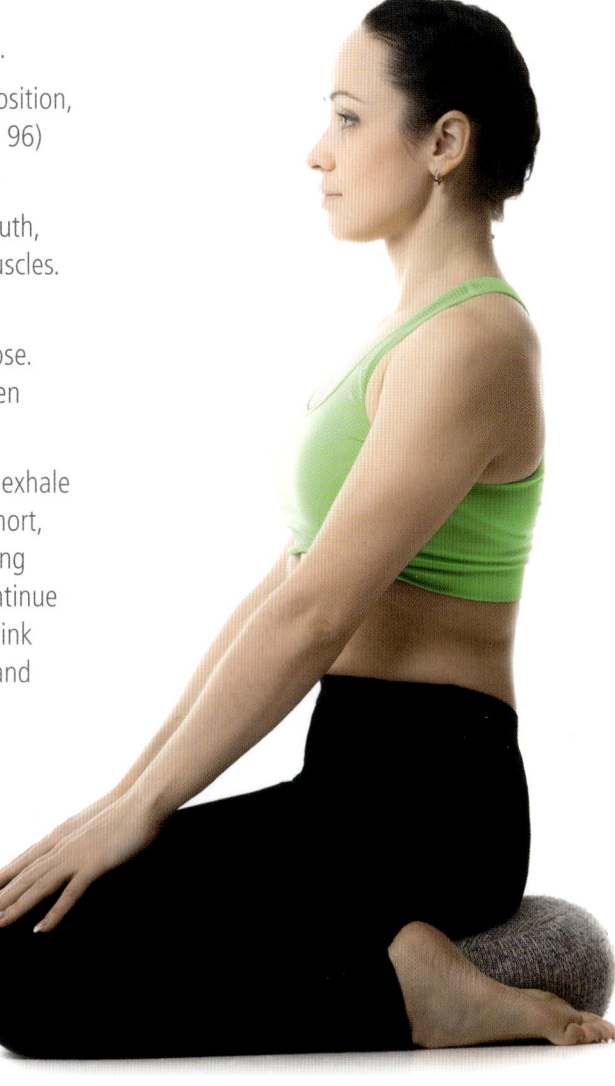

A comfortable beginner position, such as Hero Pose, allows you to concentrate on mastering your yoga breathing techniques while still maintaining good form.

25

YOGA BREATHING continued

ANULOMA VILOMA, or ALTERNATE NOSTRIL BREATHING

Anuloma viloma purifies the energy channels, or nadis, through the right and left nostrils. This stimulates the movement of prana.

To begin, position your hands in Vishnu Mudra, with the index and middle fingers curled down. Place your right thumb against the outside of your right nostril, and with your mouth closed inhale through the left nostril. Close the left nostril with your ring finger and hold for a moment. Then raise your thumb, and exhale from the right nostril. Switch hands and repeat on the opposite side. Begin with five cycles, and gradually increase the number. This method lowers your heart rate and reduces stress.

❶ To practice anuloma viloma, place your fingers in the Vishnu Mudra with your index and middle fingers curled down, keeping your ring finger and pinkie together and pointed up.

❷ Close your right nostril with your right thumb, and inhale through your left nostril.

❸ Retain your breath, squeezing the left nostril with your ring finger, and then release your thumb as you exhale through your right nostril.

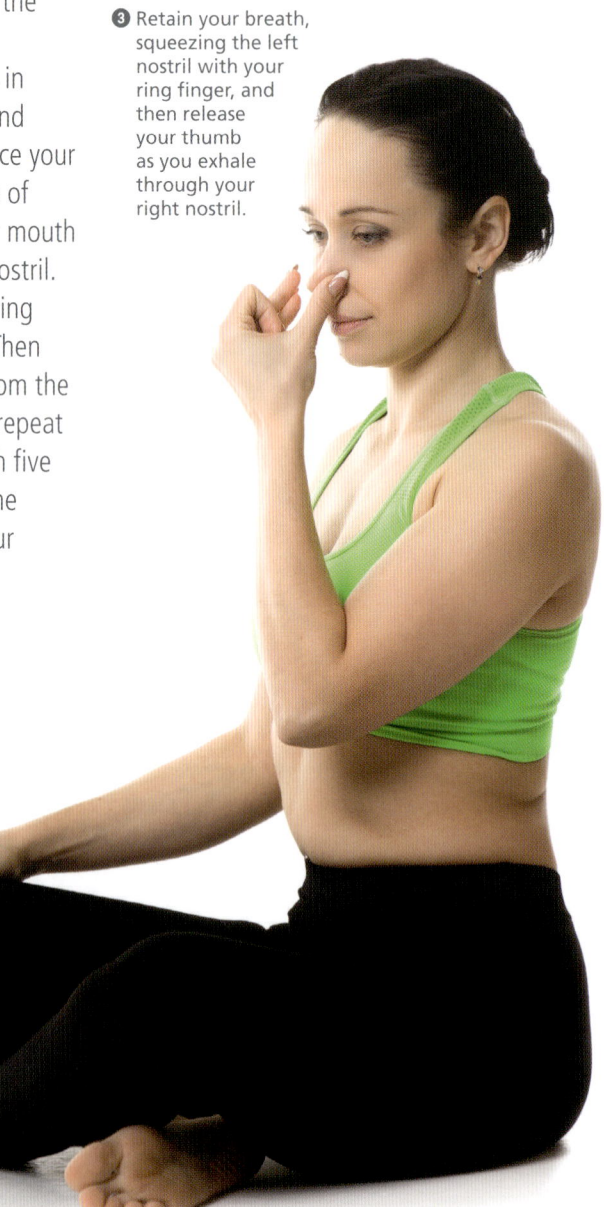

YOGA BREATHING • THE BASICS OF YOGA

SITALI, or COOLING BREATH
The Sitali technique is perfect for the end of a rigorous yoga session because it cools the body, hence the name, Cooling Breath. Unlike nearly all other yoga breathing techniques, which call for you to breathe through your nostrils, Sithali calls for you to breathe through your mouth. To practice Sithali, follow these steps.

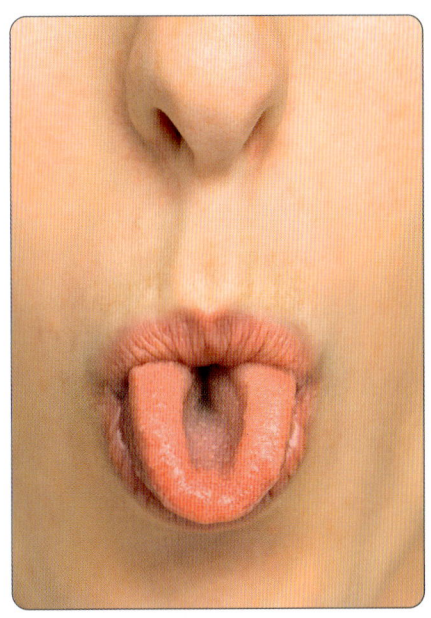

1. Sit up tall in a comfortable position, either in Easy Pose (see page 96) or Hero Pose (see page 139), and take two or three deep inhales and exhales through your nose to prepare.

2. Purse your lips, and then curl your tongue, rolling the sides upward to form a tube. Stick the end of the tongue out between your pursed lips. (If you can't curl your tongue, just make a small O shape with your mouth, or try the sitkari breathing technique.)

3. Inhale through the tube of your tongue.

4. Exhale through both nostrils.

5. Keeping your tongue curled, repeat 5 to 10 times until you feel the cool-down effect.

SITKARI
Many of us simply cannot curl our tongues, so sitkari can have the same cooling effect for those without this lingual dexterity. To prepare, sit up tall in a comfortable position, either in Easy Pose (see page 96) or Hero Pose (see page 139), making sure your spine is neutral.

1. Take a few natural breaths to center yourself.

2. Bring your upper and lower teeth together while keeping your lips as open as you can, and then inhale through the closed teeth to emit a soft hissing sound.

3. Release your teeth and close your mouth as you exhale through the nose. Repeat

4. Repeat steps 2 and 3 for a one or two minutes, which will allow the rejuvanating effect of a cooling breath to take effect.

HAND GESTURES

In the practice of meditative yoga, each part of the hand is said to have a reflex reaction in a specific region of the brain. The mudras, or hand gestures, are therefore used in some yoga poses to help guide energy flow and channel it to the brain. Over time, gurus have designated more than 100, but beginners will rely as small selection of these. In many seated yoga poses, the hands are relaxed, resting palms face-up on the thighs, in what is called Hands in Lap. But if the pose calls for a mudra, do try to include it.

The following are six of the most widely used mudras.

❶ GYAN (Chin Mudra)
This is one of the most common mudras used in beginner classes. Place the tips of your index finger and thumb together, while your other three fingers stretch away, relaxed. Your index finger stands for the planet Jupiter, which represents knowledge and expansion. This is an especially beneficial mudra to employ when seeking understanding or insight.

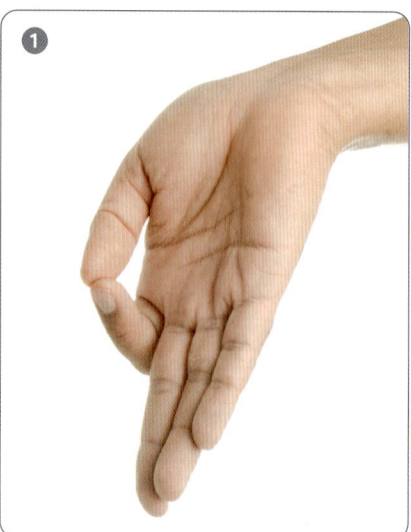

❷ ANJALI (Prayer Mudra)
With this gesture, you press your palms together, typically at your heart or behind your back.

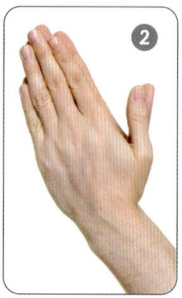

It is used to neutralize the positive (male) and the negative (female) sides of the body. It is often performed before a yoga class and again at the end. Pressing your palms together helps connect and balance the two hemispheres of your brain.

❸ SHUNI (Shoonya Mudra)
With the other fingers straight, press together the tips of your middle finger and thumb. This joining represents patience and discernment. It is used to improve intuition and awareness, as well as to purify emotions.

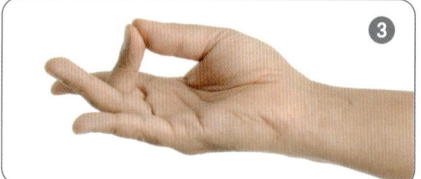

HAND GESTURES • THE BASICS OF YOGA

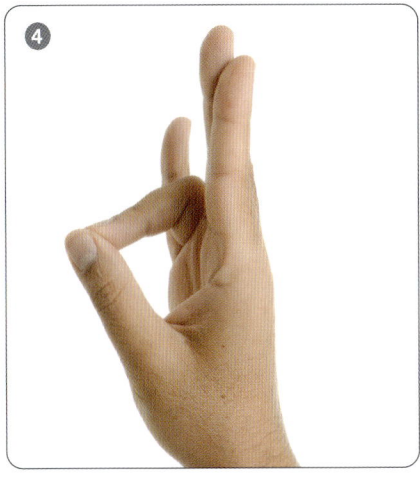

❻ VISHNU MUDRA
curl your index finger and middle finger down toward your palm, while keeping your ring finger and pinkie close together and upright. This mudra is used while practicing the breathing technique known as anuloma viloma.

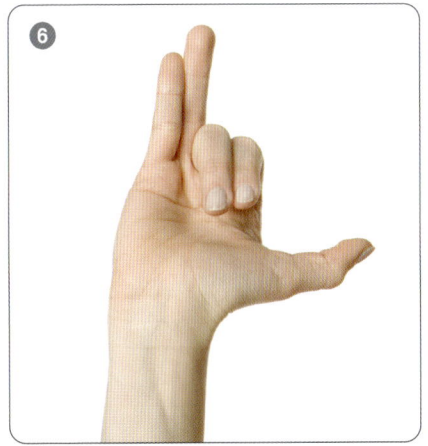

❹ SURYA RAVI MUDRA
Form a circle with your ring finger and thumb—or bend your ring finger down to the base of your thumb—keeping the other fingers straight. This pose represents courage and responsibility and is believed to improve digestion and increase metabolism.

❺ VENUS LOCK
Interlace the fingers of both hands, with the right pinkie down for women and the left pinkie down for men. This pose is said to represents both sexuality and sensuality.

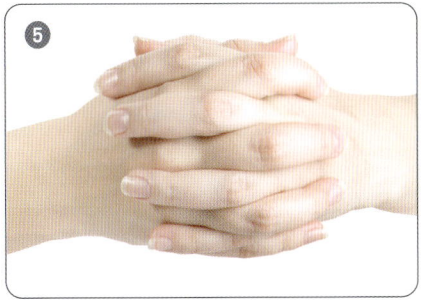

OTHER HAND GESTURES
As you progress through your yoga studies, you will come across other hand gestures. Some that you may see include Buddhi Mudra, in which the pinkie and thumb form a circle. The pinkie stands for the planet Mercury, which represents quickness and the power of communication. Prana Mudra, which activates the dormant energy inside you, calls for you to touch your ring finger and pinkie to the tip of your thumb. In Dhyana Mudra, your hands lie quietly, with your right hand resting in your left palm, thumbs touching. This pose deepens concentration. In Apana Mudra, touch your index and middle fingers to your thumb, while fanning out your outer fingers. It is used to aid both mental and physical digestion. In Ganesha, or Bear Grip Mudra, face your right palm toward your heart and your left palm outward, then curl your fingers, grip them together, and pull your arms out to your sides. This mudra stimulates your heart and intensifies concentration.

UPPER BODY
(FRONT)

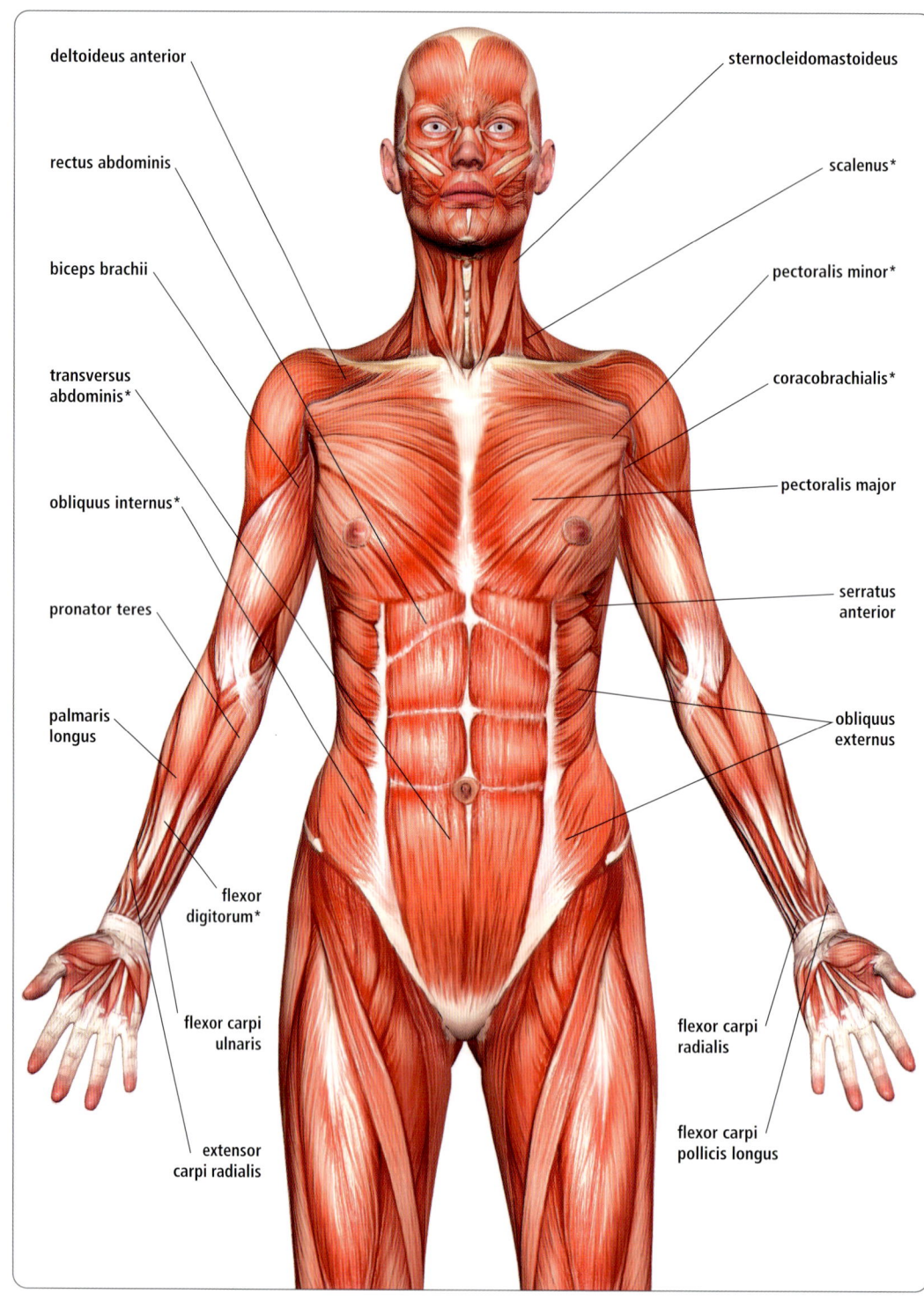

UPPER BODY
(BACK)

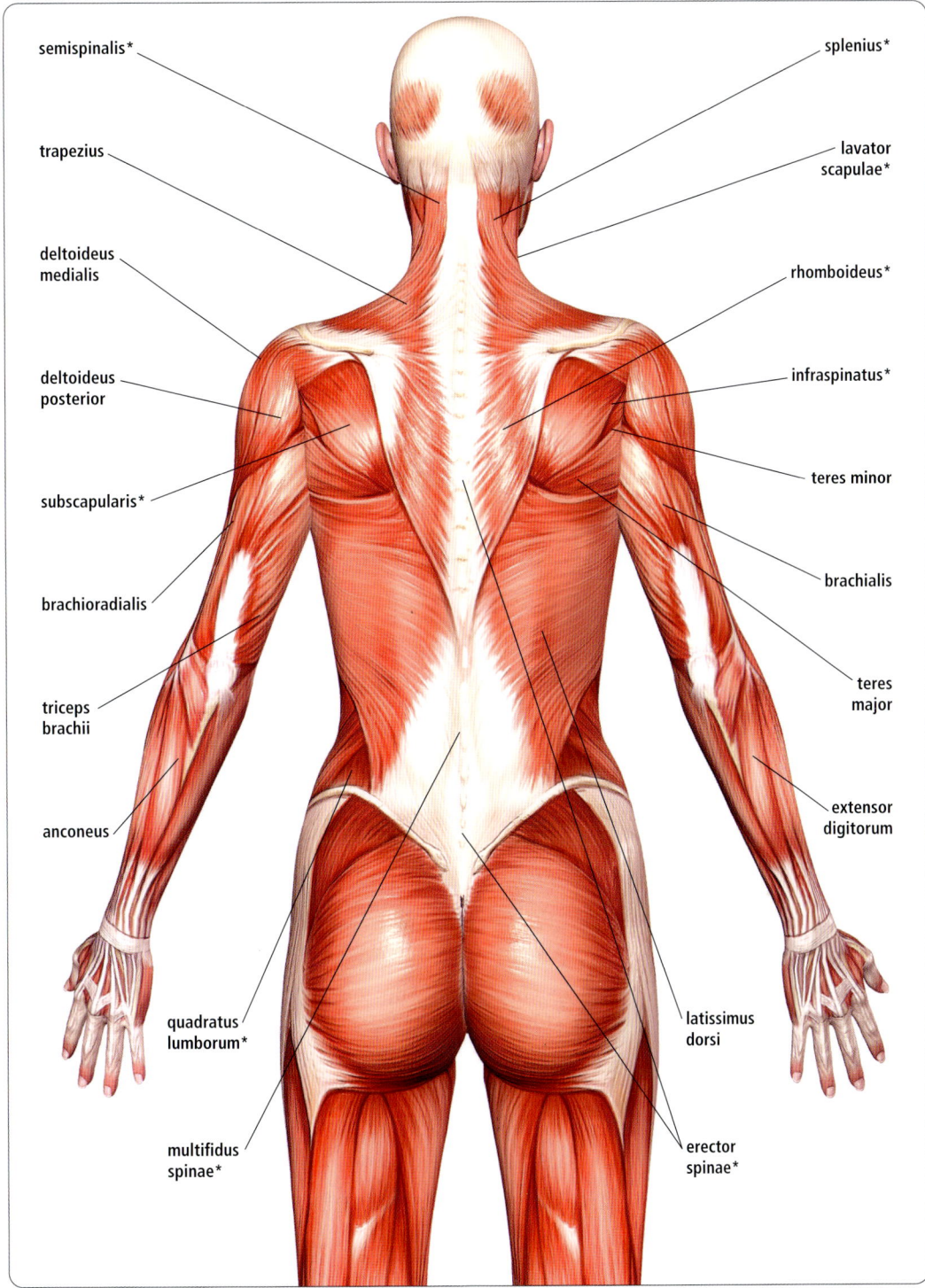

FULL-BODY ANATOMY

31

LOWER BODY
(FRONT)

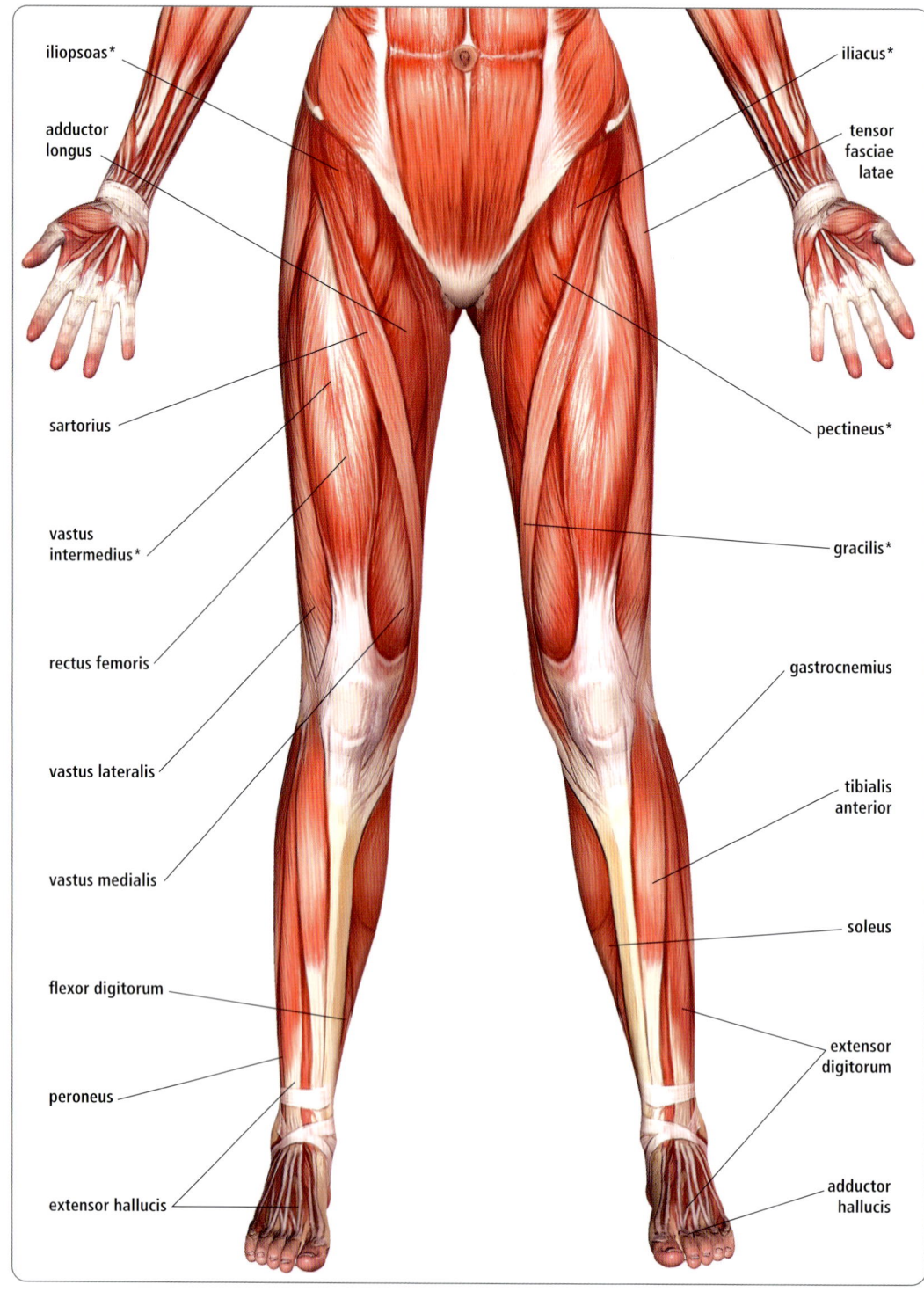

LOWER BODY
(BACK)

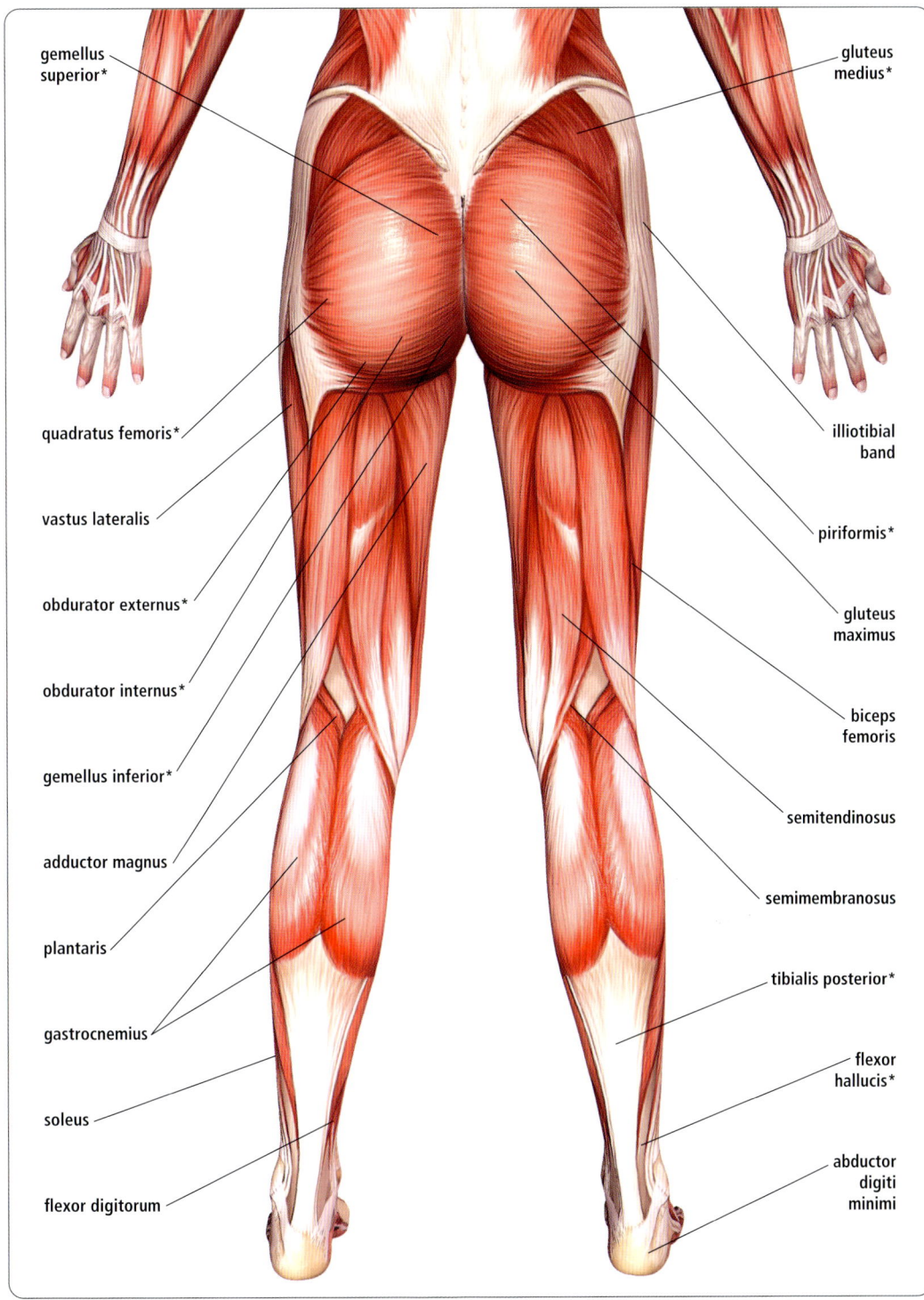

FULL-BODY ANATOMY

33

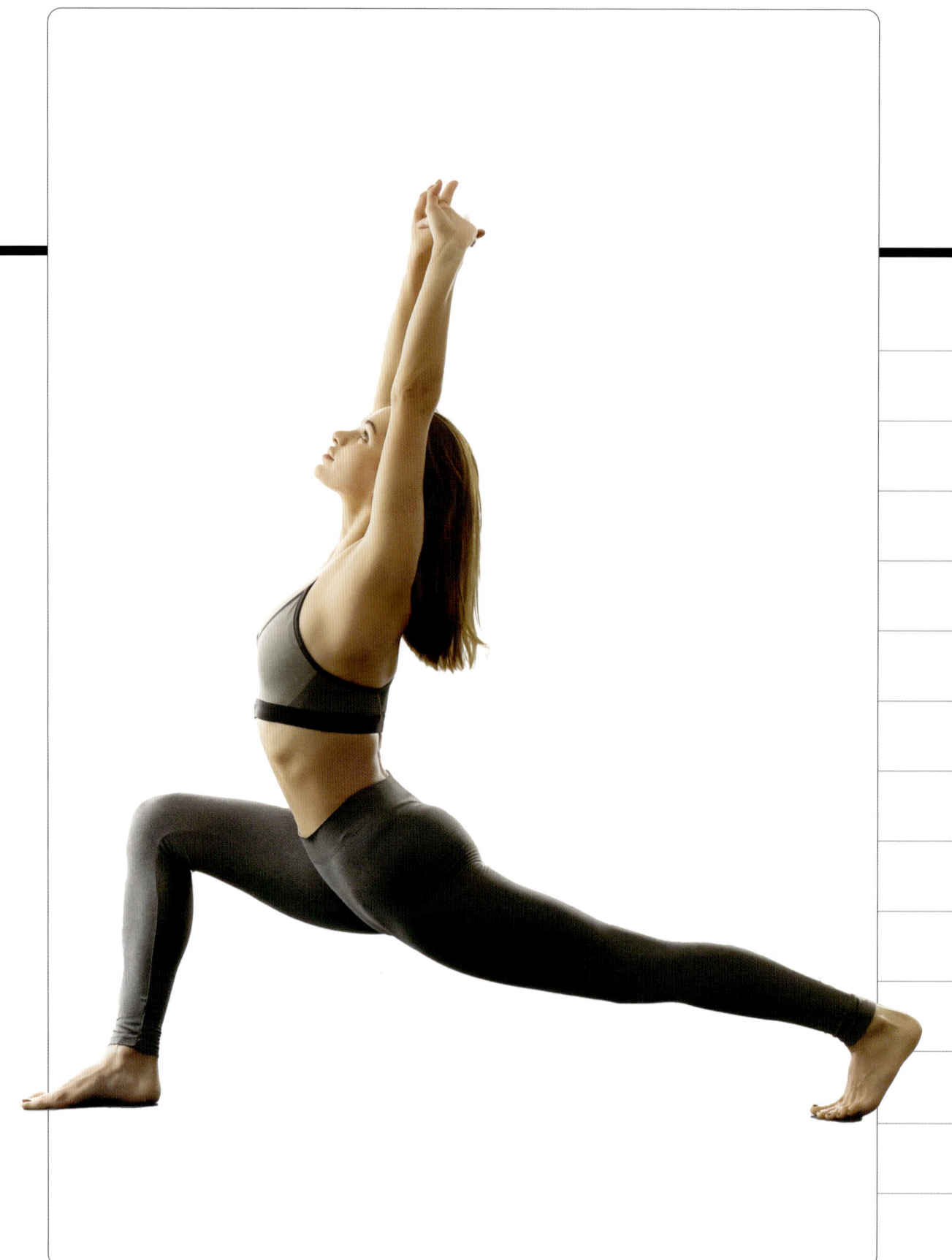

STANDING POSES

Standing poses, which are typically practiced at the start of a yoga workout, increase your understanding of the basic elements of yoga. They increase stamina, energize your body, and strengthen your legs. Standing poses reveal which areas of your body are weak or unstable, because they require strength, flexibility, and balance. When practicing these poses, keep your body's alignment in mind as you strive for a graceful balance. It is also critical that you maintain good posture and keep your feet firmly planted. Because most series of standing poses incorporate a diverse range of movements, they will help you stretch and build flexibility in every part of your body. In particular, they will help you build strength in your arms, shoulders, torso, pelvis, legs, and feet. The pelvis connects your torso and legs, so learning to stabilize your pelvis is especially important for mastering standing poses, and for preparing for other asanas that require balance and good posture.

STANDING POSES

MOUNTAIN POSE
(TADASANA)

① Stand with your feet together, with both heels and toes touching.

② Keeping your back straight and both arms pressed slightly against your sides, face your palms outward.

③ Lift all your toes and let them fan out, and then gently drop them down to create a wide, solid base.

④ Rock from side to side until you gradually bring your weight evenly onto all four corners of both feet.

⑤ While balancing your weight evenly on both feet, slightly contract the muscles in your knees and thighs, rotating both thighs inward to create a widening of the sit bones. Tuck your tailbone in between the sit bones.

⑥ Tighten your abdominals, drawing them in slightly, maintaining a firm posture.

⑦ Widen your collarbones, making sure your shoulders are parallel to your pelvis.

⑧ Lengthen your neck, so that the crown of your head rises toward the ceiling, and your shoulder blades slide down your back.

⑨ Hold for 30 seconds to 1 minute.

DO IT RIGHT
- If your ankles are knocking together uncomfortably, separate the heels slightly.
- If you are a beginner, practice the pose with your back to the wall to feel the alignment.

AVOID
- Slumping your back.
- Drooping your shoulders.

PRONUNCIATION & MEANING
- Tadasana (tah-DAHS-anna)
- *tada* = mountain

BENEFITS
- Improves posture
- Strengthens thighs

CONTRA-INDICATIONS & CAUTIONS
- Headache
- Insomnia
- Low blood pressure

MOUNTAIN POSE • STANDING POSES

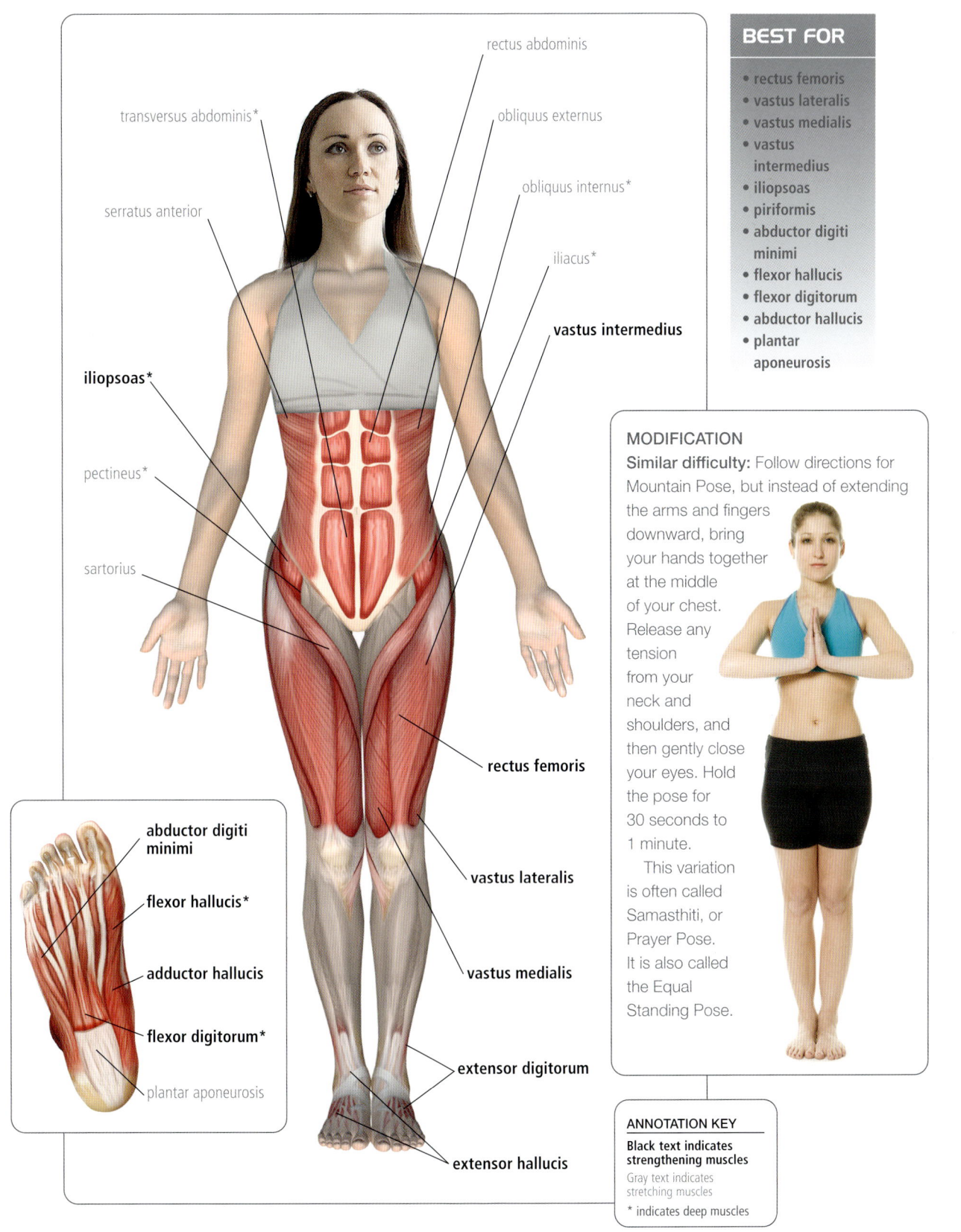

BEST FOR
- rectus femoris
- vastus lateralis
- vastus medialis
- vastus intermedius
- iliopsoas
- piriformis
- abductor digiti minimi
- flexor hallucis
- flexor digitorum
- abductor hallucis
- plantar aponeurosis

Labels on main figure:
- transversus abdominis*
- serratus anterior
- iliopsoas*
- pectineus*
- sartorius
- rectus abdominis
- obliquus externus
- obliquus internus*
- iliacus*
- **vastus intermedius**
- **rectus femoris**
- **vastus lateralis**
- **vastus medialis**
- **extensor digitorum**
- **extensor hallucis**

Foot detail labels:
- **abductor digiti minimi**
- **flexor hallucis***
- adductor hallucis
- **flexor digitorum***
- plantar aponeurosis

MODIFICATION
Similar difficulty: Follow directions for Mountain Pose, but instead of extending the arms and fingers downward, bring your hands together at the middle of your chest. Release any tension from your neck and shoulders, and then gently close your eyes. Hold the pose for 30 seconds to 1 minute.

This variation is often called Samasthiti, or Prayer Pose. It is also called the Equal Standing Pose.

ANNOTATION KEY
Black text indicates strengthening muscles
Gray text indicates stretching muscles
* indicates deep muscles

PRAYER POSE
(PRANAMASANA)

STANDING POSES

① Begin in Mountain Pose (pages 36-37), with your arms at your sides.

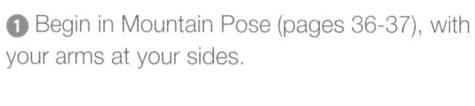

② Exhale and draw your hands together and down into prayer position at the heart.

③ Release any tension from your neck and shoulders, and then gently close your eyes. Hold for the recommended breaths.

BEST FOR
- rectus femoris
- vastus lateralis
- vastus medialis
- vastus intermedius
- iliopsoas
- piriformis
- abductor digiti minimi
- flexor hallucis
- flexor digitorum
- abductor hallucis
- **plantar aponeurosis**

PRONUNCIATION & MEANING
- Tadasana (tah-DAHS-anna)
- *tada* = mountain

BENEFITS
- Improves posture
- Strengthens thighs, knees, and ankles
- Tones abdomen and buttocks
- Relieves sciatica
- Helps to treat flat feet

CONTRA-INDICATIONS & CAUTIONS
- Headache
- Insomnia
- Low blood pressure

MODIFICATION
HARDER: To assume Reverse Prayer, bring your arms behind you, with your fingers pointing downward and your palms together. Rotate your arms so that your fingers point up to the sky.

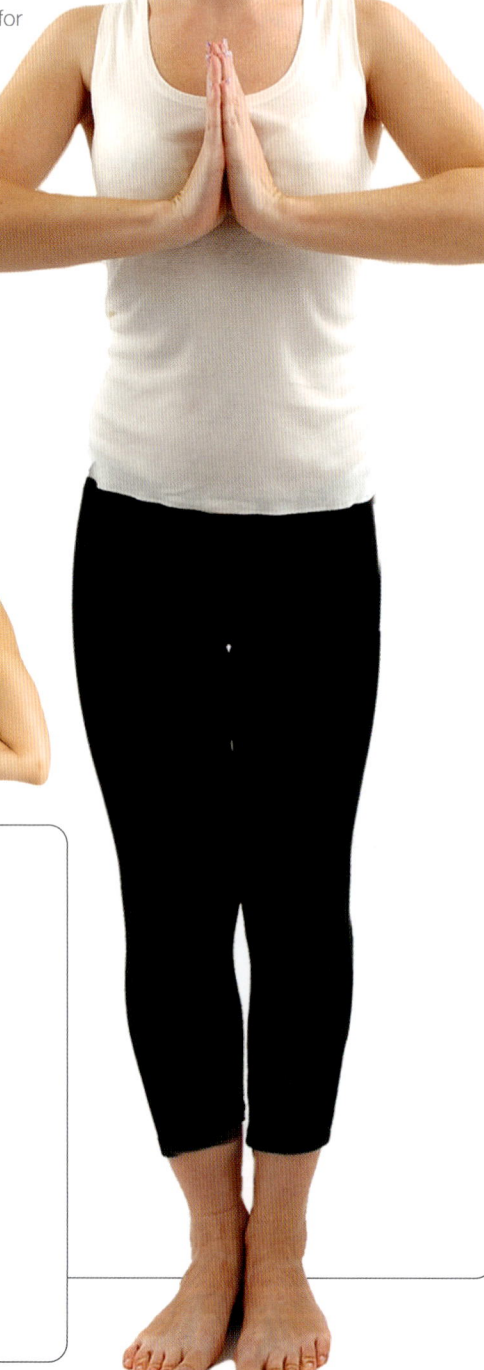

38

PRAYER POSE • STANDING POSES

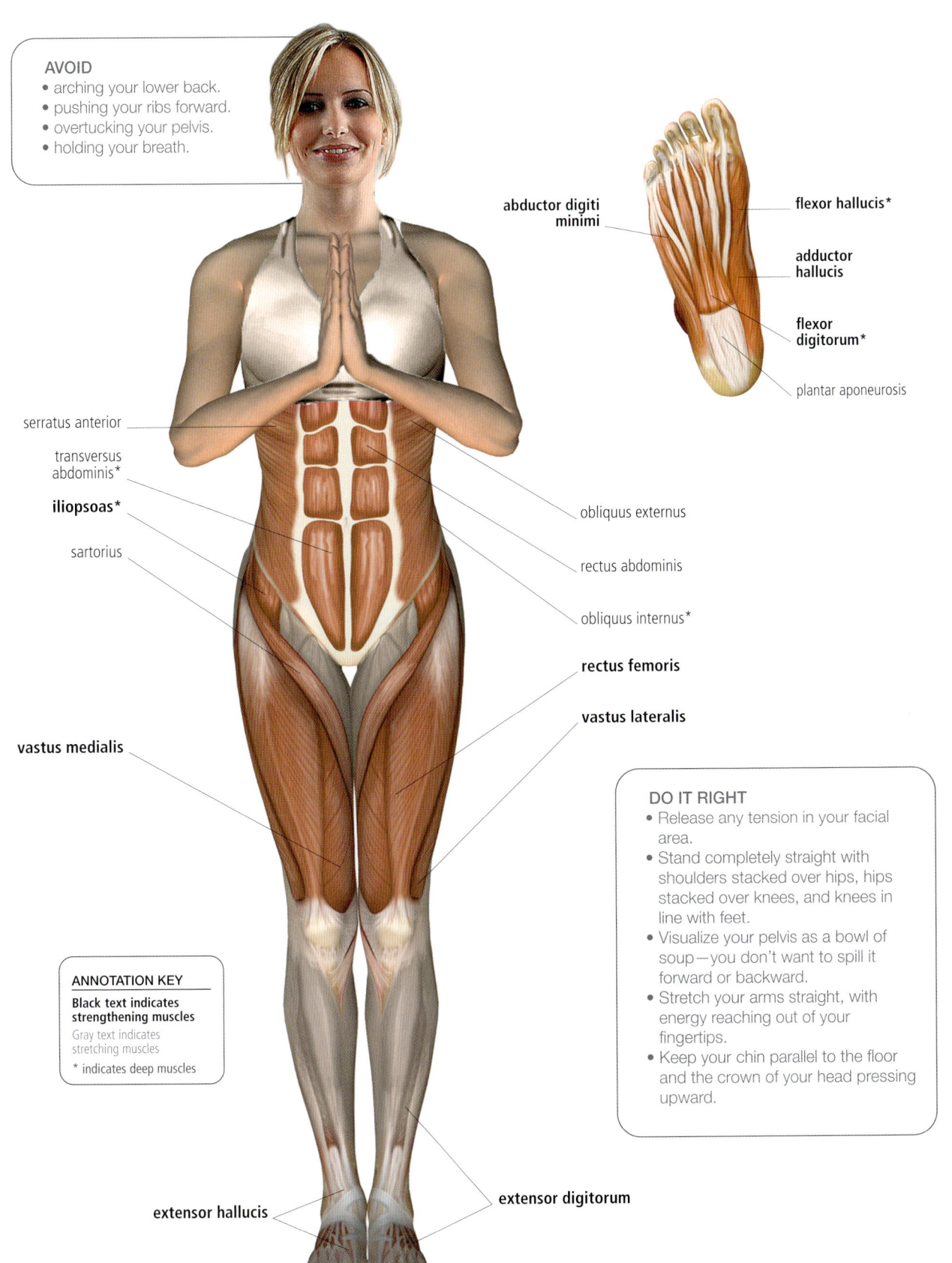

AVOID
- arching your lower back.
- pushing your ribs forward.
- overtucking your pelvis.
- holding your breath.

abductor digiti minimi

flexor hallucis*

adductor hallucis

flexor digitorum*

plantar aponeurosis

serratus anterior

transversus abdominis*

iliopsoas*

sartorius

obliquus externus

rectus abdominis

obliquus internus*

rectus femoris

vastus lateralis

vastus medialis

DO IT RIGHT
- Release any tension in your facial area.
- Stand completely straight with shoulders stacked over hips, hips stacked over knees, and knees in line with feet.
- Visualize your pelvis as a bowl of soup—you don't want to spill it forward or backward.
- Stretch your arms straight, with energy reaching out of your fingertips.
- Keep your chin parallel to the floor and the crown of your head pressing upward.

ANNOTATION KEY
Black text indicates strengthening muscles
Gray text indicates stretching muscles
* indicates deep muscles

extensor hallucis

extensor digitorum

39

UPWARD SALUTE
(URDHVA HASTASANA)

STANDING POSES

Anatomical labels (left image):
- biceps brachii
- serratus anterior
- obliquus internus*
- rectus abdominis*
- obliquus externus
- transversus abdominis*

DO IT RIGHT
- Keep your shoulders aligned directly over your hips and your hips over your heels.
- Keep back ribs broad.
- Broaden the top of your shoulder blades.
- Move your armpits down while lifting the arms upward.

AVOID
- Jutting your rib cage out of your chest.

❶ Stand in Mountain Pose (pages 36-37), with your feet shoulder-width apart and your pelvis, head, and chest aligned. Turn your palms inward.

❷ Keeping your arms parallel and palms facing each other, inhale, and sweep your arms out in front of you to the height of your shoulders, and then alongside your ears, raising them upward toward the ceiling.

❸ Spread your shoulder blades and draw your chin in slightly, as you gently tip your head back. Gaze at your thumbs.

❹ Hold for 30 seconds to 1 minute.

❺ Exhale, pulling your hands down with your palms together. As your hands lower toward your face, gently drop your head until it returns to a neutral position.

BEST FOR
- obliquus externus
- obliquus internus
- transversus abdominis
- latissimus dorsi
- teres major
- infraspinatus

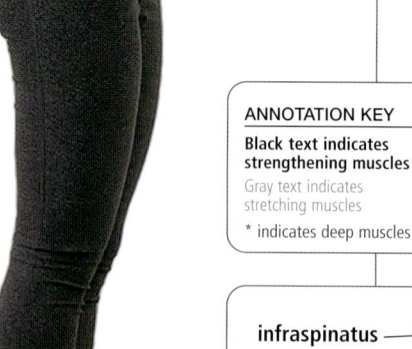

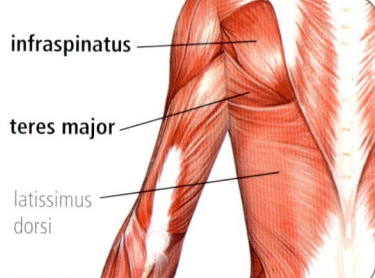

ANNOTATION KEY
Black text indicates strengthening muscles
Gray text indicates stretching muscles
* indicates deep muscles

Anatomical labels (lower right image):
- **infraspinatus**
- **teres major**
- latissimus dorsi

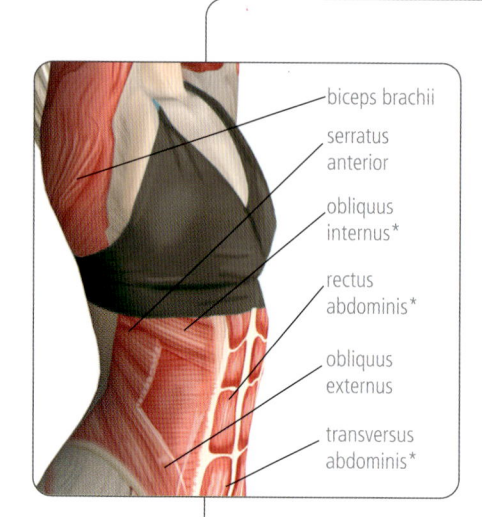

PRONUNCIATION & MEANING
- Urdhva Hastasana (oord-vah hahs-TAHS-anna)
- *urdhva* = raised (or upward); *hasta* = hand
- Also called Raised Hand Pose

BENEFITS
- Fights fatigue
- Relieves indigestion
- Alleviates back aches
- Stretches abdominals
- Stretches shoulders and armpits
- Relieves mild anxiety

CONTRA-INDICATIONS & CAUTIONS
- Shoulder injury
- Neck injury

AWKWARD POSE
(UTKATASANA)

① Stand in Mountain Pose (pages 36-37). Inhale, and raise both your hands over your head, keeping your arms straight and lengthening your spine. You may clasp your hands together or keep them shoulder-width apart.

② Exhale, and bend your knees. Bend your upper body forward so that it is at a 45-degree angle to the floor, keeping your lower back straight. Relax your calf muscles, allowing the weight of your upper body to sink into your pelvis. Transfer your weight to your heels.

③ Hold for 30 seconds to 1 minute.

④ Inhale, and straighten your knees, lifting strongly through your arms. Exhale, release your arms to your side, and return to Mountain Pose.

DO IT RIGHT
- Perform the lowering motion with your thighs, knees, and hips alone to achieve the proper position in your lower body.

ANNOTATION KEY
Black text indicates strengthening muscles
Gray text indicates stretching muscles
* indicates deep muscles

BEST FOR
- erector spinae
- extensor digitorum
- triceps brachii
- deltoideus
- infraspinatus
- teres major
- gluteus medius
- biceps femoris
- semitendinosus
- semimembranosus
- soleus
- tibialis anterior
- rectus femoris
- vastus lateralis
- vastus medialis
- vastus intermedius

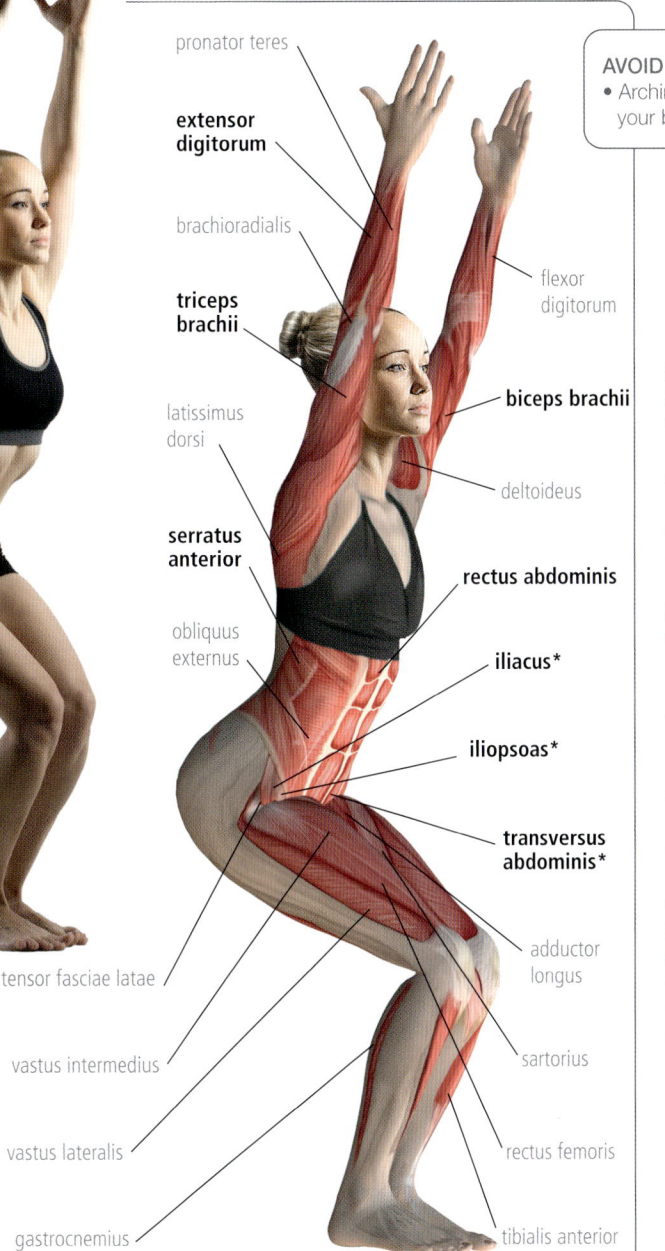

AVOID
- Arching your back.

Annotations: pronator teres, **extensor digitorum**, brachioradialis, **triceps brachii**, latissimus dorsi, **serratus anterior**, obliquus externus, tensor fasciae latae, vastus intermedius, vastus lateralis, gastrocnemius, flexor digitorum, **biceps brachii**, deltoideus, **rectus abdominis**, **iliacus***, **iliopsoas***, **transversus abdominis***, adductor longus, sartorius, rectus femoris, tibialis anterior

STANDING POSES

PRONUNCIATION & MEANING
- Utkatasana (OOT-kah-TAHS-anna)
- *utkata* = powerful, fierce
- Also called Fierce Pose or Chair Pose

BENEFITS
- Strengthens lower back and quadriceps
- Stretches chest, shoulders, arms, and hamstrings
- Relieves stress and tension
- Reduces flat feet

CONTRA-INDICATIONS & CAUTIONS
- Headache
- Insomnia
- Low blood pressure

STANDING POSES

TWISTING CHAIR POSE
(PARIVRTTA UTKATASANA)

① Stand in Mountain Pose (pages 36-37), and then squat down in Awkward Pose (Utkatasana, see page 37), with your arms extended up toward the ceiling. Lean back slightly, so that your weight rests on your heels.

BEST FOR
- rectus abdominis
- obliquus internus
- transversus abdominis
- biceps femoris
- rectus femoris
- obliquus externus
- gluteus medius
- gluteus maximus

② Squeezing your legs together, inhale, and bring your hands down to your chest. Press your palms together in prayer position.

③ Exhale, and twist toward the right, lengthening your spine as you remain in the squatting position. Rotate through your spine, torso, and shoulders, and place your left elbow on the outside of your right thigh. Look up toward the ceiling.

④ With each exhalation, deepen the twist, using your left elbow to guide your rotation.

⑤ Hold for 10 to 30 seconds. Inhale as you untwist, returning to Mountain Pose before twisting to the other side.

PRONUNCIATION & MEANING
- Parivrtta Utkatasana (par-ee-vrt-tah OOT-kah-TAHS-anna)
- *parivrtta* = twist, revolve; *utkatasana* = chair

BENEFITS
- Stimulates digestion
- Stretches spine
- Strengthens thighs, buttocks, and abdominals

CONTRA-INDICATIONS & CAUTIONS
- Back injury

AVOID
- Lessening your squatted position as you twist.
- Forcing a deep twist too aggressively with your elbow.

TWISTING CHAIR POSE • STANDING POSES

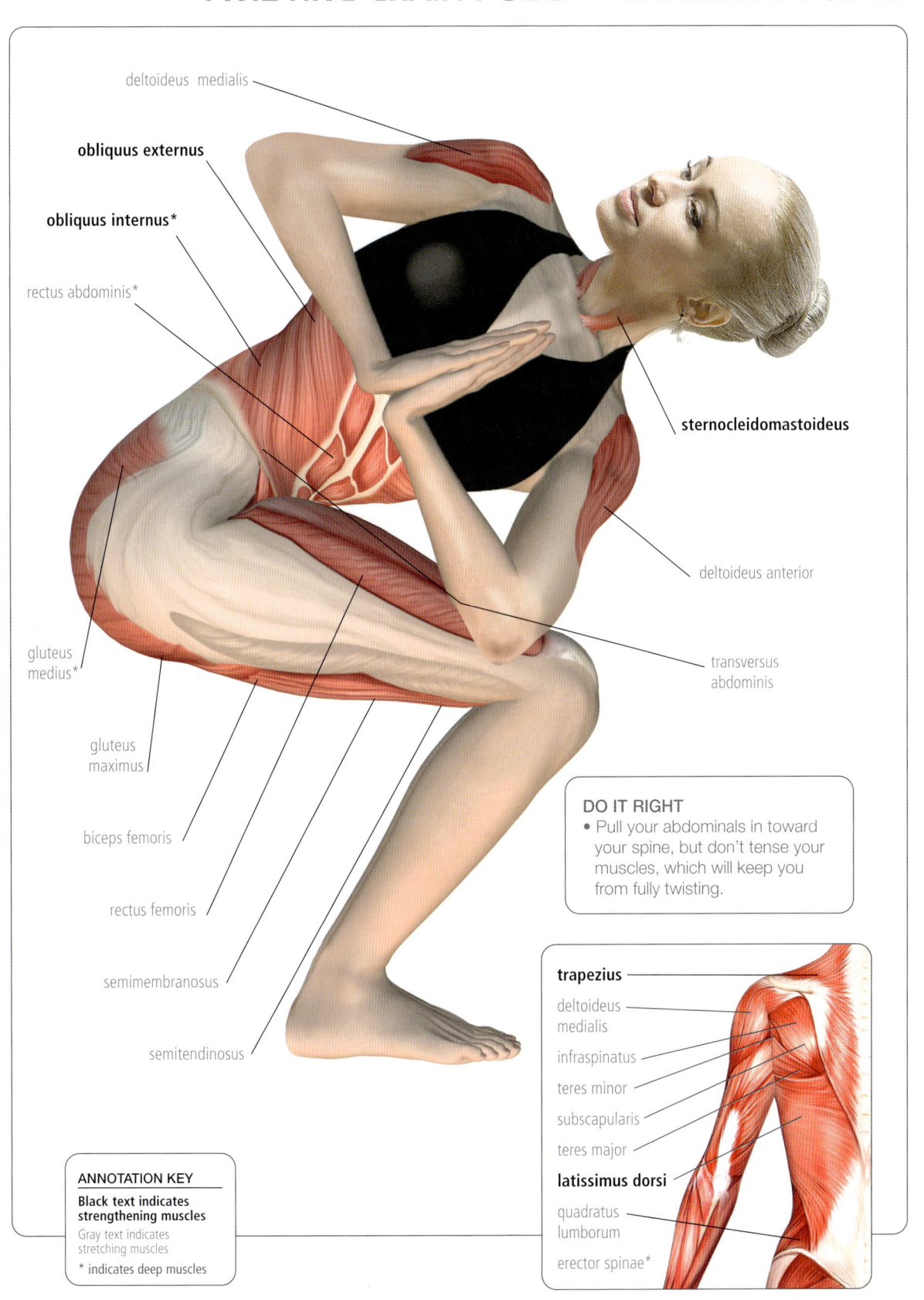

- deltoideus medialis
- **obliquus externus**
- **obliquus internus***
- rectus abdominis*
- **sternocleidomastoideus**
- deltoideus anterior
- transversus abdominis
- gluteus medius*
- gluteus maximus
- biceps femoris
- rectus femoris
- semimembranosus
- semitendinosus

DO IT RIGHT
- Pull your abdominals in toward your spine, but don't tense your muscles, which will keep you from fully twisting.

- **trapezius**
- deltoideus medialis
- infraspinatus
- teres minor
- subscapularis
- teres major
- **latissimus dorsi**
- quadratus lumborum
- erector spinae*

ANNOTATION KEY
Black text indicates strengthening muscles
Gray text indicates stretching muscles
* indicates deep muscles

43

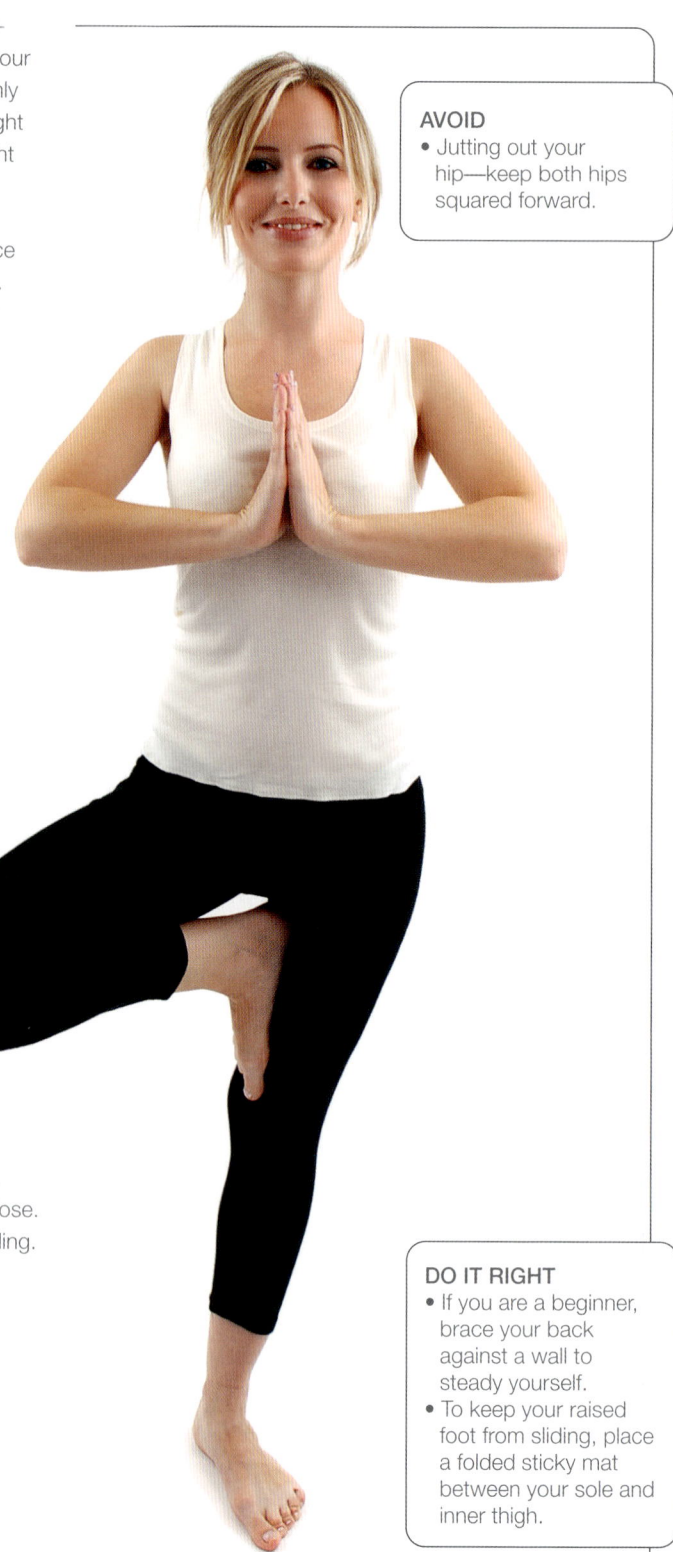

STANDING POSES

TREE POSE
(VRKSASANA)

1 Stand in Prayer Pose (pages 38-39). Shift your weight slightly onto your left foot, keeping your inner foot firmly grounded on the floor. Bend your right knee, and reach down with your right hand and grasp your right ankle.

2 Draw your right foot up, and place the sole against your inner left thigh. Press your right heel into your inner left groin, while pointing your toes toward the floor. The center of your pelvis should be directly over the left foot.

3 Rest your hands on the top rim of your pelvis. Make sure the pelvis is in a neutral position, with the top rim parallel to the floor.

4 Lengthen your tailbone toward the floor. Firmly press the sole of your right foot against your inner thigh while resisting with your outer left leg. Press your hands together, and gaze at a fixed point in front of you on the floor about 4 feet to 5 feet away.

5 Hold for 30 seconds to 1 minute. Exhale, and step back into Prayer Pose. Repeat with your opposite leg standing.

PRONUNCIATION & MEANING
- Vrksasana (vrik-SHAHS-anna)
- *vrksa* = tree

BENEFITS
- Strengthens thighs, calves, ankles, and spine
- Stretches groins, inner thighs, chest, and shoulders
- Improves sense of balance
- Relieves sciatica
- Reduces flat feet

CONTRA-INDICATIONS & CAUTIONS
- Headache
- Insomnia
- High or low blood pressure

AVOID
- Jutting out your hip—keep both hips squared forward.

DO IT RIGHT
- If you are a beginner, brace your back against a wall to steady yourself.
- To keep your raised foot from sliding, place a folded sticky mat between your sole and inner thigh.

TREE POSE • STANDING POSES

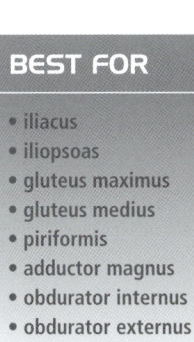

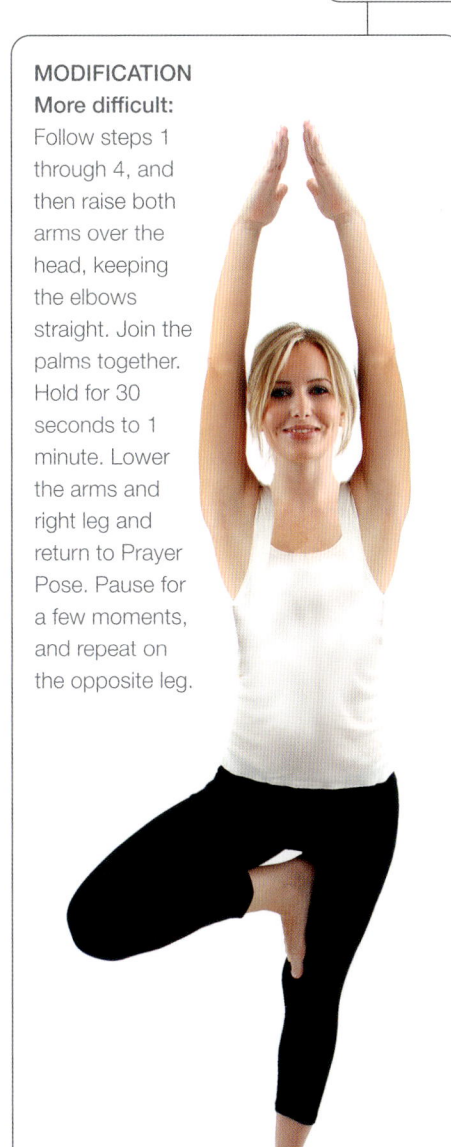

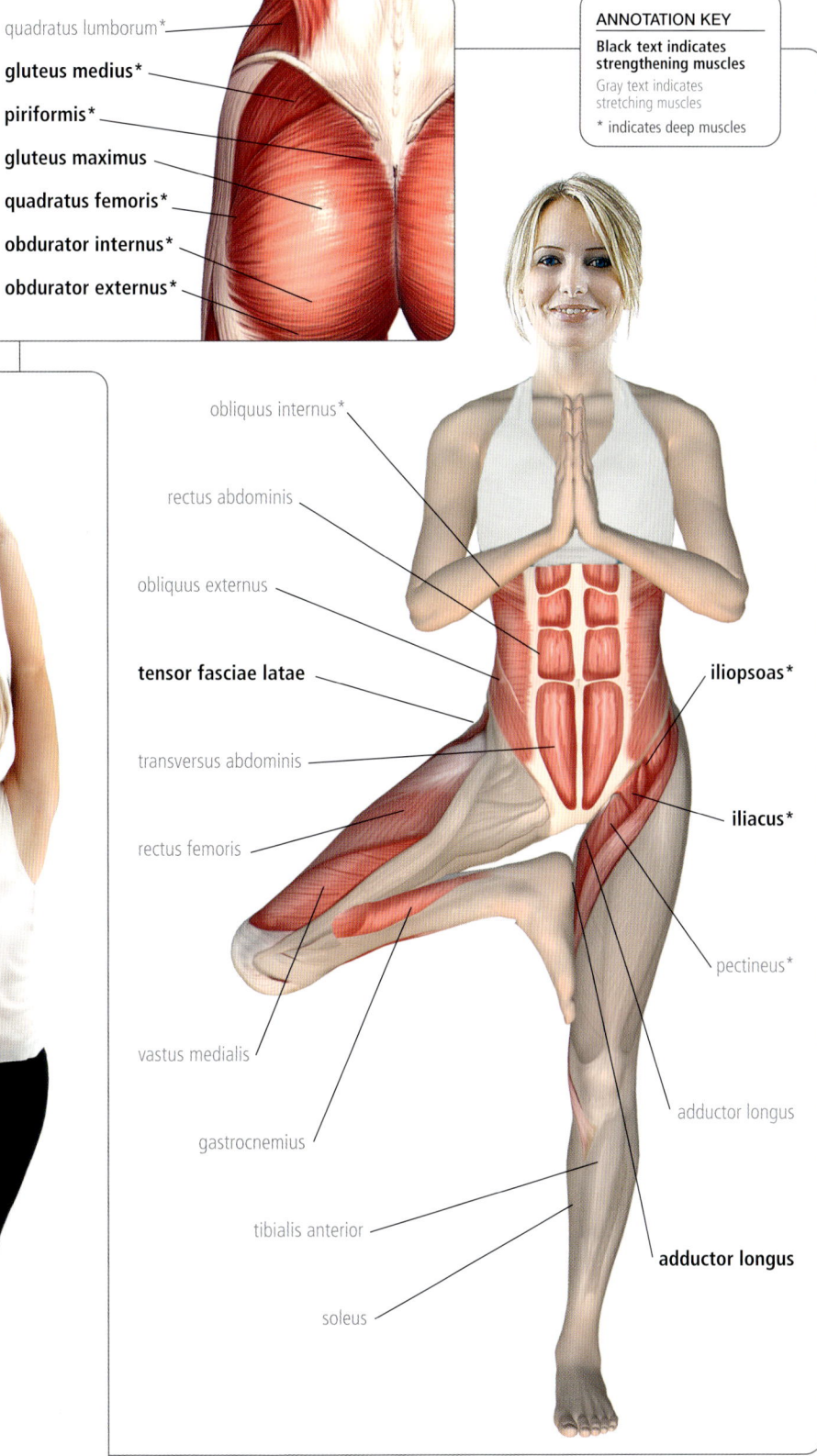

BEST FOR

- iliacus
- iliopsoas
- gluteus maximus
- gluteus medius
- piriformis
- adductor magnus
- obdurator internus
- obdurator externus
- tensor fasciae latae
- rectus femoris

ANNOTATION KEY

Black text indicates strengthening muscles
Gray text indicates stretching muscles
* indicates deep muscles

quadratus lumborum*
gluteus medius*
piriformis*
gluteus maximus
quadratus femoris*
obdurator internus*
obdurator externus*

MODIFICATION

More difficult:
Follow steps 1 through 4, and then raise both arms over the head, keeping the elbows straight. Join the palms together. Hold for 30 seconds to 1 minute. Lower the arms and right leg and return to Prayer Pose. Pause for a few moments, and repeat on the opposite leg.

obliquus internus*
rectus abdominis
obliquus externus
tensor fasciae latae
transversus abdominis
rectus femoris
vastus medialis
gastrocnemius
tibialis anterior
soleus
iliopsoas*
iliacus*
pectineus*
adductor longus
adductor longus

45

STANDING POSES

GARLAND POSE
(MALASANA)

① Stand in Mountain Pose (pages 36-37), with feet shoulder-width apart and your pelvis, head, and chest aligned.

② Keeping your heels on the floor, extend your arms straight out in front of you. Bend your knees, folding your body forward and down by dropping your pelvis.

③ Slightly separate your thighs wider than your torso. Exhale, and lean your body forward, fitting it snugly in the space between your thighs.

④ Press your elbows against the back of your knees, and join your palms together, as if in prayer, and then press your knees into your elbows.

⑤ Hold for 30 seconds to 1 minute. Exhale, and straighten your knees, slowly standing up.

AVOID
- Leaning forward.
- Drooping your shoulders.

DO IT RIGHT
- If your heels come up as you reach the squatting position, place a folded blanket under them, and squat again.
- If squatting is difficult, you can get a similar stretch by sitting on the front edge of a chair seat, with your thighs forming a right angle to your torso. Place your heels on the floor slightly in front of your knees, and lean your torso forward between the thighs.

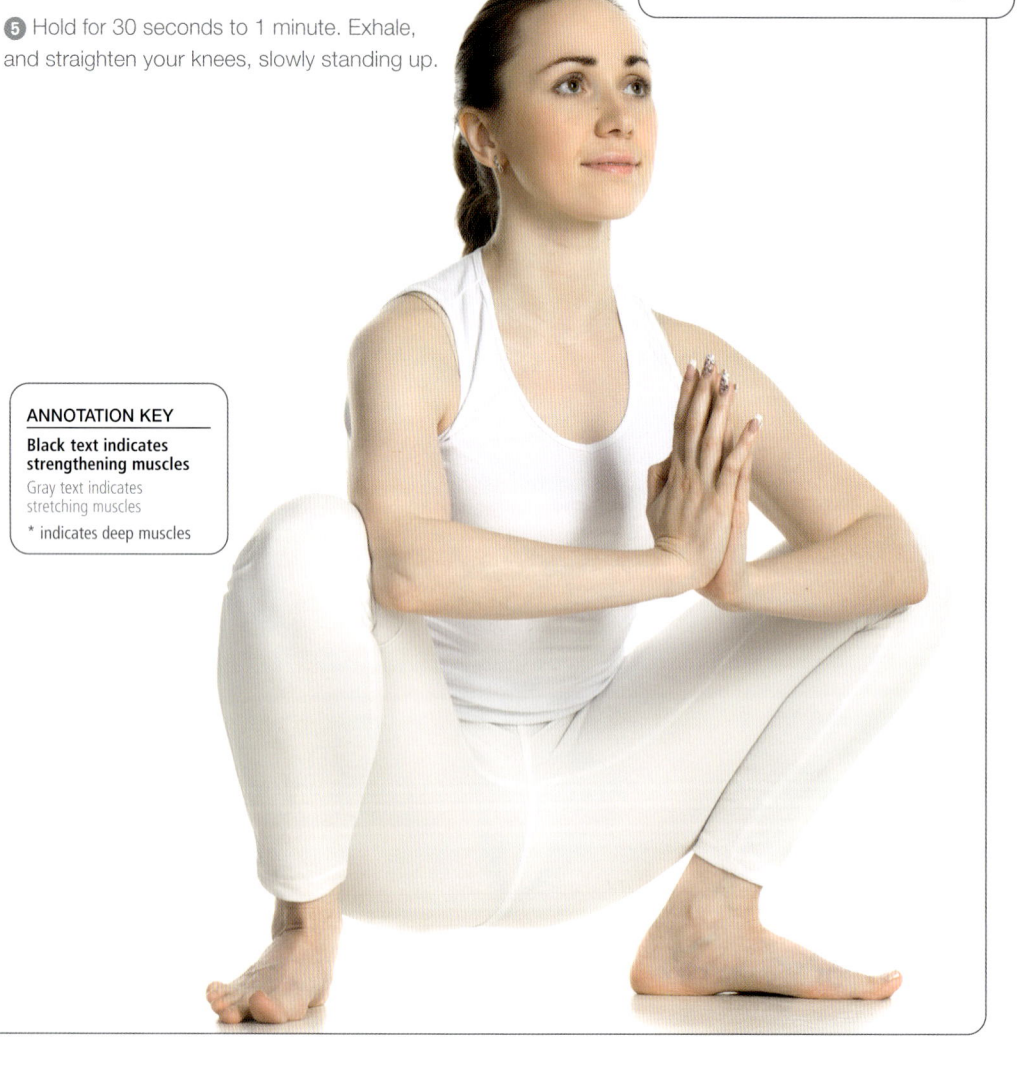

PRONUNCIATION & MEANING
- Malasana (ma-LAHS-anna)
- *mala* = garland
- Also called Wide Squat or Frog Pose

BENEFITS
- Stretches ankles, groins, lower legs, and back torso
- Tones pelvic-floor muscles
- Tones abdominals

CONTRA-INDICATIONS & CAUTIONS
- Headache
- Insomnia
- Low blood pressure

ANNOTATION KEY
Black text indicates strengthening muscles
Gray text indicates stretching muscles
* indicates deep muscles

GARLAND POSE • STANDING POSES

BEST FOR

- quadratus lumborum*
- quadratus femoris
- transversus abdominis
- biceps femoris
- sartorius
- vastus intermedius
- vastus medialis
- vastus lateralis
- semitendonosus
- semimembranosus

quadratus lumborum*
gluteus medius*
gemellus superior*
piriformis*
gluteus maximus
quadratus femoris*
obdurator internus*
obdurator externus*
gemellus inferior*

obliquus internus*
adductor longus
adductor magnus
obliquus externus
transversus abdominis*
vastus lateralis
tibialis anterior
extensor digitorum longus
peroneus longus
peroneus brevis
flexor digitorum longus*
extensor hallucis longus

rectus abdominis
vastus medialis
sartorius
biceps femoris
semitendinosus
semimembranosus
gastrocnemius
tibilialis posterior*
soleus
abductor digiti minimi
adductor hallucis

ANNOTATION KEY

Black text indicates strengthening muscles
Gray text indicates stretching muscles
* indicates deep muscles

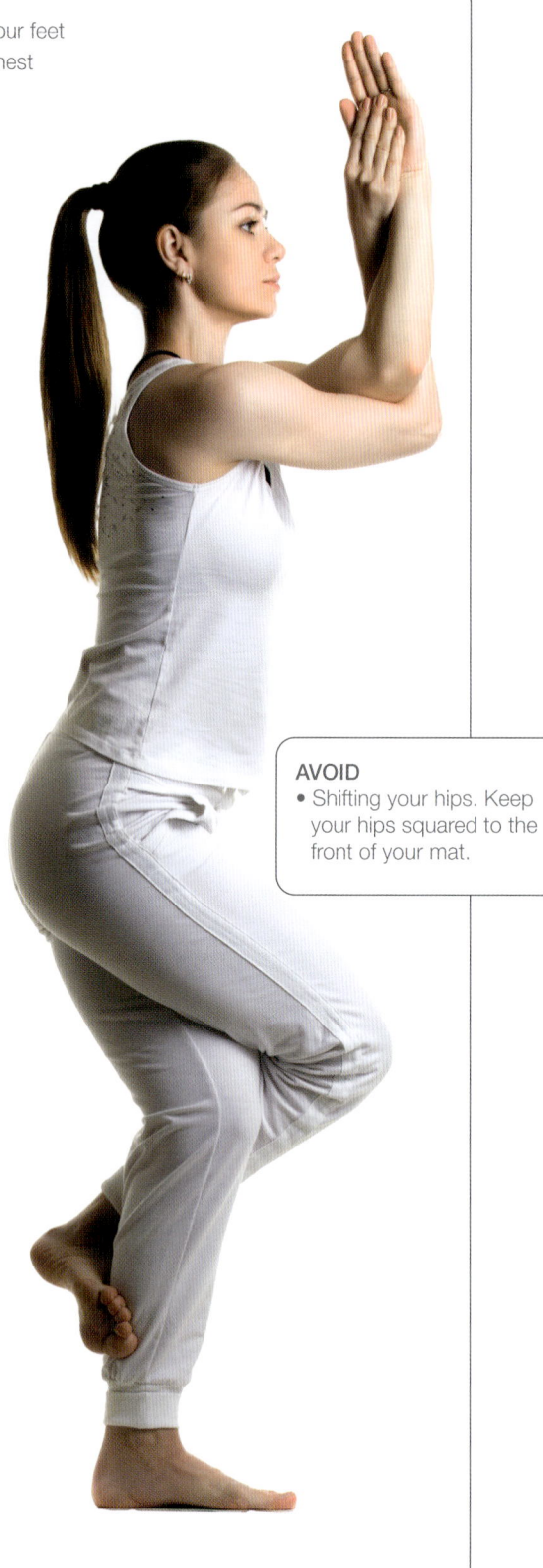

STANDING POSES

EAGLE POSE
(GARUDASANA)

① Stand in Mountain Pose (pages 36-37), with your feet shoulder-width apart and your pelvis, head, and chest aligned.

② Shift your weight to your right leg, and then bend your knees slightly. Lift your left foot as you balance on your right foot, and cross your left thigh over the right.

③ Point your left toes toward the floor, press your foot back, and then hook the top of your foot behind your lower right calf. Maintain your balance on your right foot.

④ Inhale, and stretch your arms straight forward, keeping them parallel to the floor, and spread your scapulas wide across your back. Cross the arms in front of your torso so that your right arm is above the left, and then bend your elbows. Bring your right elbow into the crook of the left, and raise your forearms so that they are perpendicular to the floor. The backs of your hands should be facing each other.

⑤ Press your right hand to the right and your left hand to the left, so that your palms face each other. Your right-hand thumb should pass in front of the little finger of your left hand. Press your palms together, lift your elbows up, and stretch your fingers toward the ceiling.

⑥ Hold for 15 to 60 seconds.

⑦ Slowly unwind your legs and arms, and return to Mountain Pose. Repeat with your arms and legs reversed.

PRONUNCIATION & MEANING
- Garudasana (gah-rue-DAHS-anna)
- *garuda* = eagle, or the name of a mythic king of birds

BENEFITS
- Strengthens ankles and calves
- Stretches ankles, calves, thighs, hips, shoulders, and upper back
- Improves concentration
- Improves sense of balance

CONTRA-INDICATIONS & CAUTIONS
- Arm injury
- Hip injury
- Knee injury

AVOID
- Shifting your hips. Keep your hips squared to the front of your mat.

EAGLE POSE • STANDING POSES

DO IT RIGHT
- If you find it difficult to wrap your arms around each other until your palms touch, stretch your arms straight forward, parallel to the floor, while holding onto the ends of a strap.
- If you find it difficult to maintain your balance as you hook the foot of your raised leg behind the calf of your standing leg, press the big toe of your raised-leg foot against the floor.

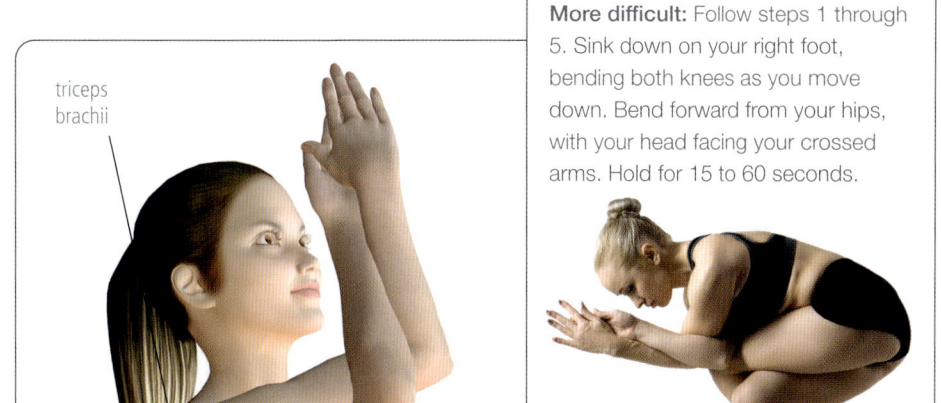

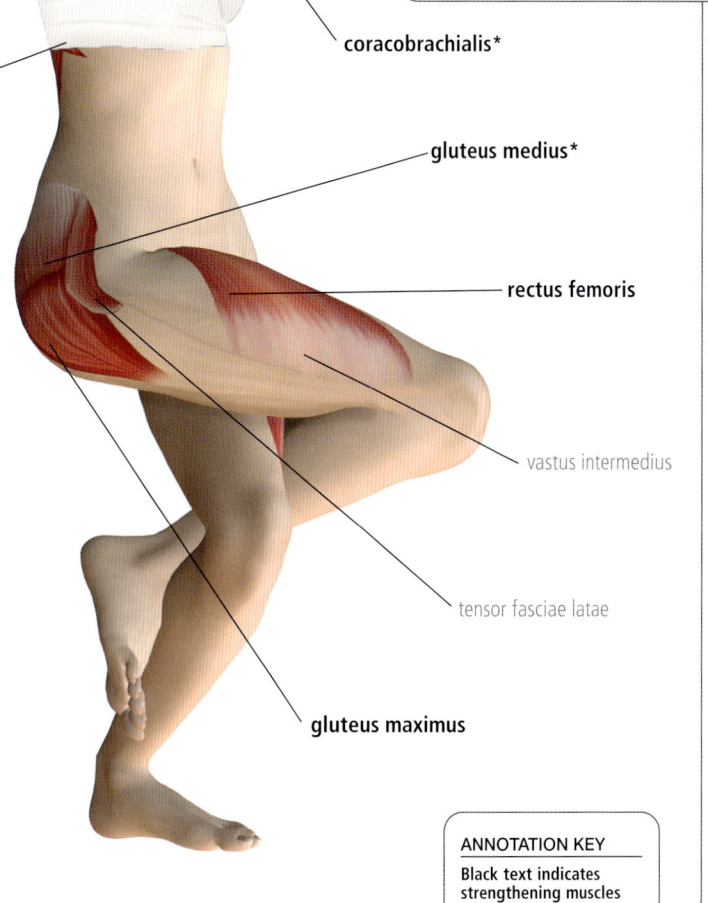

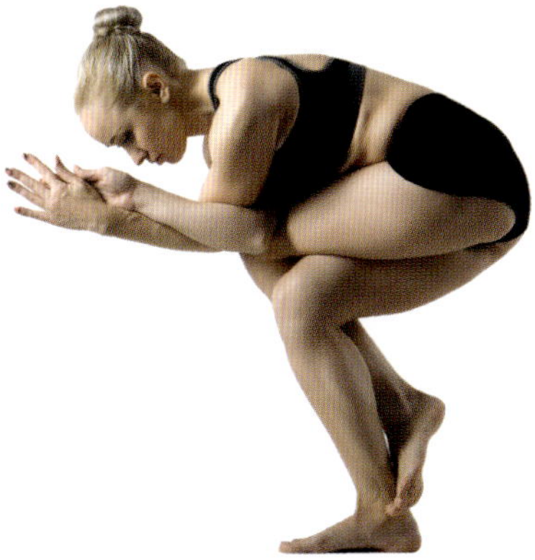

BEST FOR
- trapezius
- infraspinatus
- teres major
- teres minor
- latissimus dorsi
- gluteus medius
- adductor magnus
- quadratus lumborum
- serratus anterior

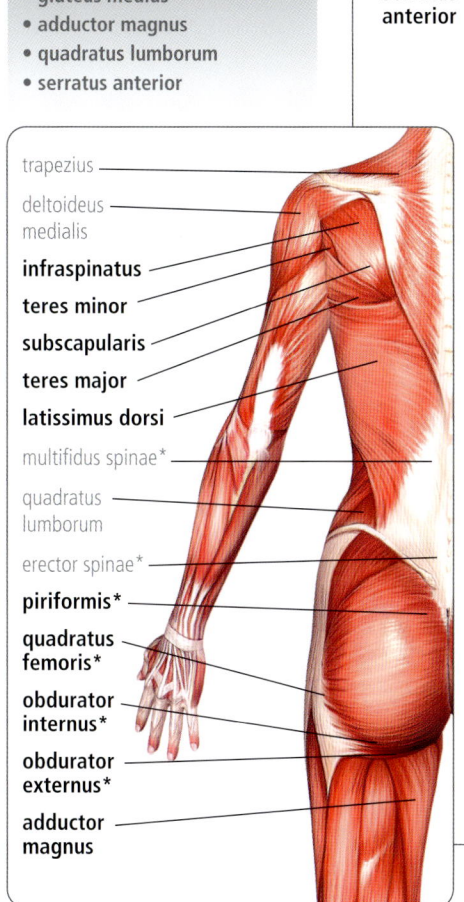

MODIFICATION
More difficult: Follow steps 1 through 5. Sink down on your right foot, bending both knees as you move down. Bend forward from your hips, with your head facing your crossed arms. Hold for 15 to 60 seconds.

triceps brachii
serratus anterior
coracobrachialis*
gluteus medius*
rectus femoris
vastus intermedius
tensor fasciae latae
gluteus maximus

trapezius
deltoideus medialis
infraspinatus
teres minor
subscapularis
teres major
latissimus dorsi
multifidus spinae*
quadratus lumborum
erector spinae*
piriformis*
quadratus femoris*
obdurator internus*
obdurator externus*
adductor magnus

ANNOTATION KEY
Black text indicates strengthening muscles
Gray text indicates stretching muscles
* indicates deep muscles

49

STANDING POSES

TRIANGLE POSE
(TRIKONASANA)

① Stand in Mountain Pose (pages 36-37), with your pelvis, head, and chest aligned.

② Separate your feet slightly farther than the width of your shoulders.

③ Inhale, and raise both arms straight out to the side, keeping them parallel to the floor with your palms facing down.

④ Exhale slowly, and without bending your knees, pivot on your heels to turn your right foot all the way to the right and your left foot slightly toward the right, keeping your heels in line with each other.

⑤ Drop your torso as far as is comfortable to the right side, keeping your arms parallel to the floor.

⑥ Once the torso is fully extended to the right, drop your right arm so that your right hand rests on your shin or on the front of your ankle. At the same time, extend your left arm straight up toward the ceiling. Gently twist your spine and torso counterclockwise, using your extended arms as a lever, while your spinal axis remains parallel to the ground. Extend your arms apart from each other in opposite directions.

⑦ Turn your head to gaze at your left thumb, slightly intensifying the twist in your spine. Hold for 30 seconds to 1 minute.

⑧ Inhale, and return to a standing position with the arms outstretched, strongly pressing the back heel into the floor. Reverse the feet, and repeat on the other side.

AVOID
- Twisting your hips.

PRONUNCIATION & MEANING
- Trikonasana (trik-cone-AHS-anna)
- *trikona* = three angles, or triangle

BENEFITS
- Stretches thighs, knees, ankles, hips, groins, hamstrings, calves, shoulders, chest, and spine
- Relieves stress
- Stimulates digestion
- Relieves the symptoms of menopause
- Relieves backache

CONTRA-INDICATIONS & CAUTIONS
- Diarrhea
- Headache
- High or low blood pressure
- Neck issues

TRIANGLE POSE • STANDING POSES

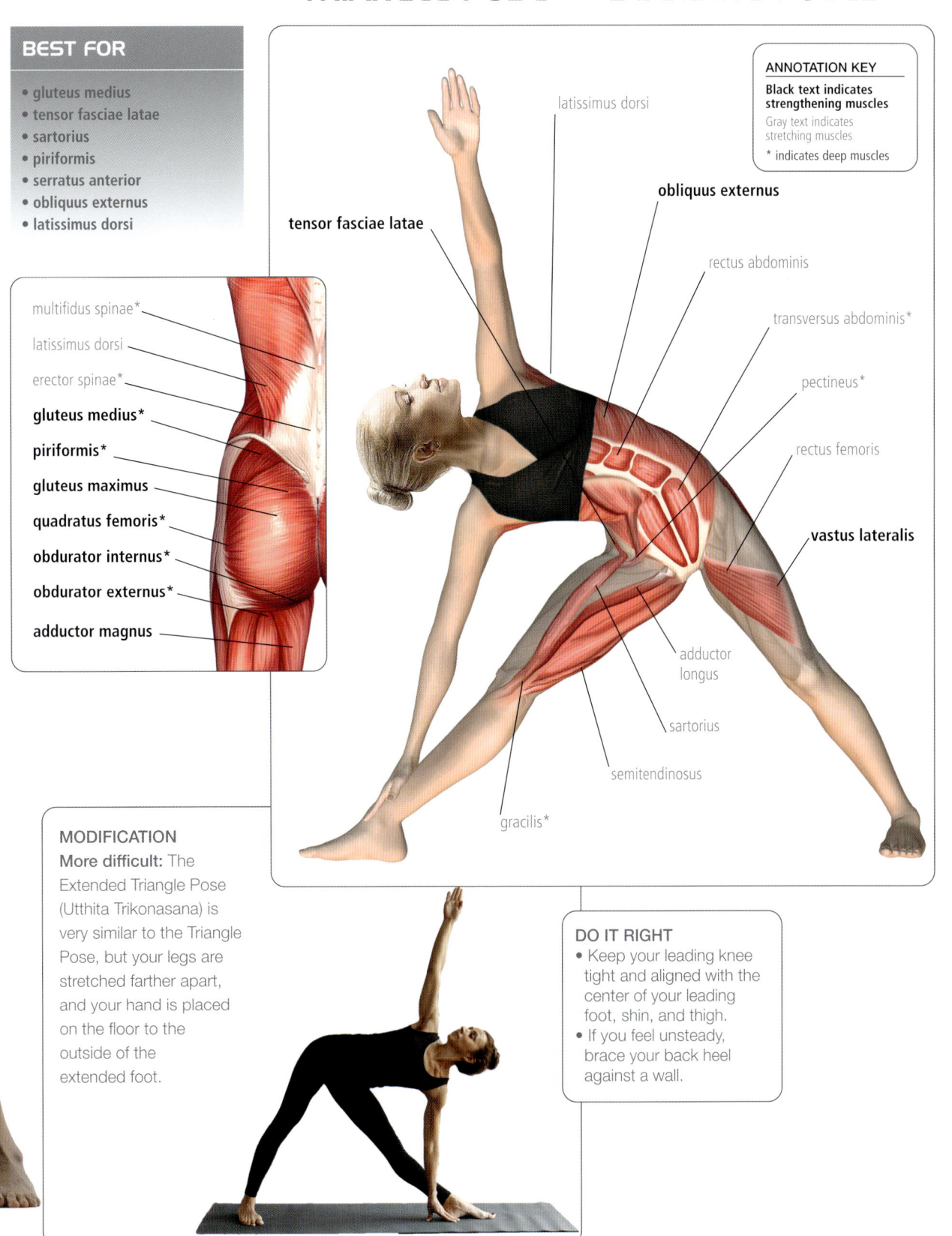

BEST FOR
- gluteus medius
- tensor fasciae latae
- sartorius
- piriformis
- serratus anterior
- obliquus externus
- latissimus dorsi

ANNOTATION KEY
Black text indicates strengthening muscles
Gray text indicates stretching muscles
* indicates deep muscles

Labels on main figure:
- latissimus dorsi
- **obliquus externus**
- **tensor fasciae latae**
- rectus abdominis
- transversus abdominis*
- pectineus*
- rectus femoris
- **vastus lateralis**
- adductor longus
- sartorius
- semitendinosus
- gracilis*

Labels on inset:
- multifidus spinae*
- latissimus dorsi
- erector spinae*
- **gluteus medius***
- **piriformis***
- gluteus maximus
- quadratus femoris*
- obdurator internus*
- obdurator externus*
- adductor magnus

MODIFICATION
More difficult: The Extended Triangle Pose (Utthita Trikonasana) is very similar to the Triangle Pose, but your legs are stretched farther apart, and your hand is placed on the floor to the outside of the extended foot.

DO IT RIGHT
- Keep your leading knee tight and aligned with the center of your leading foot, shin, and thigh.
- If you feel unsteady, brace your back heel against a wall.

51

EXTENDED SIDE ANGLE POSE
(UTTHITA PARSVAKONASANA)

STANDING POSES

① Stand in Warrior II Pose (pages 60-61) with your right leg bent, your left leg extended, and your arms raised to the sides, parallel to the floor.

② Anchor your left heel to the floor. Your right knee should be bent over your right ankle, so that your shin is perpendicular to the floor. Aim the inside of your knee toward the outside of your foot. Bring your right thigh parallel to the floor.

AVOID
- Sagging at the middle—your forward thigh should remain parallel to the floor.
- Lifting the heel of your extended leg.

③ Firm your shoulder blades against your back ribs. Extend your left arm straight up toward the ceiling, and then turn your left palm to face toward your head. Inhale, and reach your left arm over the back of your left ear, palm facing the floor, stretching from your left heel through your left fingertips to lengthen the entire left side of your body. Make sure your elbow remains straight.

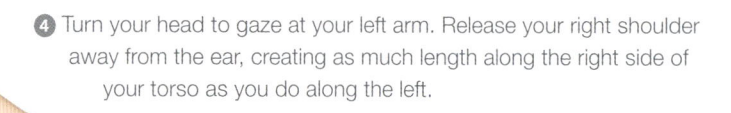

④ Turn your head to gaze at your left arm. Release your right shoulder away from the ear, creating as much length along the right side of your torso as you do along the left.

⑤ Continue to ground your left heel to the floor, exhale, and lay the right side of your torso down onto the top of your right thigh. Press your right fingertips or palm on the floor just outside of your right foot. Push your right knee back against your inner arm, while tucking your tailbone toward your pubis and pressing your hips forward.

⑥ Hold for 30 seconds to 1 minute.

⑦ Inhale, and begin to rise. Push both heels strongly into the floor, and reach your left arm toward the ceiling to lighten the upward movement. Reverse your feet, and repeat on the other side.

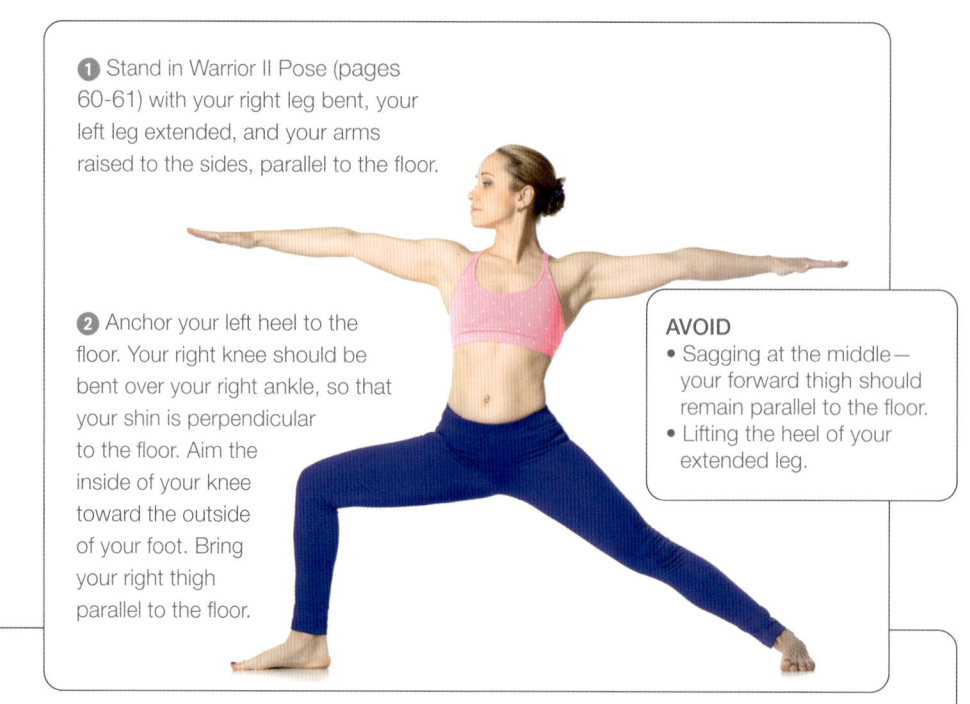

PRONUNCIATION & MEANING
- Utthita Parsvakonasana (oo-TEE-tah parsh-vah-cone-AHS-anna)
- *utthita* = extended; *parsva* = side, flank; *kona* = angle

BENEFITS
- Strengthens legs, knees, and ankles
- Stretches legs, knees, ankles, groins, spine, waist, chest and lungs, and shoulders
- Stimulates abdominal organs
- Increases stamina

CONTRA-INDICATIONS & CAUTIONS
- Headache
- Insomnia
- High or low blood pressure

EXTENDED SIDE ANGLE POSE • STANDING POSES

DO IT RIGHT
- If you feel unsteady, brace your back heel against a wall.
- If you have trouble reaching the floor with your hand, place your right hand on a block, or bend your elbow and place your forearm on your right thigh, hand facing up, and shoulder still away from ear.

BEST FOR
- semitendinosus
- semimembranosus
- obliquus internus
- transversus abdominis
- biceps femoris
- sartorius
- obliquus externus
- piriformis
- gracilis
- tensor fasciae latae

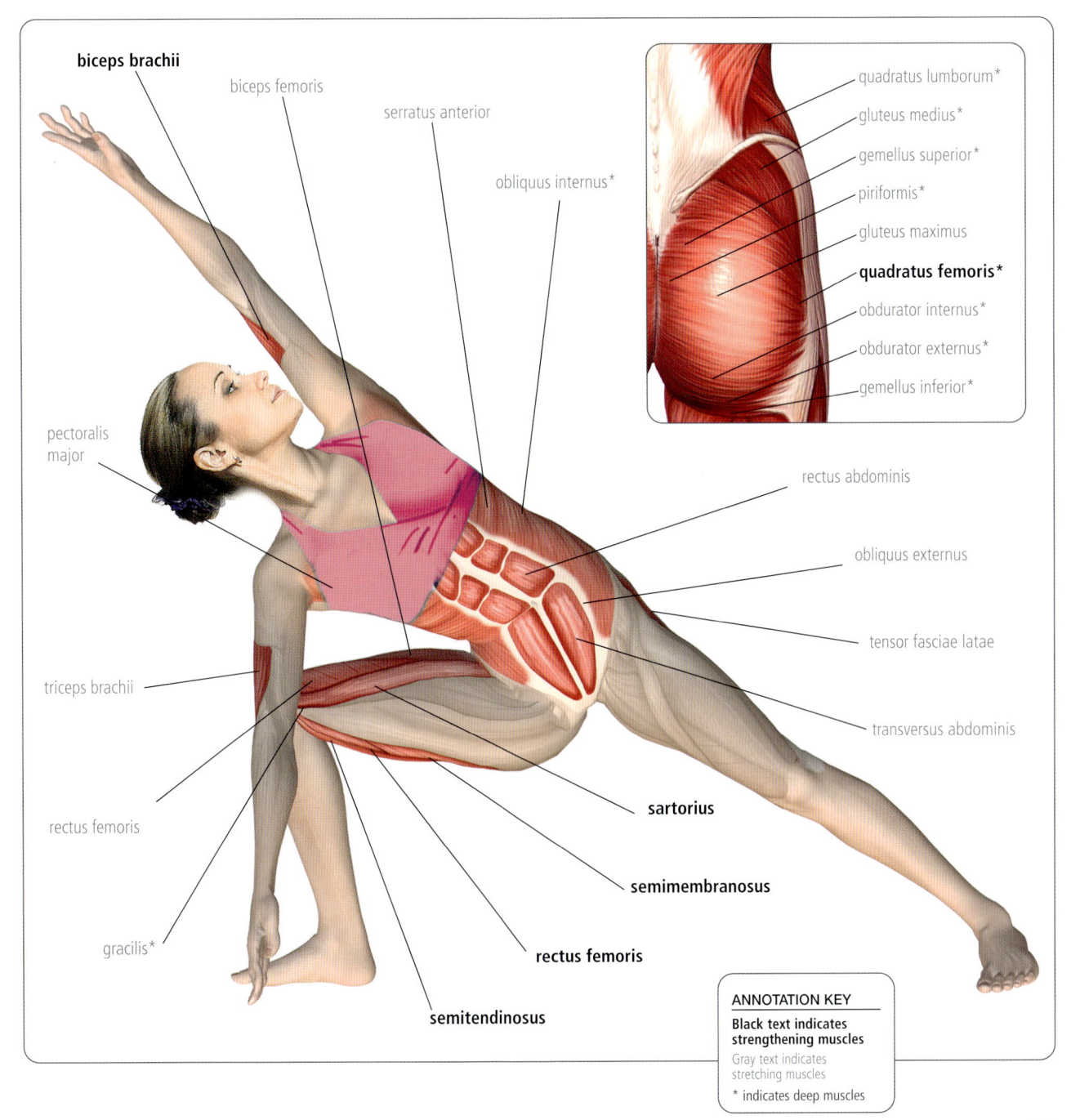

biceps brachii

biceps femoris

serratus anterior

obliquus internus*

quadratus lumborum*
gluteus medius*
gemellus superior*
piriformis*
gluteus maximus
quadratus femoris*
obdurator internus*
obdurator externus*
gemellus inferior*

pectoralis major

rectus abdominis

obliquus externus

triceps brachii

tensor fasciae latae

transversus abdominis

rectus femoris

sartorius

semimembranosus

gracilis*

rectus femoris

semitendinosus

ANNOTATION KEY
Black text indicates strengthening muscles
Gray text indicates stretching muscles
* indicates deep muscles

53

STANDING POSES

LOW LUNGE POSE
(ANJANEYASANA)

❶ Stand in Downward-Facing Dog Pose. Exhale, and step your right foot forward between your hands, aligning your right knee over your heel.

❷ Lower your left knee to the floor, and, keeping your right knee fixed in place, slide your left back until you feel a comfortable stretch in the front of your left thigh and groin. Rest the top of your left foot on the floor.

❸ Inhale, and lift your torso to an upright position. At the same time, sweep your arms out to the sides and up toward the ceiling. Draw your tailbone down toward the floor, and lift your pubis toward your navel.

DO IT RIGHT
- If your lowered knee feels uncomfortable, place a folded towel underneath it.

❹ Tilt your head, and gaze upward while reaching your pinkies toward the ceiling. Hold for 1 minute.

❺ Exhale, and fold your torso back down to your right thigh. Place your hands on the floor, and flip your toes so that the bottoms press against the floor. Exhale, and lift your left knee off the floor and step back to the Downward-Facing Dog Pose. Repeat on the other side.

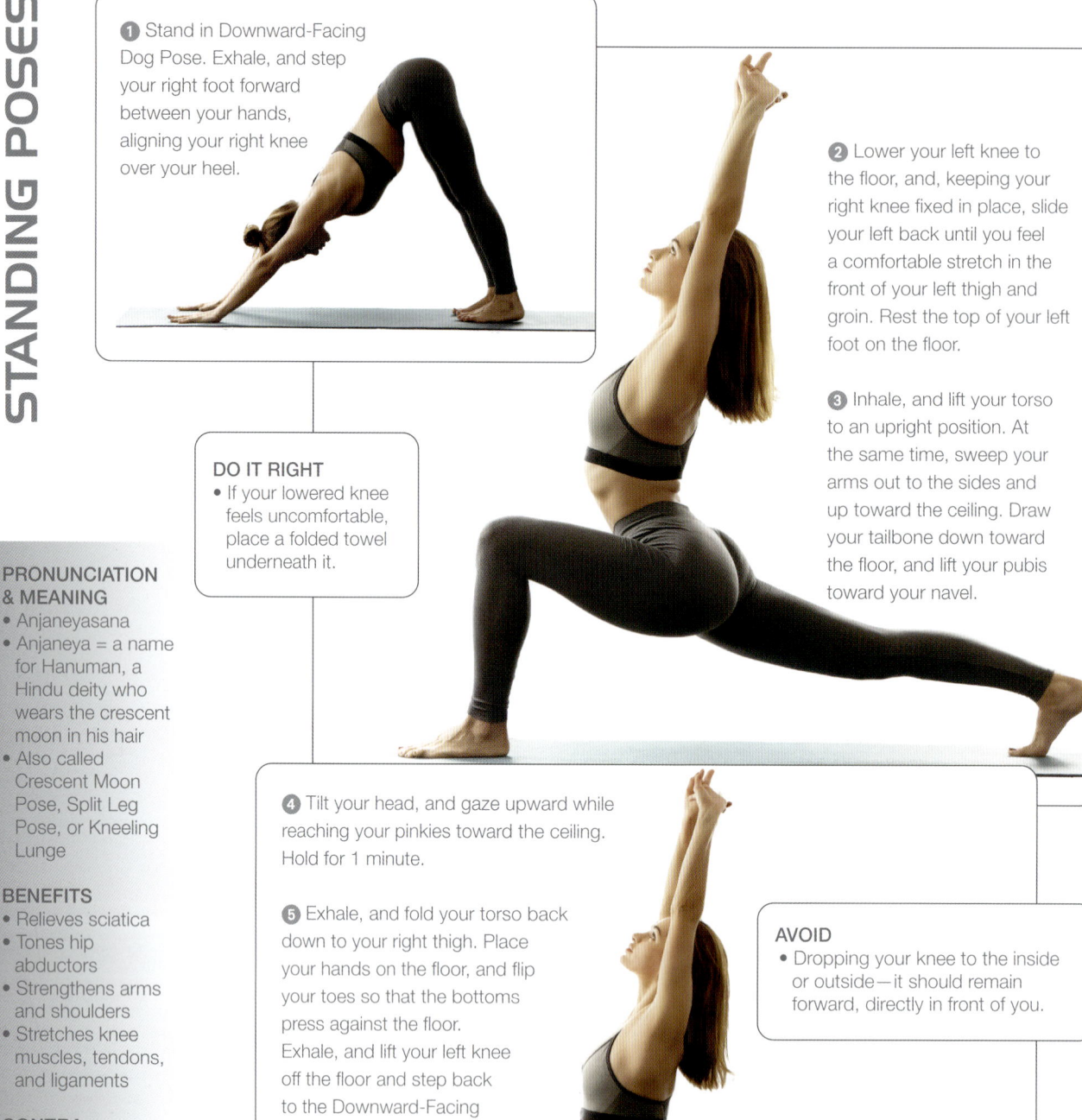

AVOID
- Dropping your knee to the inside or outside—it should remain forward, directly in front of you.

PRONUNCIATION & MEANING
- Anjaneyasana
- Anjaneya = a name for Hanuman, a Hindu deity who wears the crescent moon in his hair
- Also called Crescent Moon Pose, Split Leg Pose, or Kneeling Lunge

BENEFITS
- Relieves sciatica
- Tones hip abductors
- Strengthens arms and shoulders
- Stretches knee muscles, tendons, and ligaments

CONTRA-INDICATIONS & CAUTIONS
- Heart problems

LOW LUNGE POSE • STANDING POSES

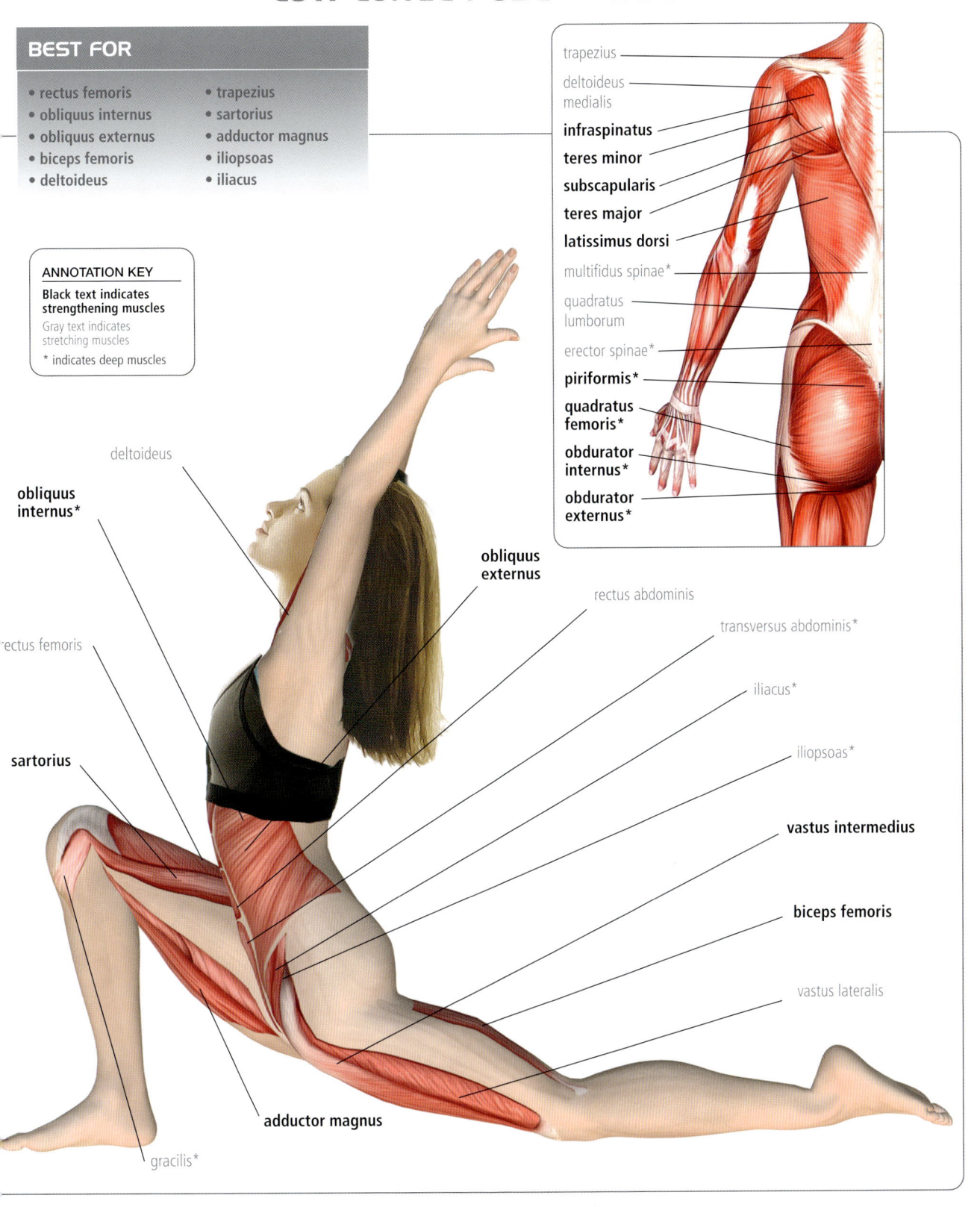

BEST FOR

- rectus femoris
- obliquus internus
- obliquus externus
- biceps femoris
- deltoideus
- trapezius
- sartorius
- adductor magnus
- iliopsoas
- iliacus

ANNOTATION KEY
Black text indicates strengthening muscles
Gray text indicates stretching muscles
* indicates deep muscles

trapezius
deltoideus medialis
infraspinatus
teres minor
subscapularis
teres major
latissimus dorsi
multifidus spinae*
quadratus lumborum
erector spinae*
piriformis*
quadratus femoris*
obdurator internus*
obdurator externus*

deltoideus

obliquus internus*

obliquus externus

rectus abdominis

transversus abdominis*

iliacus*

iliopsoas*

rectus femoris

sartorius

vastus intermedius

biceps femoris

vastus lateralis

adductor magnus

gracilis*

55

STANDING POSES

HIGH LUNGE

❶ Stand in Mountain Pose (pages 36-37), and inhale deeply. Exhale, and carefully step back with your left leg, keeping it in line with your hips as you step back. The ball of your left foot should be in contact with the floor as you do the motion.

❷ Slowly slide your left foot farther back, while bending your right knee, stacking it directly above your ankle.

❸ Position your palms or fingers on the floor on either side of your right leg, and slowly press your palms or fingers against the floor to enhance the placement of your upper body and your head.

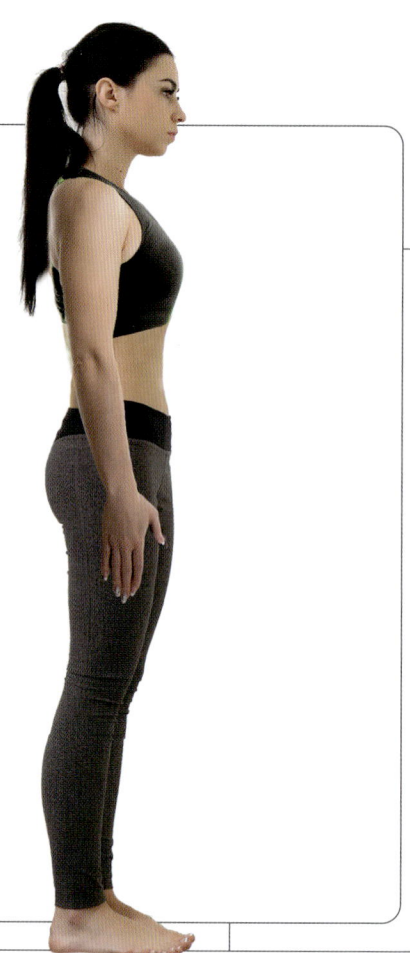

❹ Lift your head, and gaze straight forward, while leaning your upper body forward and carefully rolling your shoulders down and backward.

❺ Press the ball of your left foot gradually on the floor, contract your thigh muscles, and press up to maintain your left leg in a straight position.

❻ Hold for 5 to 6 seconds. Slowly return to Mountain Pose, and then repeat on the other side.

AVOID
- Dropping your back-extended knee to the floor.

PRONUNCIATION & MEANING
- There is no agreed-upon Sanskrit name for this pose.
- Sometimes called the Horse Rider's Pose (Ashva Sanchalanasana)

BENEFITS
- Strengthens legs and arms
- Stretches groins
- Relieves constipation

CONTRA-INDICATIONS & CAUTIONS
- Arm injury
- Shoulder injury
- Hip injury
- High or low blood pressure
- Severe headache

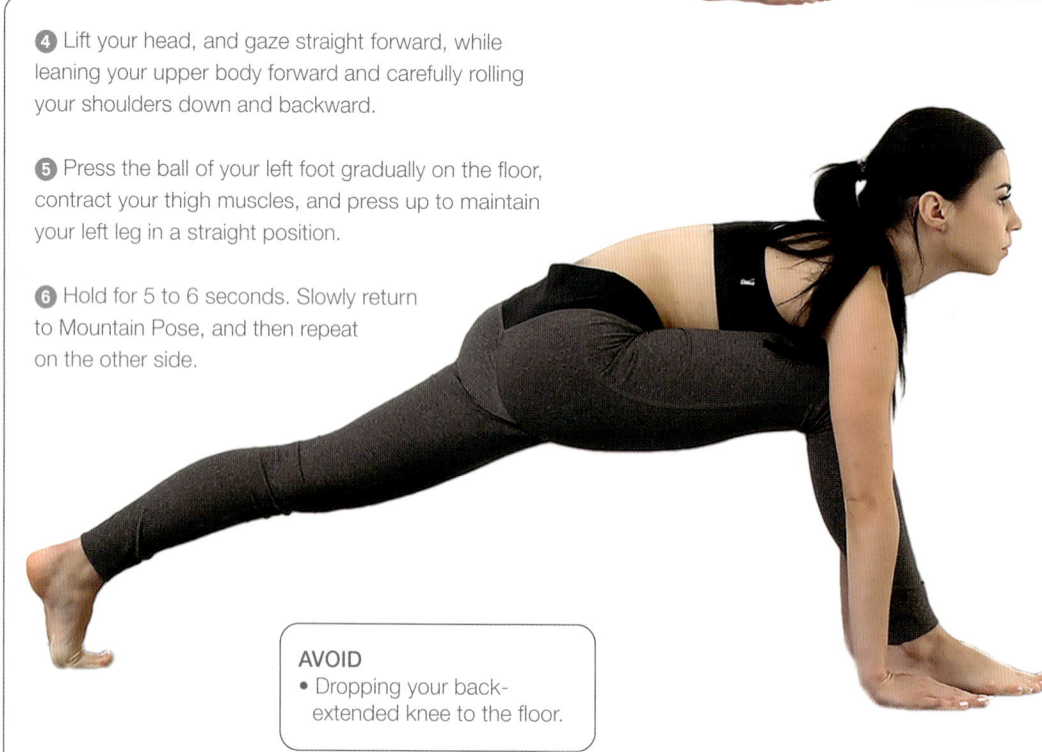

HIGH LUNGE • STANDING POSES

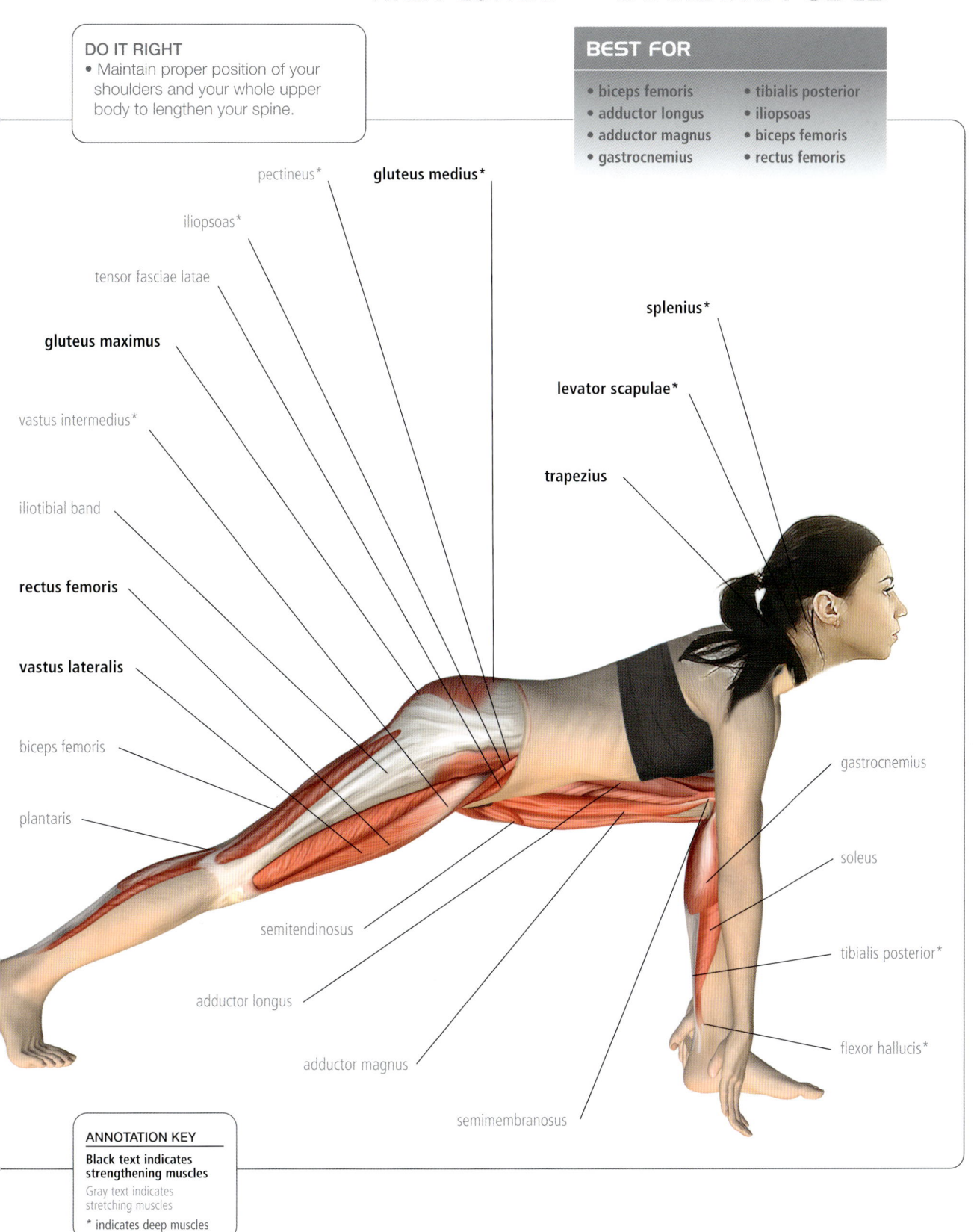

DO IT RIGHT
- Maintain proper position of your shoulders and your whole upper body to lengthen your spine.

BEST FOR
- biceps femoris
- adductor longus
- adductor magnus
- gastrocnemius
- tibialis posterior
- iliopsoas
- biceps femoris
- rectus femoris

pectineus*

gluteus medius*

iliopsoas*

tensor fasciae latae

splenius*

gluteus maximus

levator scapulae*

vastus intermedius*

trapezius

iliotibial band

rectus femoris

vastus lateralis

gastrocnemius

biceps femoris

plantaris

soleus

semitendinosus

tibialis posterior*

adductor longus

flexor hallucis*

adductor magnus

semimembranosus

ANNOTATION KEY

Black text indicates strengthening muscles

Gray text indicates stretching muscles

* indicates deep muscles

57

STANDING POSES

WARRIOR POSE I
(VIRABHADRASANA I)

1 Stand in Mountain Pose (pages 36-37). Exhale, and step your left foot back 3.5 to 4 feet apart. Align your left heel behind the right heel, and then turn your left foot out 45 degrees, keeping you right foot facing straight forward. Rotate your hips so both hipbones are squared forward and are parallel to the front of your mat.

2 Inhale, and raise your arms up toward the ceiling while keeping them parallel to each other and shoulder-width apart. Firm your shoulder blades against your back, and draw them down toward your tailbone.

3 Exhale, contract yours abdominals, and tuck your tailbone under. With your left heel firmly grounded, exhale, and then slowly bend your right knee, stacking it over your heel. Your right shin should be perpendicular to the floor and your right thigh parallel to the floor.

4 Keep your head in a neutral position, gazing forward, or tilt it back and look up at your thumbs. Hold for 30 seconds to 1 minute.

5 To come up, inhale, press the back heel firmly into the floor and reach up with your arms, straightening your right knee. Turn your feet forward, exhale, and release your arms. Take a few breaths, turn your feet to the left, and repeat on the other side.

AVOID
- Shifting your weight too far forward so that your front knee is aligned over your toes.
- Allowing your hips to shift to either side.

DO IT RIGHT
- Apply slightly more pressure in your right heel rather than in your toes to keep your right knee stable.
- If you are a beginner, to maintain balance, decrease the distance between your feet by several inches, still keeping your right knee over your heel.

PRONUNCIATION & MEANING
- Virabhadrasana I (veer-ah-bah-DRAHS-anna)
- Virabhadra = the name of a fierce warrior
- Also known as Virabhadra's Pose

BENEFITS
- Strengthens arms, shoulders, thighs, ankles, and back
- Stretches hip flexors, abdominals, and ankles
- Expands chest, lungs, and shoulders
- Develops stamina
- Improves sense of balance

CONTRA-INDICATIONS & CAUTIONS
- Heart problems
- High blood pressure
- Shoulder injury

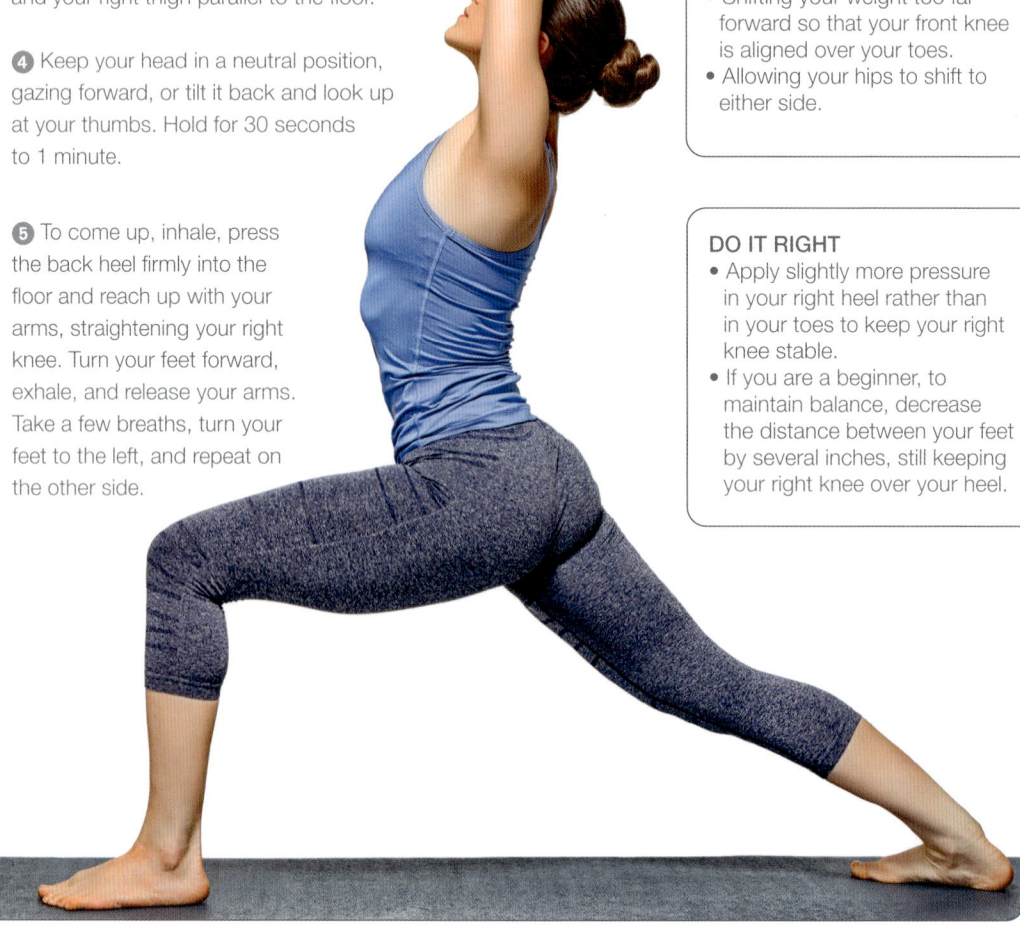

WARRIOR POSE I • STANDING POSES

BEST FOR
- rectus abdominis
- obliquus internus
- transversus abdominis
- biceps femoris
- sartorius
- obliquus externus

ANNOTATION KEY
Black text indicates strengthening muscles
Gray text indicates stretching muscles
* indicates deep muscles

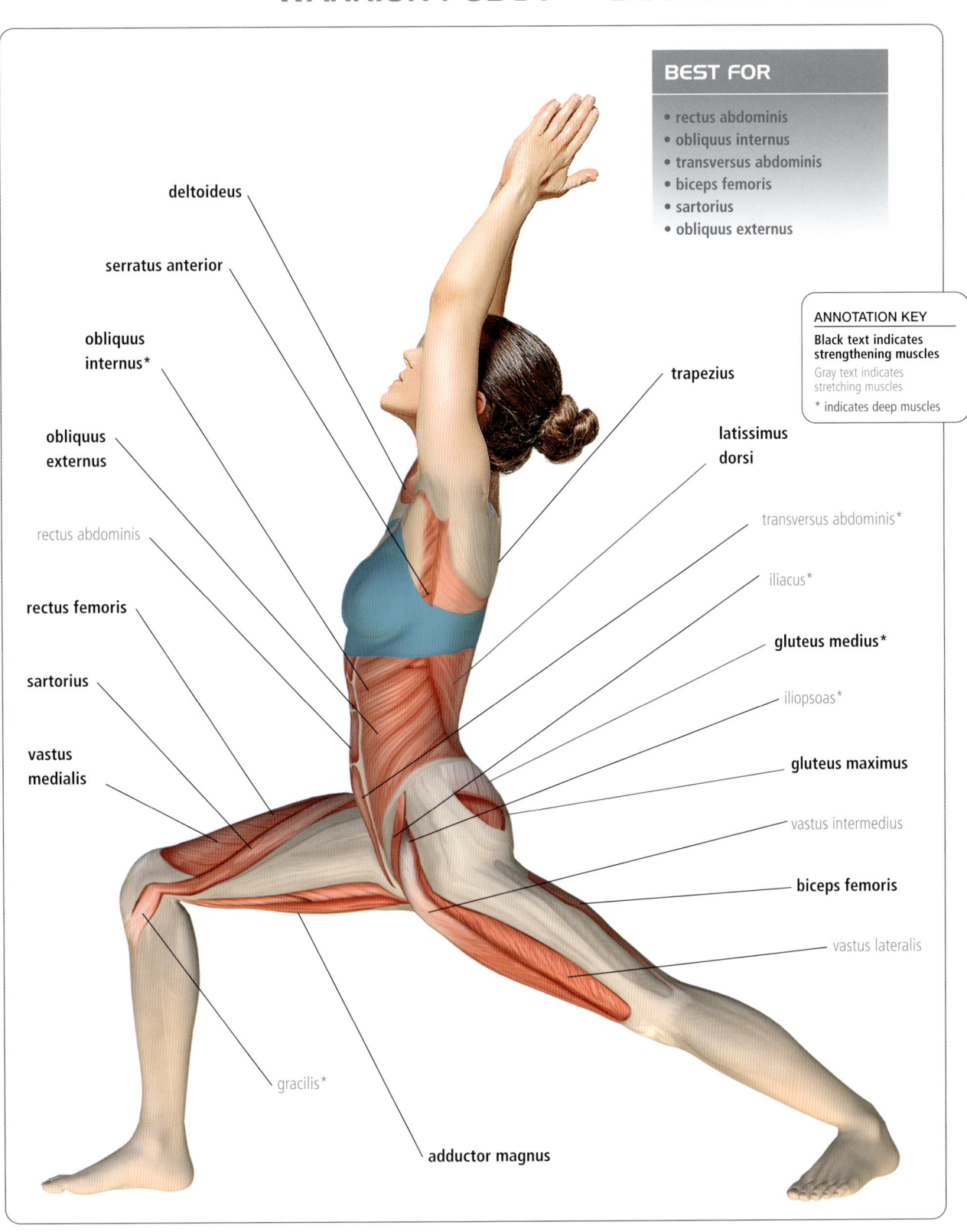

- deltoideus
- serratus anterior
- obliquus internus*
- obliquus externus
- rectus abdominis
- rectus femoris
- sartorius
- vastus medialis
- gracilis*
- adductor magnus
- trapezius
- latissimus dorsi
- transversus abdominis*
- iliacus*
- gluteus medius*
- iliopsoas*
- gluteus maximus
- vastus intermedius
- biceps femoris
- vastus lateralis

59

WARRIOR POSE II
(VIRABHADRASANA II)

STANDING POSES

① Stand in Mountain Pose (pages 36-37). Exhale, and step sideways so that your feet are 3.5 to 4 feet apart.

② Raise your arms parallel to the floor and reach them out to the sides, shoulder blades wide, palms facing downward.

DO IT RIGHT
- Focus on turning the knee of your bent leg outward, opening your hips and groins.

③ Turn your left foot in slightly to the right and your right foot out to the right 90 degrees. Align your right heel with your left heel. Firm your thighs and turn your right thigh outward so that the center of your right kneecap is in line with the center of your right ankle.

④ Exhale, and bend your right knee, so that your shin is perpendicular to the floor. Bring your right thigh parallel to the floor, anchoring your right knee by contracting the muscles of your left leg and pressing the outside of your left heel firmly to the floor. Keep the sides of your torso equally long and your shoulders aligned directly over your pelvis. Press your tailbone slightly toward your pubis.

⑤ Turn your head to the right and look out over your fingers.

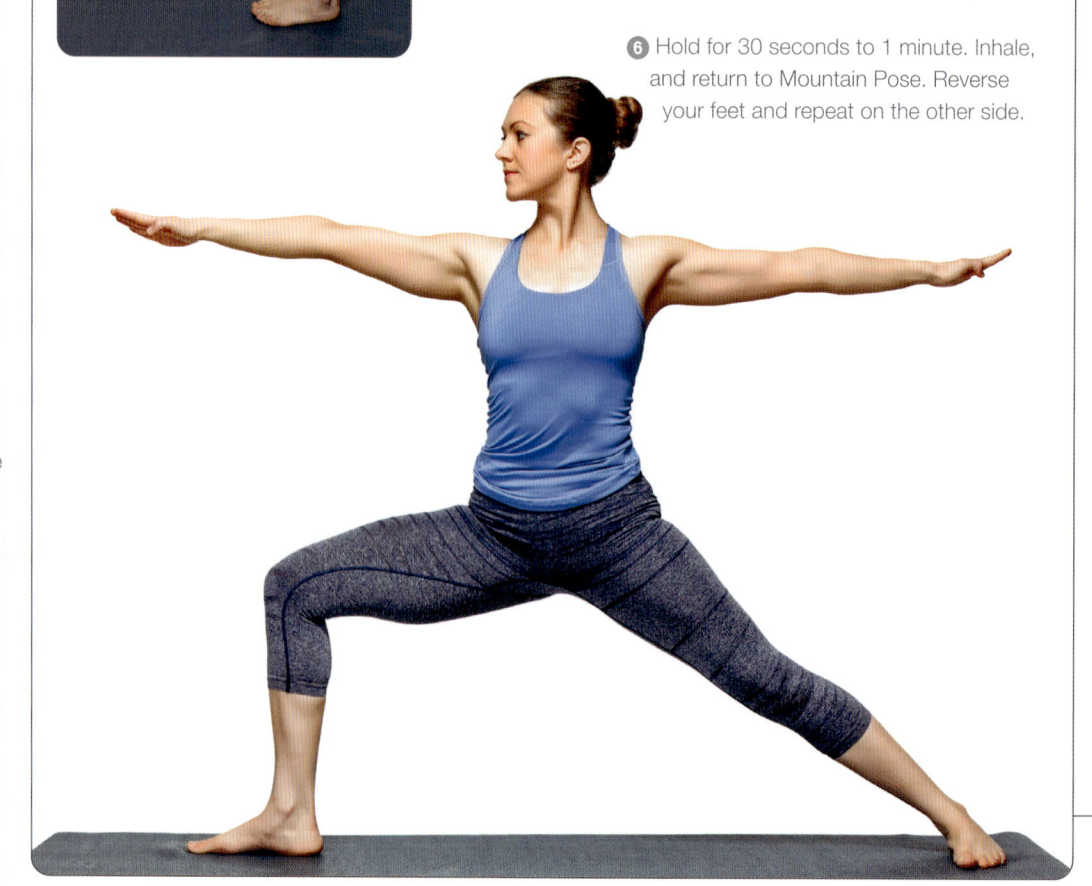

⑥ Hold for 30 seconds to 1 minute. Inhale, and return to Mountain Pose. Reverse your feet and repeat on the other side.

PRONUNCIATION & MEANING
- Virabhadrasana II (veer-ah-bah-DRAHS-anna)
- Virabhadra = the name of a fierce warrior

BENEFITS
- Strengthens legs and ankles
- Stretches legs, ankles, groins, chest, and shoulders
- Stimulates digestion
- Increases stamina
- Relieves backache
- Relieves carpal tunnel syndrome
- Relieves sciatica

CONTRA-INDICATIONS & CAUTIONS
- Diarrhea
- High blood pressure
- Neck issues

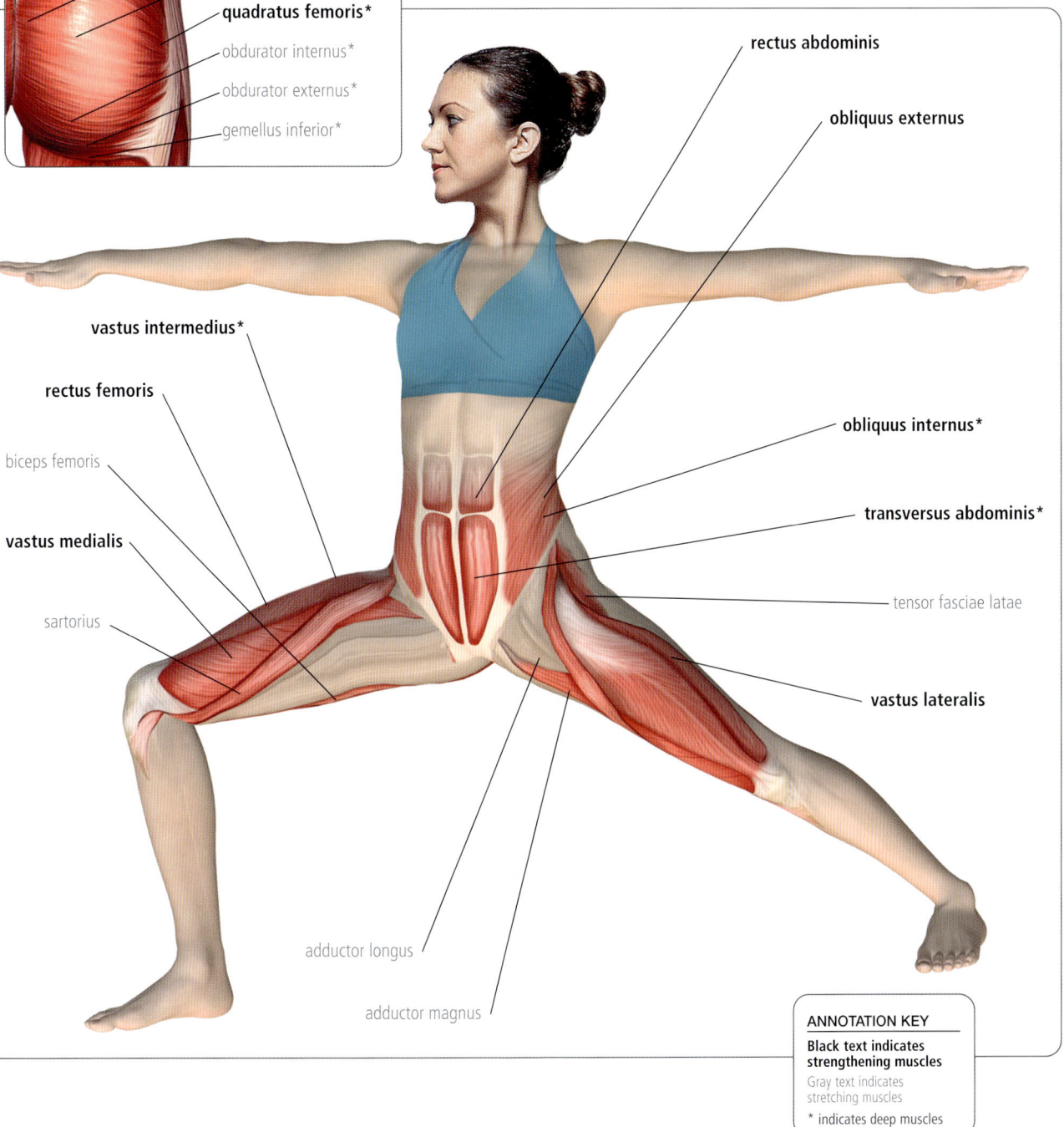

WARRIOR POSE II • STANDING POSES

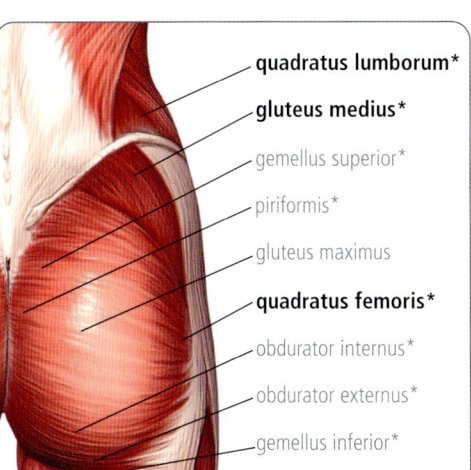

AVOID
- Allowing the knee to drift over to either side.
- Leaning your torso over your bent leg.

BEST FOR
- gluteus maximus
- gluteus medius
- obliquus externus
- biceps femoris
- sartorius
- adductor longus
- adductor magnus
- sartorius

quadratus lumborum*
gluteus medius*
gemellus superior*
piriformis*
gluteus maximus
quadratus femoris*
obdurator internus*
obdurator externus*
gemellus inferior*

rectus abdominis
obliquus externus
vastus intermedius*
rectus femoris
biceps femoris
vastus medialis
sartorius
obliquus internus*
transversus abdominis*
tensor fasciae latae
vastus lateralis
adductor longus
adductor magnus

ANNOTATION KEY
Black text indicates strengthening muscles
Gray text indicates stretching muscles
* indicates deep muscles

61

STANDING POSES

WARRIOR POSE III
(VIRABHADRASANA III)

① Stand in Mountain Pose (pages 36-37). Exhale, and step your right foot 1 foot forward, and shift all of your weight onto your right leg.

② Inhale, and raise your arms over your head, interlacing your fingers and pointing your index fingers upward.

③ Exhale, and lift your left leg up behind you, hinging at your hips to lower your arms and torso down toward the floor.

④ Gaze down at a point on the floor for balance. Elongate your body from your left toes through the crown of your head to your fingers, making one straight line.

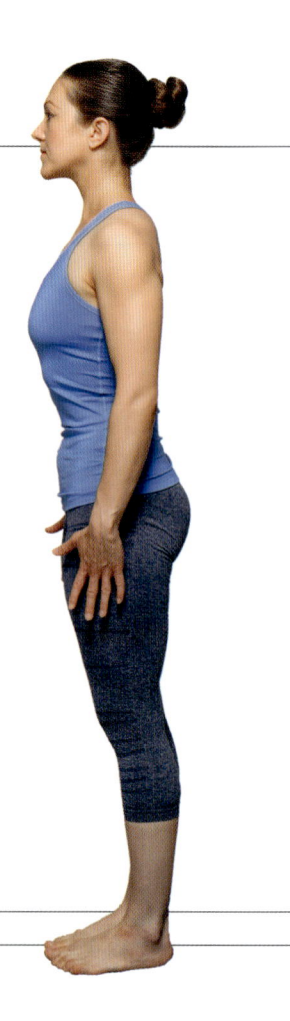

⑤ Hold for 30 seconds to 1 minute.

⑥ Inhale, and raise your arms upward as you lower your left leg back to the floor. Bring both feet together into the Mountain Pose.

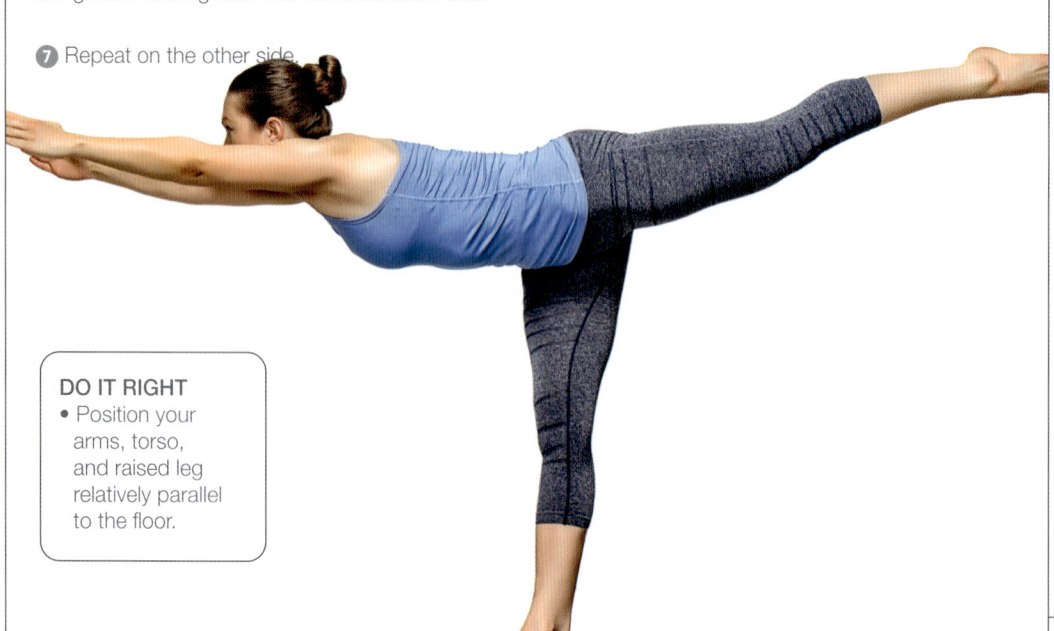

⑦ Repeat on the other side.

PRONUNCIATION & MEANING
- Virabhadrasana III (veer-ah-bah-DRAHS-anna)
- Virabhadra = the name of a fierce warrior

BENEFITS
- Strengthens ankles, legs, shoulders, and back muscles
- Tones abdominals
- Improves sense of balance
- Improves posture

CONTRA-INDICATIONS & CAUTIONS
- High blood pressure

DO IT RIGHT
- Position your arms, torso, and raised leg relatively parallel to the floor.

62

WARRIOR POSE III • STANDING POSES

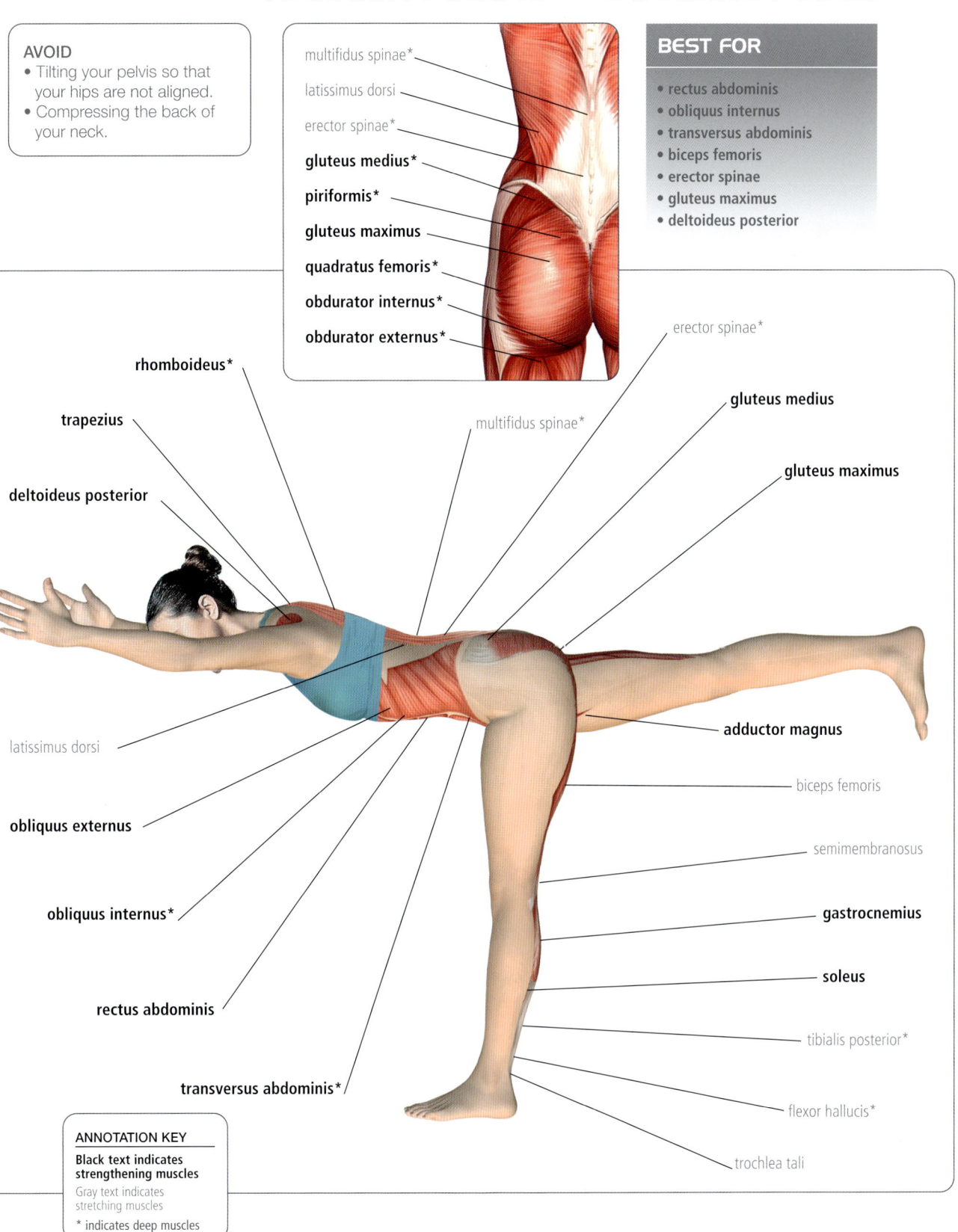

AVOID
- Tilting your pelvis so that your hips are not aligned.
- Compressing the back of your neck.

BEST FOR
- rectus abdominis
- obliquus internus
- transversus abdominis
- biceps femoris
- erector spinae
- gluteus maximus
- deltoideus posterior

multifidus spinae*
latissimus dorsi
erector spinae*
gluteus medius*
piriformis*
gluteus maximus
quadratus femoris*
obdurator internus*
obdurator externus*

rhomboideus*
trapezius
deltoideus posterior
multifidus spinae*
erector spinae*
gluteus medius
gluteus maximus
latissimus dorsi
adductor magnus
obliquus externus
biceps femoris
semimembranosus
gastrocnemius
obliquus internus*
soleus
tibialis posterior*
rectus abdominis
flexor hallucis*
transversus abdominis*
trochlea tali

ANNOTATION KEY
Black text indicates strengthening muscles
Gray text indicates stretching muscles
* indicates deep muscles

63

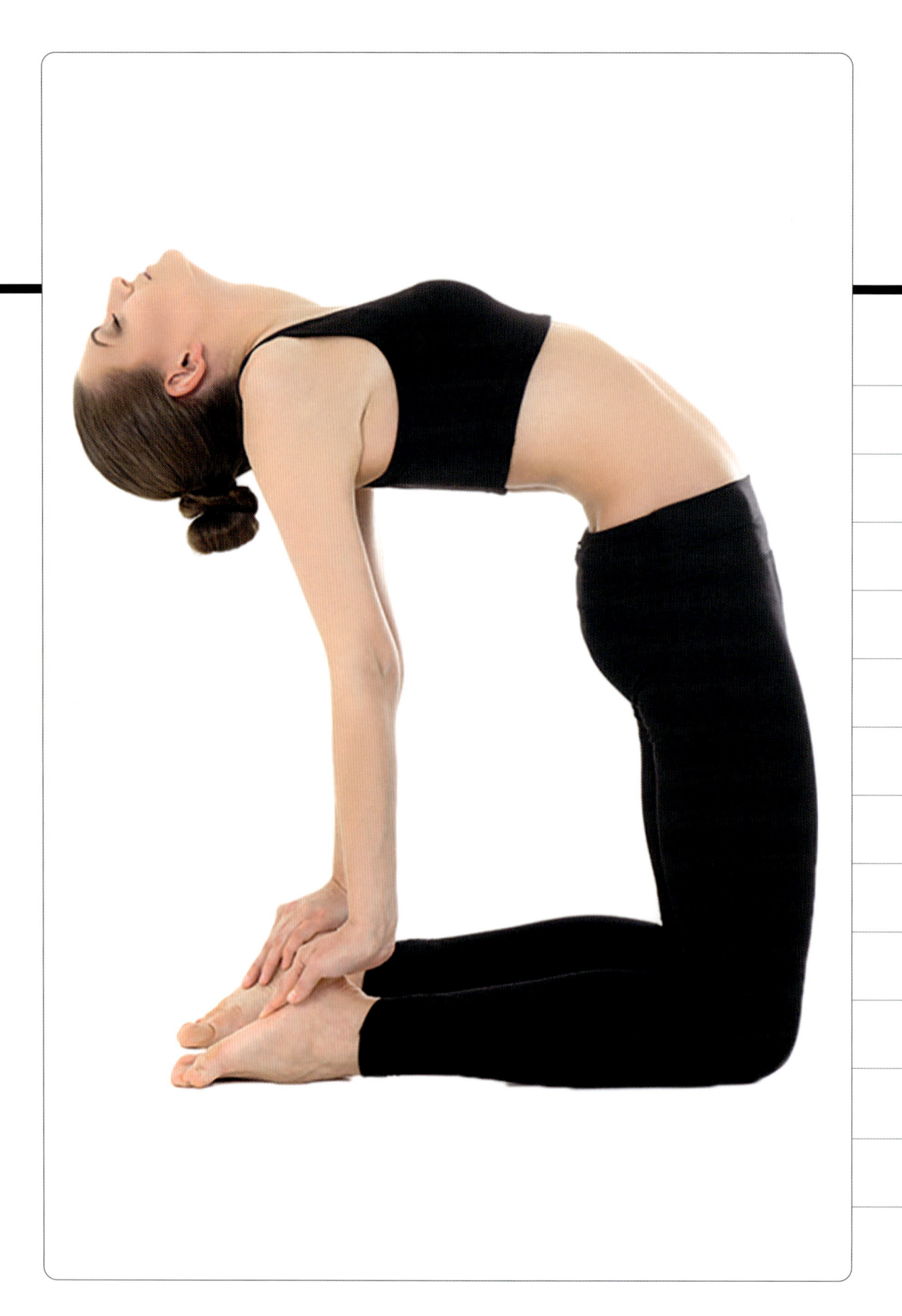

FORWARD BENDS & BACKBENDS

Forward bends are one of the most basic yoga poses, although they are not without variety. They can include standing or sitting poses. Forward bends release your spine by stretching your hamstrings and your back, increasing overall flexibility. To avoid straining your back, make sure to bend at the hips, not the waist.

Many newcomers to yoga tend to find backbends uncomfortable. These poses help correct the bad posture caused by sitting or slouching for several hours a day. However, these poses don't just impact your posture; they incorporate the entire body. They will open your chest, strengthen your back, and give your hips and spine mobility in addition to stretching your shoulders, abdominals, and tops of your legs.

STANDING TOE TOUCH

FORWARD BENDS & BACKBENDS

① Stand with your legs and feet parallel and shoulder-width apart. Bend your knees slightly.

② Slowly round your spine downward, from your neck through your lower back, and lower your arms down along the sides of your legs as you reach for your toes.

③ Continue to lower your torso downward as you bend at your waist, and let the weight of your body draw your head toward the floor as you stretch.

④ Hold for the recommended breaths.

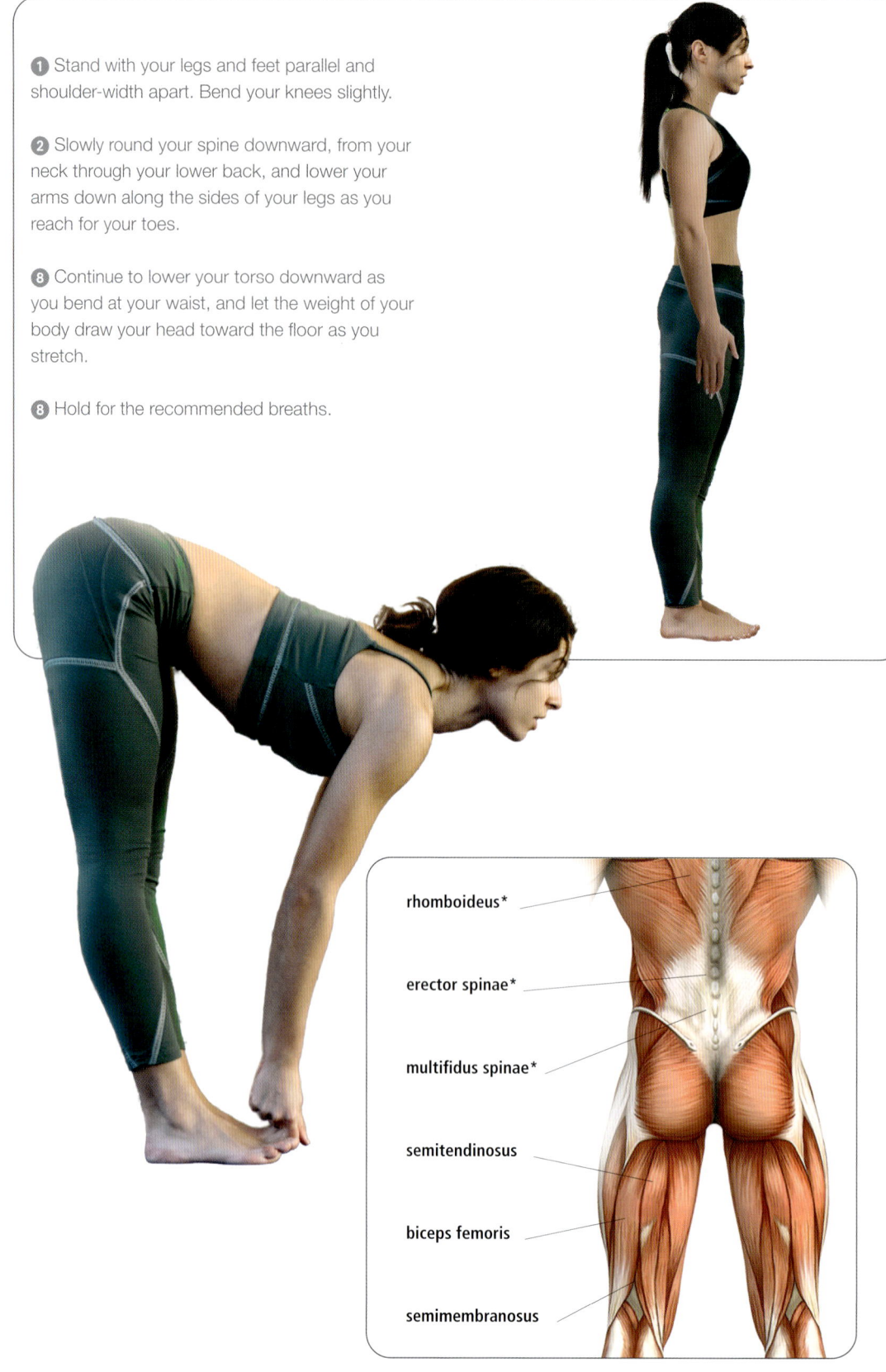

PRONUNCIATION & MEANING
- No name has been given

BENEFITS
- Strengthens ankles, legs, shoulders, and back muscles
- Tones abdominals
- Improves sense of balance
- Improves posture

CONTRA-INDICATIONS & CAUTIONS
- High blood pressure

rhomboideus*

erector spinae*

multifidus spinae*

semitendinosus

biceps femoris

semimembranosus

STANDING HALF FORWARD BEND
(ARDHA UTTANASANA)

6 From Standing Forward Bend, move into Standing Half Forward Bend (Ardha Uttanasana) by placing your hands beside your feet. Inhale, and lift your head and upper torso away from your legs. Your back should be flat. Straighten your elbows and use your fingertips to guide your lift.

7 Lift your chest forward, and elongate your spine into a slight arch. Lengthen the back of your neck as you gaze forward.

8 Hold for 10 to 30 seconds. Lower yourself back down to Standing Forward Bend, or inhale, and lift your torso all the way back up to Mountain Pose.

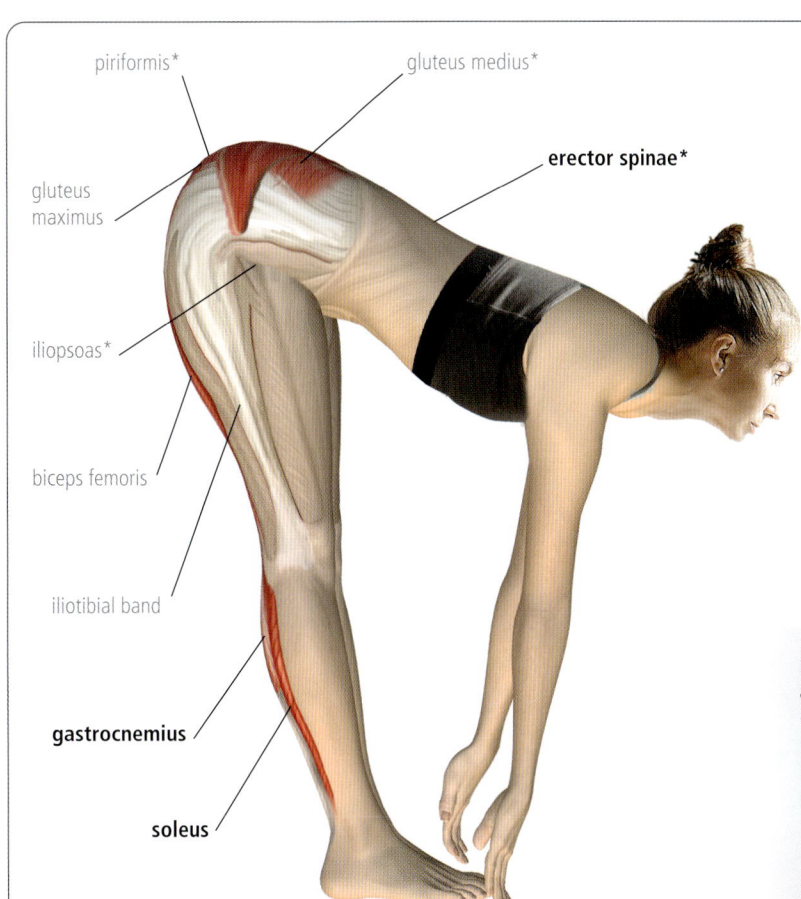

Muscle labels:
- piriformis*
- gluteus medius*
- erector spinae*
- gluteus maximus
- iliopsoas*
- biceps femoris
- iliotibial band
- **gastrocnemius**
- **soleus**

FORWARD BENDS & BACKBENDS

ANNOTATION KEY
Black text indicates strengthening muscles
Gray text indicates stretching muscles
* indicates deep muscles

BEST FOR
- biceps femoris
- iliotibial band
- gluteus maximus
- gluteus medius
- erector spinae

PRONUNCIATION & MEANING
- Virabhadrasana III (veer-ah-bah-DRAHS-anna)
- Virabhadra = the name of a fierce warrior

LEVEL
- Intermediate

BENEFITS
- Strengthens ankles, legs, shoulders, and back muscles
- Tones abdominals
- Improves sense of balance
- Improves posture

CONTRA-INDICATIONS & CAUTIONS
- High blood pressure

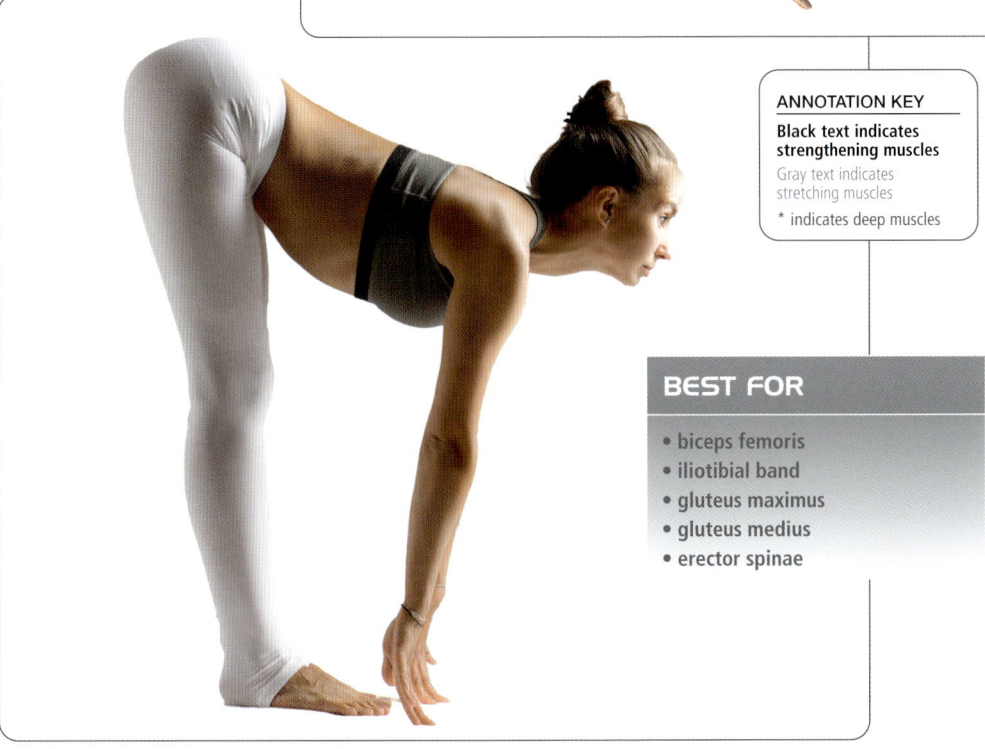

HEAD-TO-KNEE FORWARD BEND
(JANU SIRSASANA)

FORWARD BENDS & BACKBENDS

❶ Begin in Staff Pose (pages 98-99). Bend your left knee, and draw your heel toward your groin, placing the sole of your foot on your right inner thigh. Lower your left knee to the floor. Your right leg should sit at a right angle to your left shin. Draw both sit bones to the floor.

❷ Inhale, and lift up through your spine. Turn your torso slightly to your right as you exhale so that it aligns with your right leg. Flex your foot, and contract the muscles in your right thigh to push the back of your leg toward the floor.

❸ With another exhalation, stretch your sternum forward as you fold your torso over your right leg. Grasp the inside of your right foot with your left hand. Use your right hand to guide your torso to the right.

❹ Extend your right arm forward toward your right foot. You may grasp your foot with both hands or place your hands on the floor on either side of your foot with your elbows bent. If possible, place your forehead on your right shin. With each inhalation, lengthen your spine, and with each exhalation, deepen the stretch.

❺ Hold for 1 to 3 minutes. Repeat with your left leg straight and your right leg bent.

PRONUNCIATION & MEANING
- Janu Sirsasana (JAH-new shear-SHAHS-anna)
- *janu* = knee; *sirsa* = head

BENEFITS
- Stretches hamstrings, groins, and spine
- Stimulates digestion
- Relieves headaches
- Alleviates high blood pressure

CONTRA-INDICATIONS & CAUTIONS
- Knee injury
- Lower-back injury
- Diarrhea

DO IT RIGHT
- Your abdominals should be the first part of your body to touch your thigh; your head should be the last.
- To help guide the forward bend from your hips, place a folded blanket beneath your buttocks.
- Avoid rounding your back or allowing the foot of your bent leg to shift beneath your straight leg.

AVOID
- Allowing the foot of your bent leg to shift beneath your straight leg.

HEAD-TO-KNEE FORWARD BEND
FORWARD BENDS & BACKBENDS

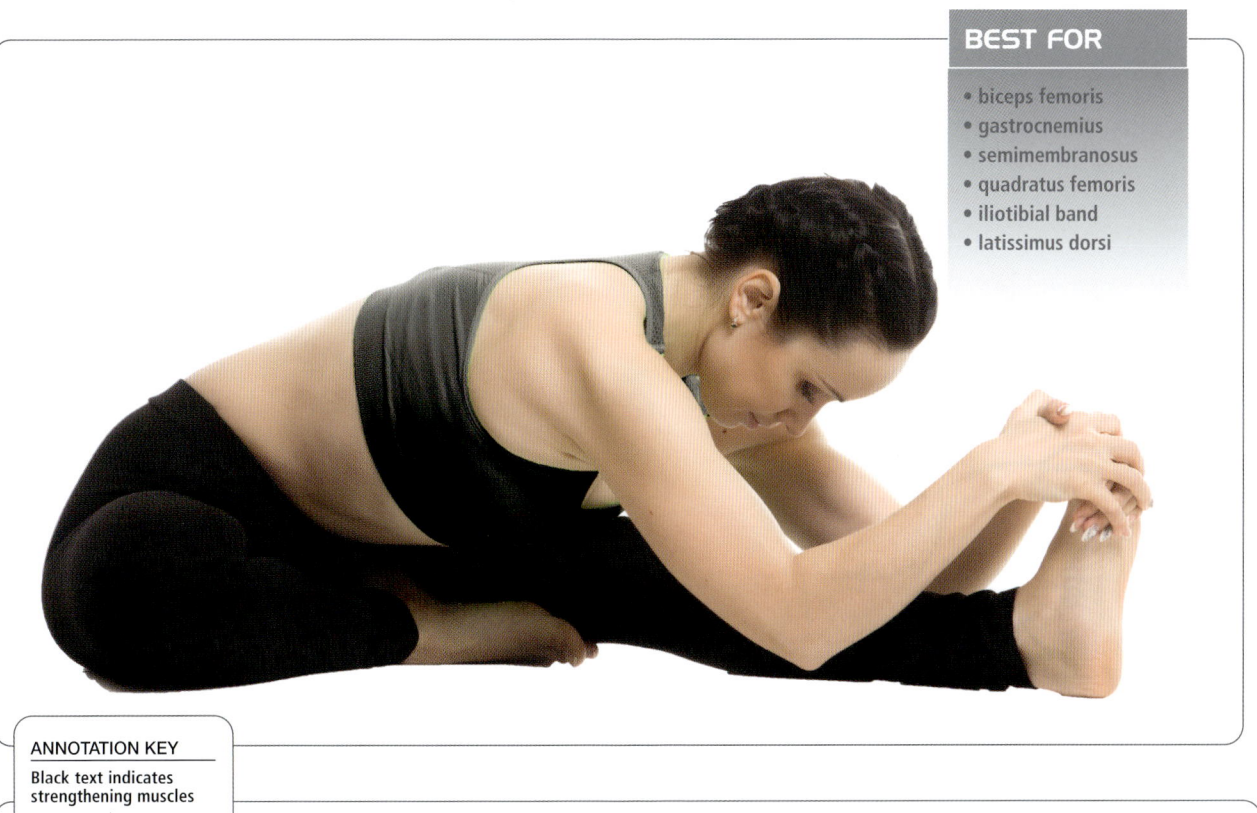

BEST FOR
- biceps femoris
- gastrocnemius
- semimembranosus
- quadratus femoris
- iliotibial band
- latissimus dorsi

ANNOTATION KEY
Black text indicates strengthening muscles
Gray text indicates stretching muscles
* indicates deep muscles

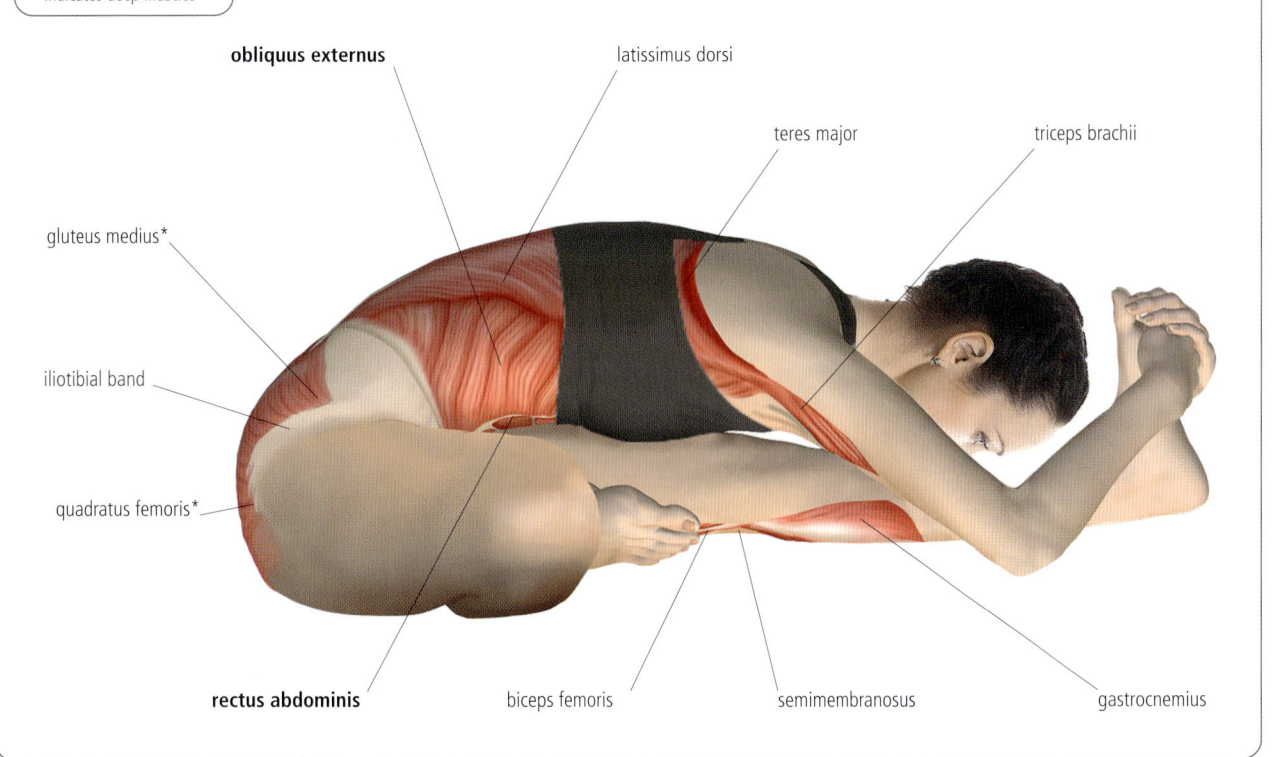

obliquus externus

latissimus dorsi

teres major

triceps brachii

gluteus medius*

iliotibial band

quadratus femoris*

rectus abdominis

biceps femoris

semimembranosus

gastrocnemius

69

SEATED FORWARD BEND
(PASCHIMOTTANASANA)

FORWARD BENDS & BACKBENDS

① Sitting in Staff Pose (pages 36-37)), rock back and forth slightly to draw your sit bones as far away from your heels as possible. Flex your feet, and contract your thighs to press the backs of your legs against the floor.

② Inhale, and lift your arms straight up toward the ceiling, lengthening your spine. Exhale, and stretch your sternum forward, bending from your hips.

③ With your head forward, lower your abdominals to your thighs. Grasp the soles of your feet or your ankles with your hands.

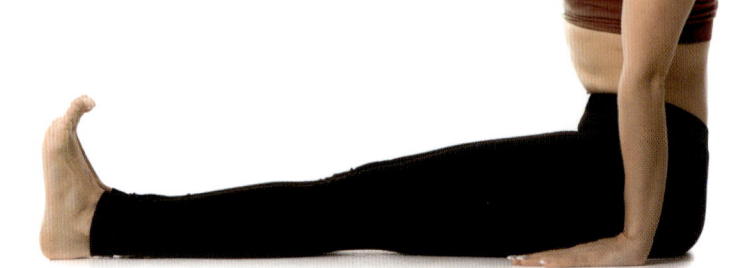

④ With each inhalation, lengthen your spine. With each exhalation, deepen the stretch. If possible, bend your elbows to gently lengthen your torso forward, and place your forehead on your shins.

⑤ Hold for 1 to 3 minutes.

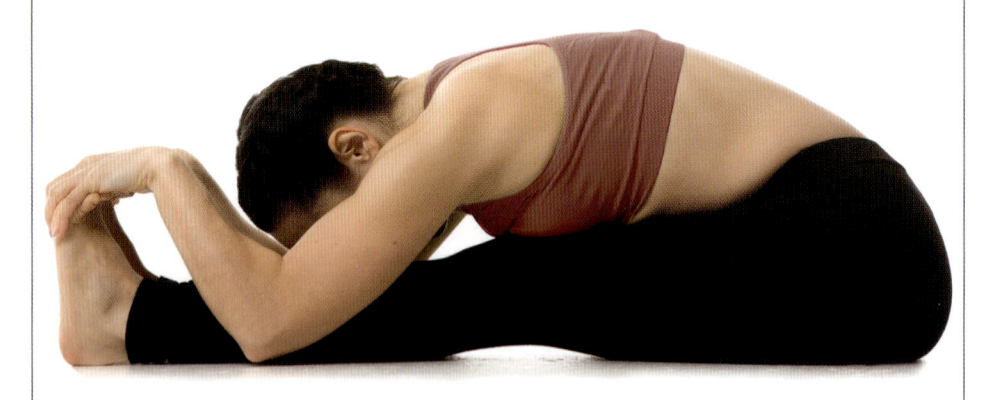

PRONUNCIATION & MEANING
- Paschimottanasana (POSH-ee-moh-tan-AHS-anna)
- *pascha* = behind, west, after; *uttana* = intense stretch

BENEFITS
- Stretches hamstrings, shoulders, and spine
- Stimulates digestion
- Relieves headache and stress
- Alleviates high blood pressure

CONTRA-INDICATIONS & CAUTIONS
- Back injury
- Diarrhea

BEST FOR
- biceps femoris
- semitendinosus
- semimembranosus
- quadratus femoris
- erector spinae
- obdurator externus

DO IT RIGHT
- Keep your feet flexed.
- Try sitting on a folded blanket if desired.
- To help you fold deeper onto your thighs, think of having a slight arch in your lower back as you root your thighs into the floor.
- Close your eyes if you feel comfortable doing so.
- Try to lengthen your exhalations so that they are longer than your inhalations.
- Avoid letting your big toes move closer to you than the other toes; as you flex, your feet should be straight, as if you were standing on the floor.

SEATED FORWARD BEND • FORWARD BENDS & BACKBENDS

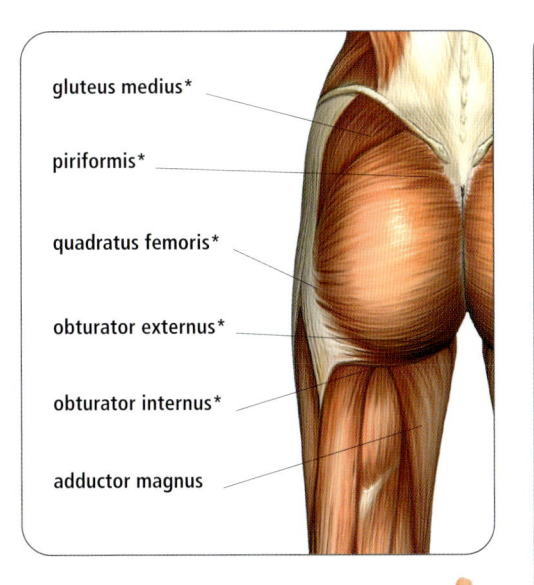

- gluteus medius*
- piriformis*
- quadratus femoris*
- obturator externus*
- obturator internus*
- adductor magnus

MODIFICATION
Easier: If your hamstrings and/or lower back feel tight, try placing a yoga strap around the balls of your feet instead of reaching all the way to your feet.

AVOID
- Rounding your back.
- Forcing your torso downward.

ANNOTATION KEY
Black text indicates strengthening muscles
Gray text indicates stretching muscles
* indicates deep muscles

- erector spinae*
- quadratus lumborum*
- semimembranosus
- biceps femoris
- semitendinosus
- obturator externus

71

WIDE-LEGGED FORWARD BEND
(PRASARITA PADOTTANASANA)

FORWARD BENDS & BACKBENDS

① Stand in Mountain Pose (pages 36-37). Take a large step—about 3 to 4 feet—to the side. Your feet should be parallel to each other. Lift up through your spine, and contract your thigh muscles.

② Exhale, and bend forward from your hips, keeping your back flat. Draw your sternum forward as you lower your torso, gazing straight ahead. With your elbows straight, place your fingertips on the floor.

③ With another exhalation, place your hands on the floor in between your feet, and lower your torso into a full forward bend. Lengthen your spine by pulling your sit bones up toward the ceiling and drawing your head to the floor. If possible, bend your elbows and place your forehead on the floor.

④ Hold for 30 seconds to 1 minute. To come out of the pose, straighten your elbows and raise your torso while keeping your back flat.

AVOID
- Bending forward from your waist.
- Compressing the back of your neck as you look forward.

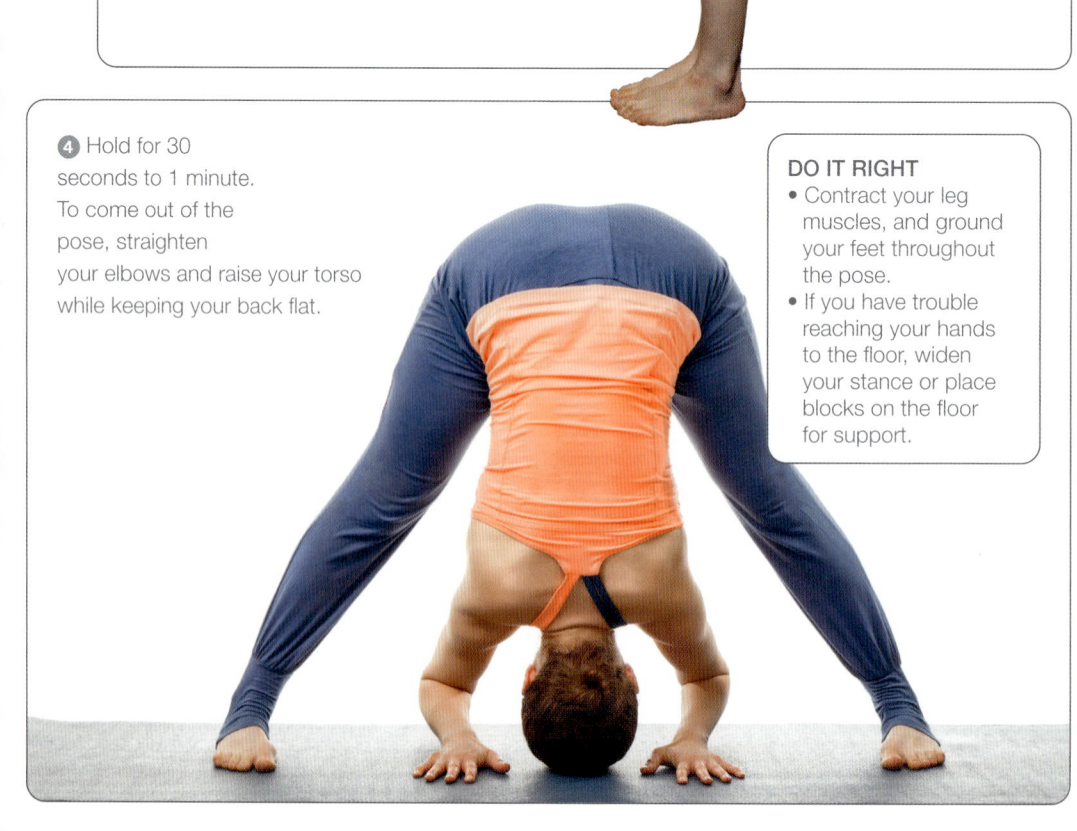

DO IT RIGHT
- Contract your leg muscles, and ground your feet throughout the pose.
- If you have trouble reaching your hands to the floor, widen your stance or place blocks on the floor for support.

PRONUNCIATION & MEANING
- Prasarita Padottanasana (pra-sa-REE-tah pah-doh-tahn-AHS-anna)
- *prasarita* = spread, expanded; *pada* = foot; *ut* = intense; *tan* = to stretch or extend

BENEFITS
- Stretches and strengthens hamstrings, groins, and spine

CONTRA-INDICATIONS & CAUTIONS
- Lower-back issues

WIDE-LEGGED FORWARD BEND • FORWARD BENDS & BACKBENDS

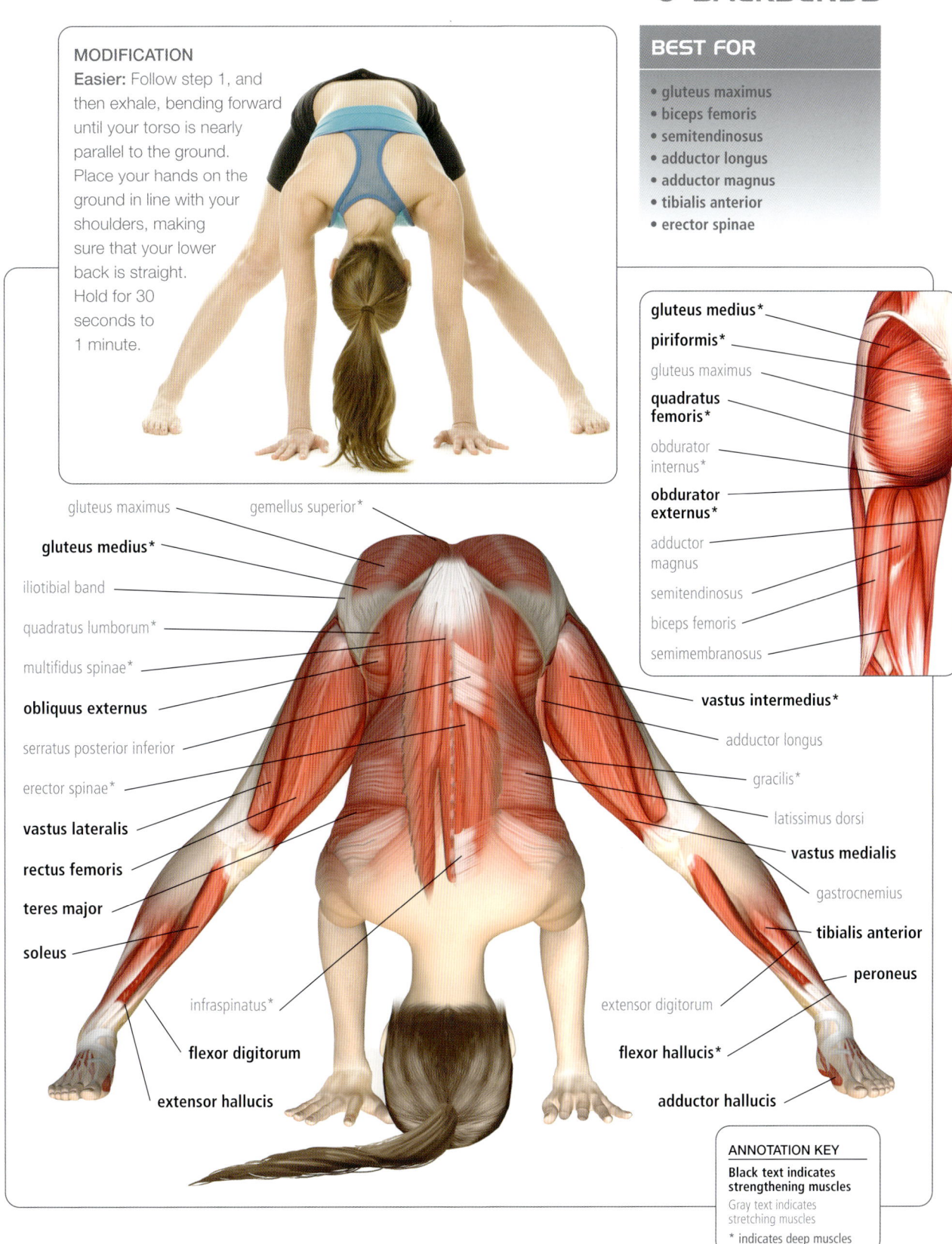

MODIFICATION
Easier: Follow step 1, and then exhale, bending forward until your torso is nearly parallel to the ground. Place your hands on the ground in line with your shoulders, making sure that your lower back is straight. Hold for 30 seconds to 1 minute.

BEST FOR
- gluteus maximus
- biceps femoris
- semitendinosus
- adductor longus
- adductor magnus
- tibialis anterior
- erector spinae

Muscle labels (side view)
- gluteus medius*
- piriformis*
- gluteus maximus
- quadratus femoris*
- obdurator internus*
- obdurator externus*
- adductor magnus
- semitendinosus
- biceps femoris
- semimembranosus

Muscle labels (main view)
- gluteus maximus
- gemellus superior*
- gluteus medius*
- iliotibial band
- quadratus lumborum*
- multifidus spinae*
- obliquus externus
- serratus posterior inferior
- erector spinae*
- vastus lateralis
- rectus femoris
- teres major
- soleus
- infraspinatus*
- flexor digitorum
- extensor hallucis
- vastus intermedius*
- adductor longus
- gracilis*
- latissimus dorsi
- vastus medialis
- gastrocnemius
- tibialis anterior
- peroneus
- extensor digitorum
- flexor hallucis*
- adductor hallucis

ANNOTATION KEY
Black text indicates strengthening muscles
Gray text indicates stretching muscles
* indicates deep muscles

73

EXTENDED PUPPY POSE
(UTTANA SHISHOSANA)

FORWARD BENDS & BACKBENDS

PRONUNCIATION & MEANING
- Uttana Shishosana (oo-TAH-na shee-SHOWS-anna)
- *uttana* = intense stretch; *shishu* = baby

BENEFITS
- Stretches the shoulders and spine

CONTRA-INDICATIONS & CAUTIONS
- Knee injury

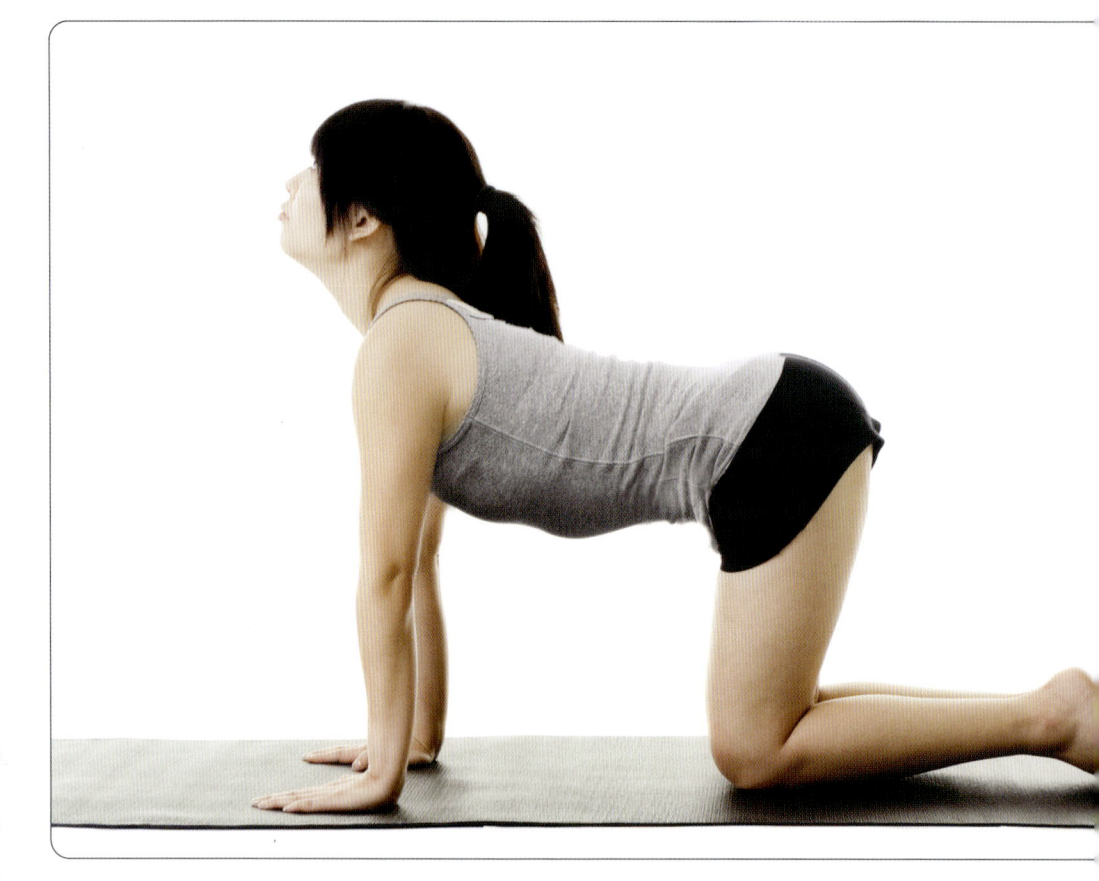

❶ Kneel on your knees, with your knees directly below your hips. Your fingertips should be facing forward with your hands one shoulder-width apart.

❷ Bend forward to your hands and knees, with your wrists directly below your shoulders.

❸ Exhale, and press your hips back while lowering your chest toward the floor. Keep your elbows straight and lifted off the floor.

❹ Relax your forehead on the floor. Stretch forward through your arms and back through your sit bones to deepen the stretch through your spine.

❺ Hold for 30 seconds to 1 minute.

DO IT RIGHT
- Slightly arch your upper back, providing your shoulders and spine with a gentle and stress-relieving stretch.
- Aim to stretch your spine in both directions to get the most from this pose.

AVOID
- Resting your elbows on the floor.
- Allowing your torso to sink at the middle.
- Releasing from the pose too quickly—as with an inverted pose, fast-changing blood flow can cause dizziness.

EXTENDED PUPPY POSE • FORWARD BENDS & BACKBENDS

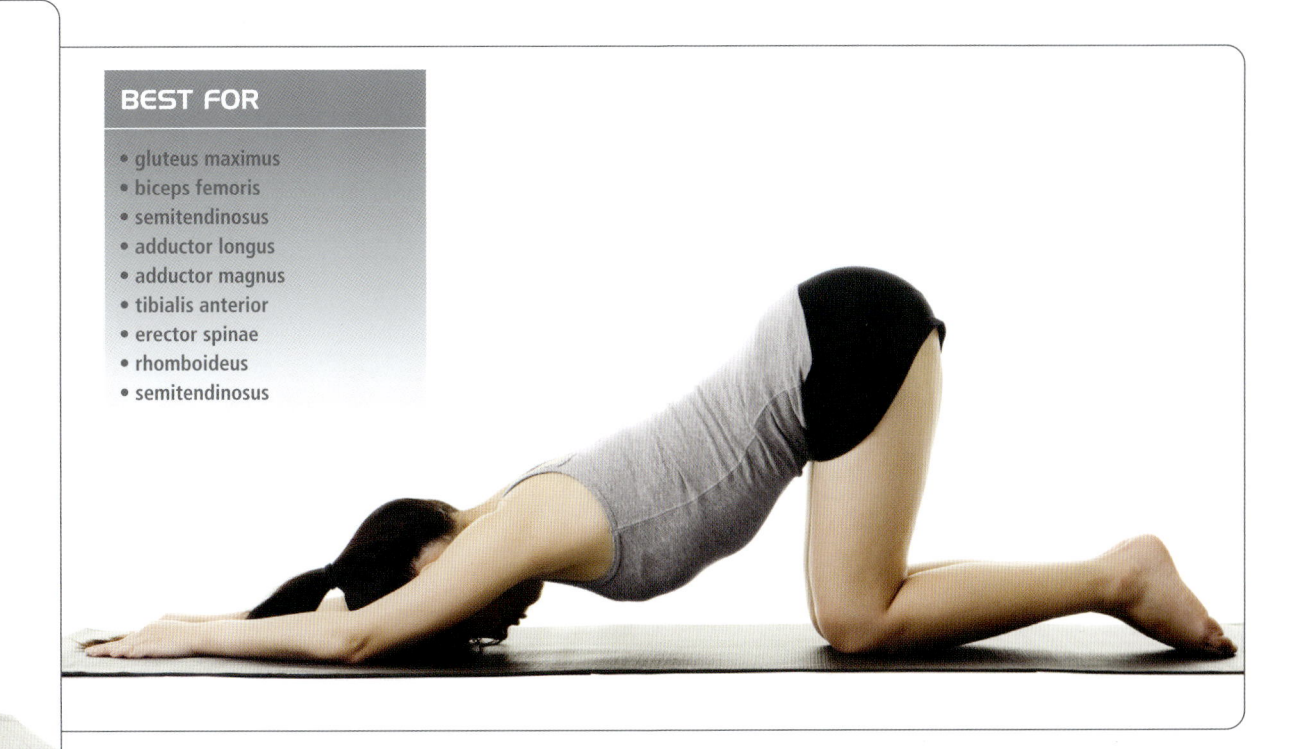

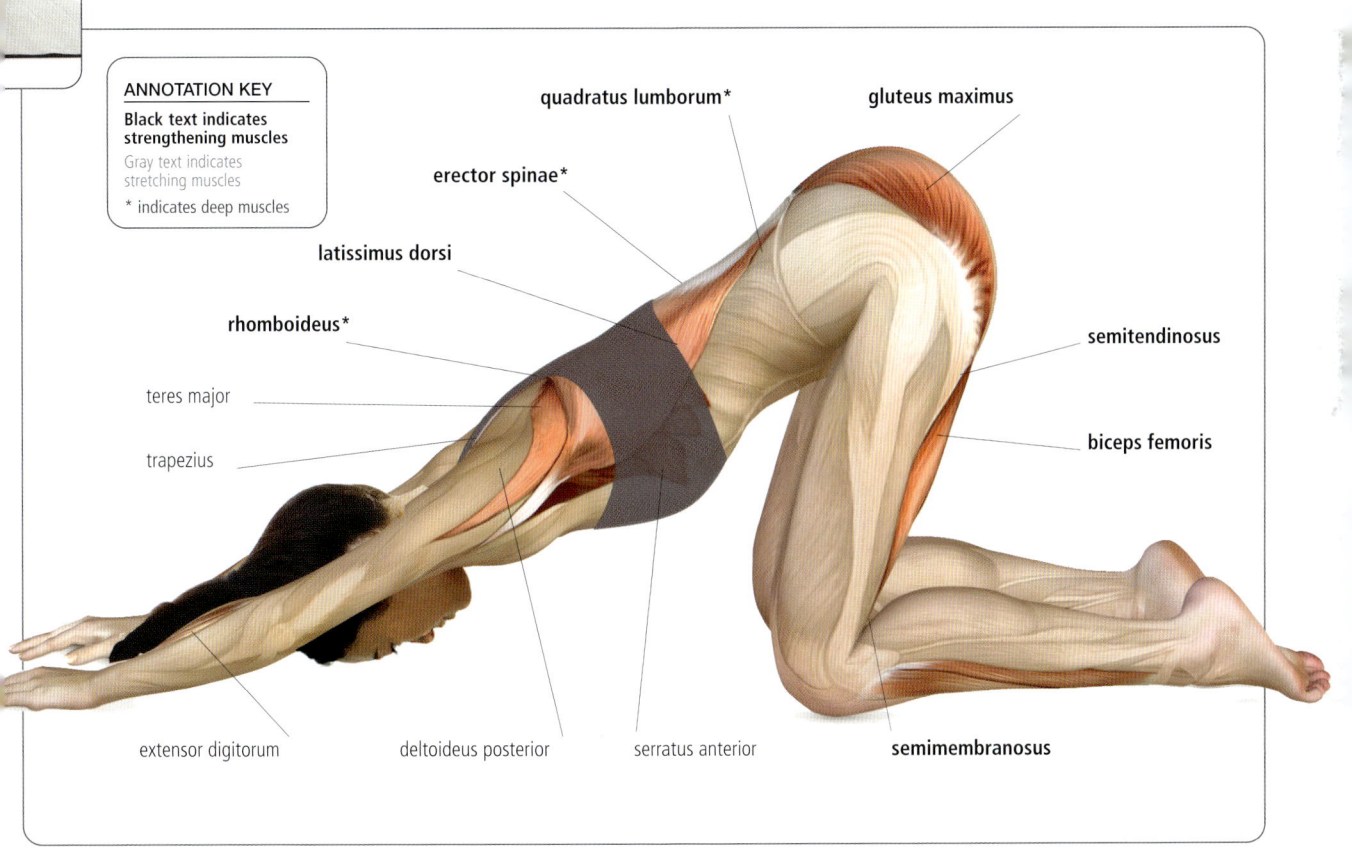

BEST FOR
- gluteus maximus
- biceps femoris
- semitendinosus
- adductor longus
- adductor magnus
- tibialis anterior
- erector spinae
- rhomboideus
- semitendinosus

ANNOTATION KEY
Black text indicates strengthening muscles
Gray text indicates stretching muscles
* indicates deep muscles

- quadratus lumborum*
- gluteus maximus
- erector spinae*
- latissimus dorsi
- rhomboideus*
- semitendinosus
- teres major
- biceps femoris
- trapezius
- extensor digitorum
- deltoideus posterior
- serratus anterior
- semimembranosus

75

FORWARD BENDS & BACKBENDS

CAT POSE TO COW POSE
(MARJARYASANA TO BITILASANA)

① Begin on your hands and knees, with your wrists directly below your shoulders and your knees directly below your hips. Your fingertips should be facing forward with your hands one shoulder-width apart. Gaze at the floor, keeping your head in a neutral position.

② Exhale, and round your spine up toward the ceiling, dropping your head. Draw your abdominals in toward your spine. Keep your hips lifted and your shoulders in the same position.

③ Inhale, and uncurl your spine. Remain on your hands and knees.

④ With your next inhalation, arch your spine, lifting your chest forward and your sit bones up toward the ceiling. Gaze forward.

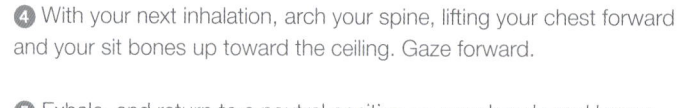

⑤ Exhale, and return to a neutral position on your hands and knees.

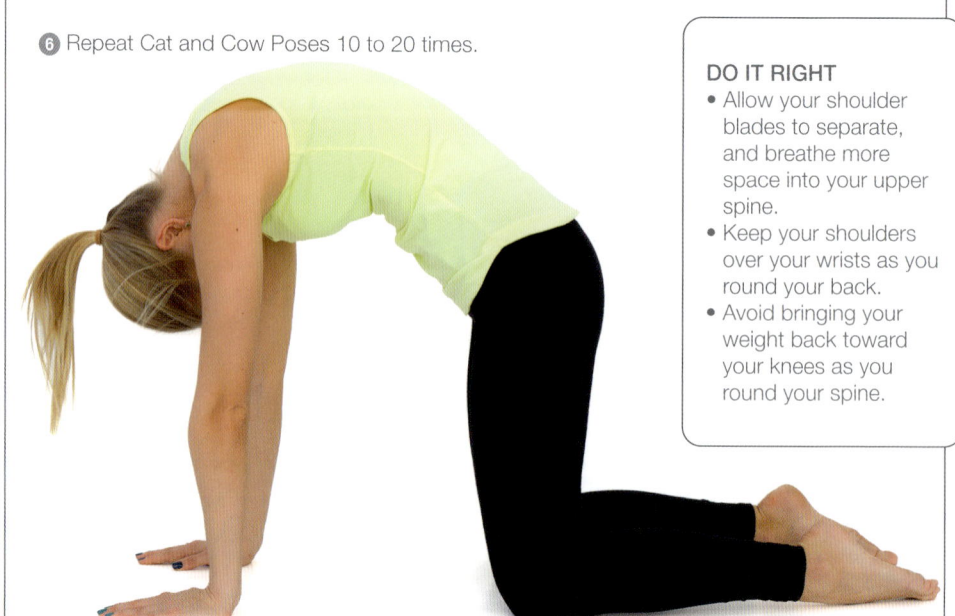

⑥ Repeat Cat and Cow Poses 10 to 20 times.

PRONUNCIATION & MEANING
- Marjaryasana (mar-jar-ee-AHS-anna) *marjari* = cat
- Bitilasana (bit-il-AHS-anna)

BENEFITS
- Stretches shoulders, chest, abdominals, neck, and spine
- Relieves stress

CONTRA-INDICATIONS & CAUTIONS
- Knee injury

DO IT RIGHT
- Allow your shoulder blades to separate, and breathe more space into your upper spine.
- Keep your shoulders over your wrists as you round your back.
- Avoid bringing your weight back toward your knees as you round your spine.

CAT POSE TO COW POSE • FORWARD BENDS & BACKBENDS

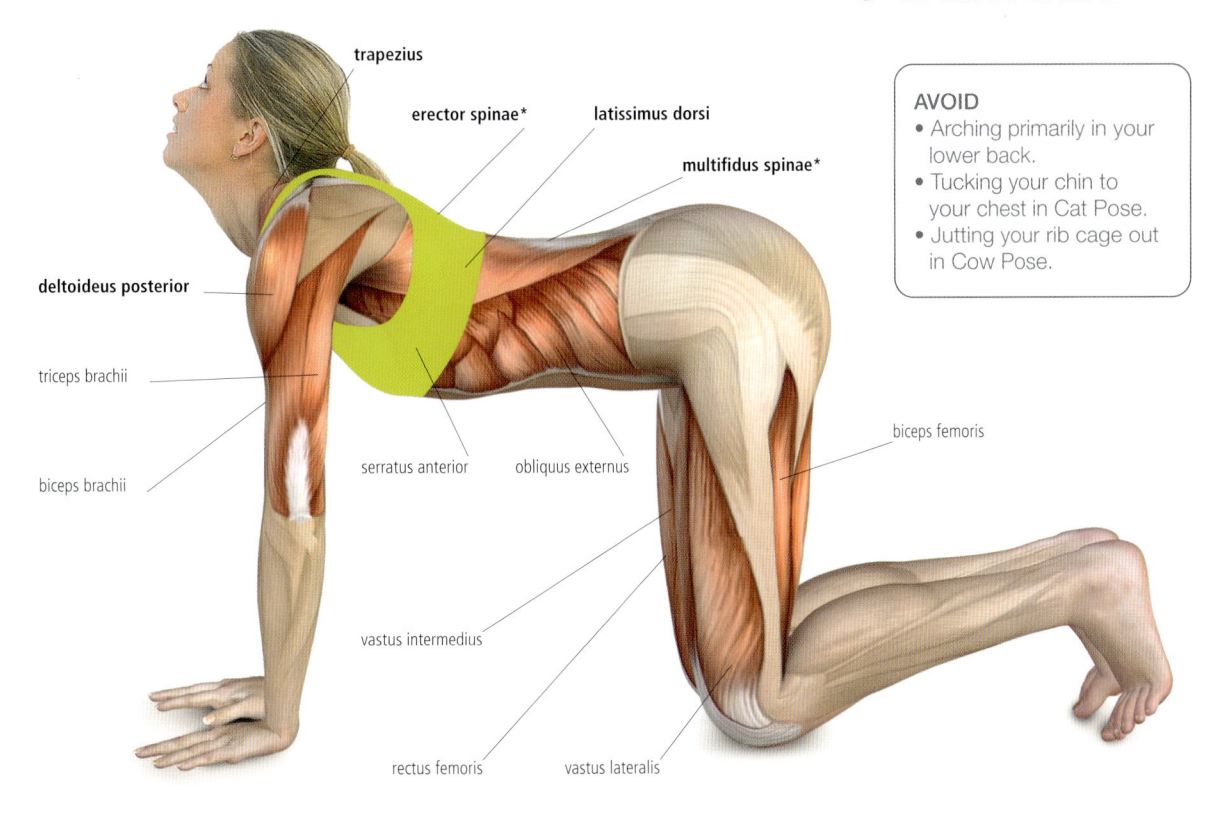

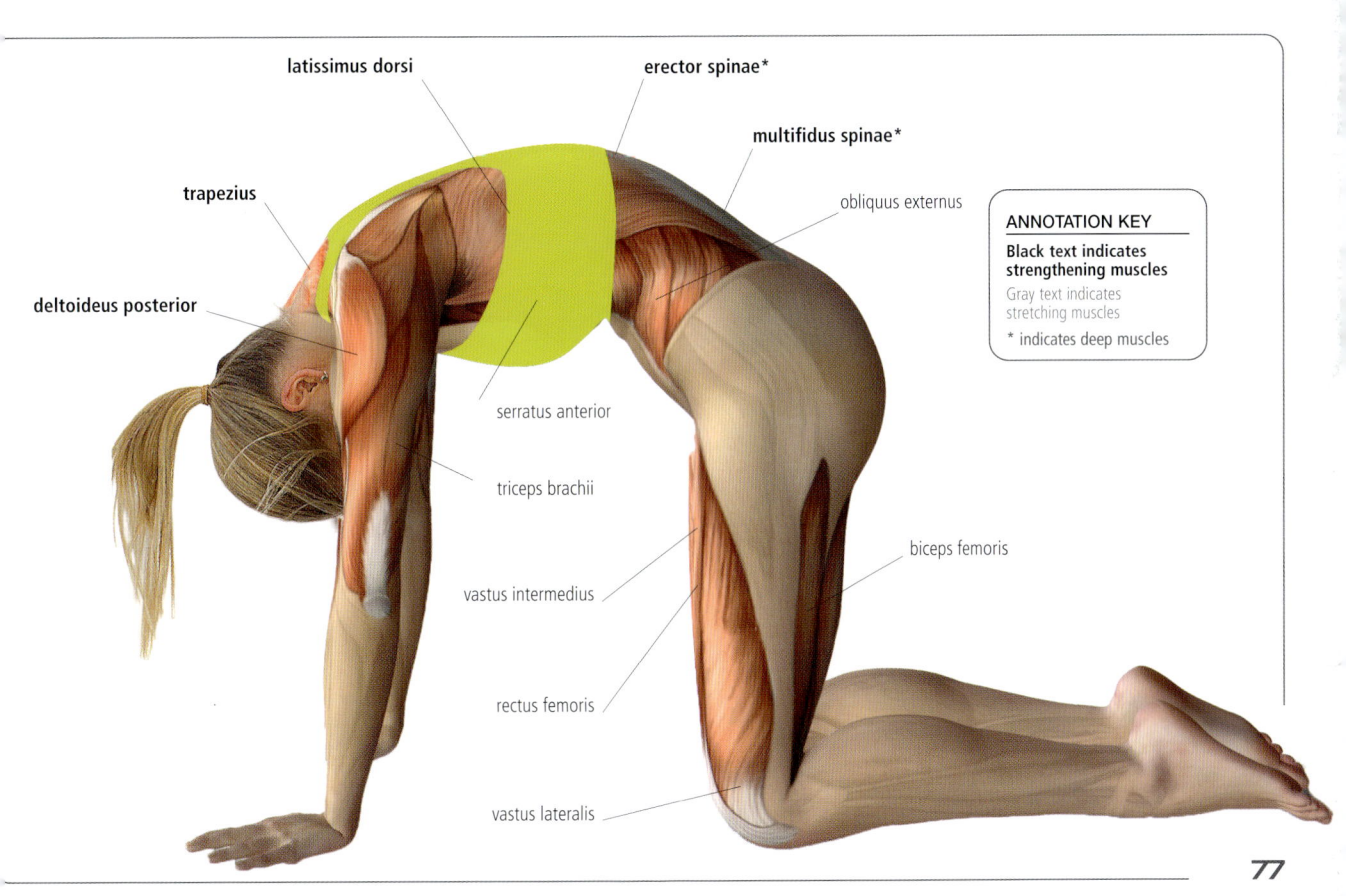

Cow Pose labels:
- trapezius
- erector spinae*
- latissimus dorsi
- multifidus spinae*
- deltoideus posterior
- triceps brachii
- biceps brachii
- serratus anterior
- obliquus externus
- biceps femoris
- vastus intermedius
- rectus femoris
- vastus lateralis

AVOID
- Arching primarily in your lower back.
- Tucking your chin to your chest in Cat Pose.
- Jutting your rib cage out in Cow Pose.

Cat Pose labels:
- latissimus dorsi
- erector spinae*
- multifidus spinae*
- trapezius
- obliquus externus
- deltoideus posterior
- serratus anterior
- triceps brachii
- vastus intermedius
- biceps femoris
- rectus femoris
- vastus lateralis

ANNOTATION KEY
Black text indicates strengthening muscles
Gray text indicates stretching muscles
* indicates deep muscles

UPWARD-FACING DOG POSE
(URDHVA MUKHA SVANASANA)

FORWARD BENDS & BACKBENDS

❶ Lie prone on the floor. Bend your elbows, placing your hands flat on the floor on either side of your chest. Keep your elbows pulled in toward your body. Separate your legs one hip-width apart, and extend through your toes. The tops of your feet should be touching the floor.

❷ Inhale, and press against the floor with your hands and the tops of your feet, lifting your torso and hips off the floor. Contract your thighs, and tuck your tailbone toward your pubis.

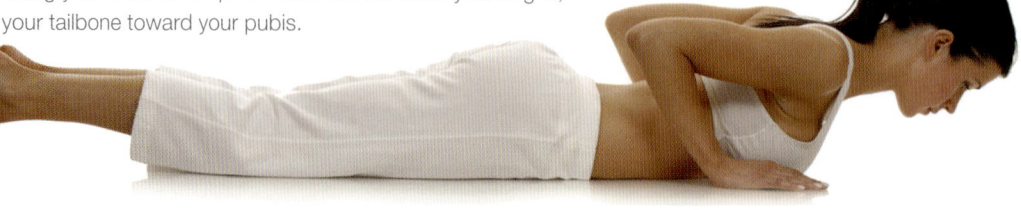

❸ Lift through the top of your chest, fully extending your arms and creating an arch in your back from your upper torso. Push your shoulders down and back, and elongate your neck as you gaze slightly upward.

❹ Hold for 15 to 30 seconds, and exhale as you lower yourself to the floor.

PRONUNCIATION & MEANING
- Urdhva Mukha Svanasana (OORD-vah MOO-kah shvon-AHS-anna
- *urdhva* = rising upward, elevated; *mukha* = face; *shvana* = dog

BENEFITS
- Strengthens spine, arms, and wrists
- Stretches chest and abdominals
- Improves posture

CONTRA-INDICATIONS & CAUTIONS
- Back injury
- Wrist injury or carpal tunnel syndrome

DO IT RIGHT
- Elongate your legs and arms to create full extension.
- Make sure that your wrists are positioned directly below your shoulders so that you don't exert too much pressure on your lower back.

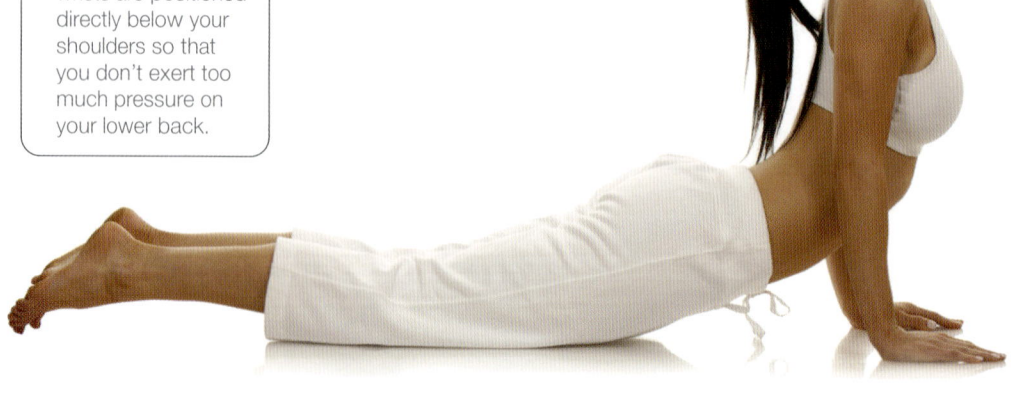

UPWARD-FACING DOG POSE • FORWARD BENDS & BACKBENDS

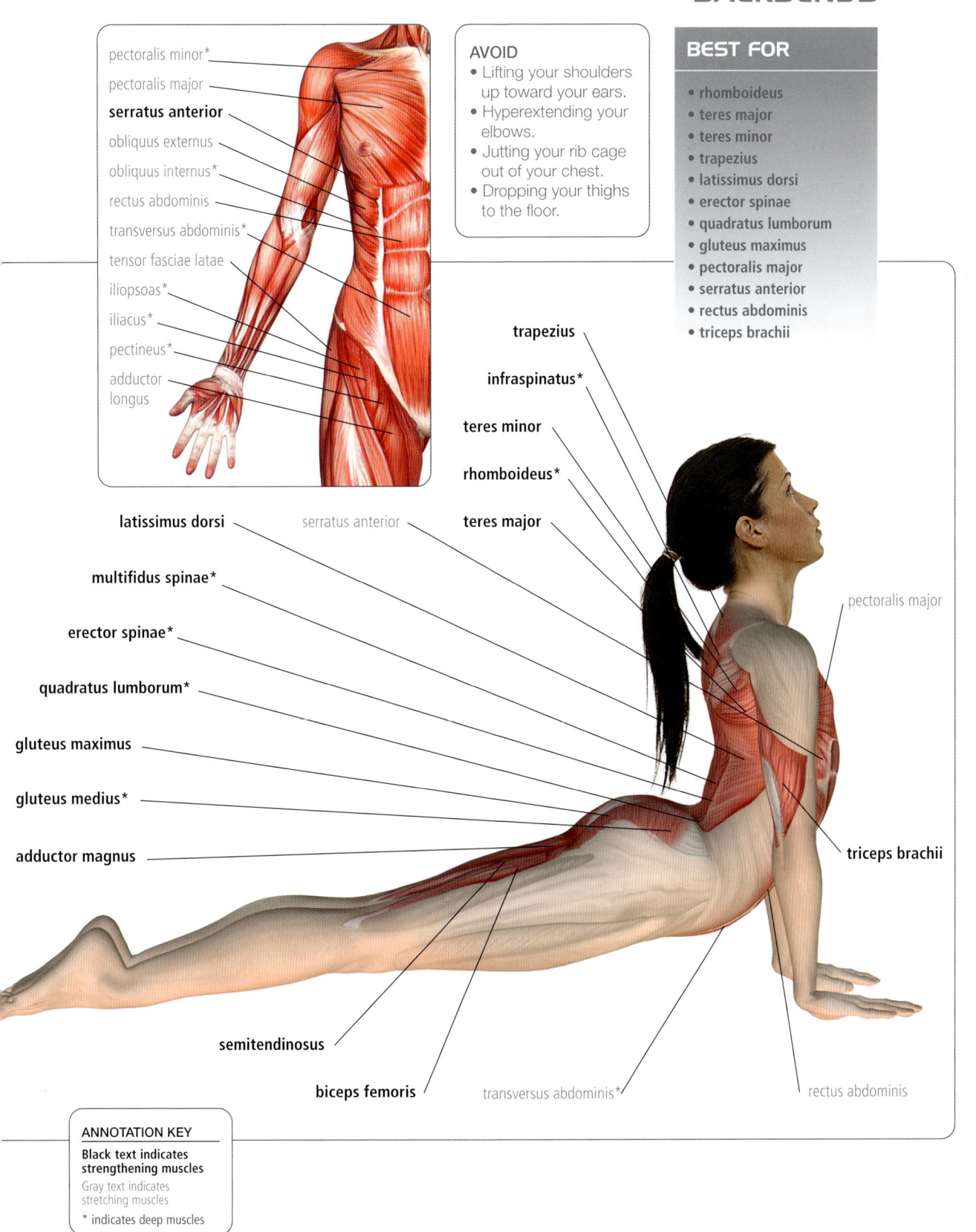

AVOID
- Lifting your shoulders up toward your ears.
- Hyperextending your elbows.
- Jutting your rib cage out of your chest.
- Dropping your thighs to the floor.

BEST FOR
- rhomboideus
- teres major
- teres minor
- trapezius
- latissimus dorsi
- erector spinae
- quadratus lumborum
- gluteus maximus
- pectoralis major
- serratus anterior
- rectus abdominis
- triceps brachii

Labels on figure:

pectoralis minor*
pectoralis major
serratus anterior
obliquus externus
obliquus internus*
rectus abdominis
transversus abdominis*
tensor fasciae latae
iliopsoas*
iliacus*
pectineus*
adductor longus

trapezius
infraspinatus*
teres minor
rhomboideus*
teres major

latissimus dorsi   serratus anterior
multifidus spinae*
erector spinae*
quadratus lumborum*
gluteus maximus
gluteus medius*
adductor magnus
semitendinosus
biceps femoris   transversus abdominis*   rectus abdominis

pectoralis major
triceps brachii

ANNOTATION KEY
Black text indicates strengthening muscles
Gray text indicates stretching muscles
* indicates deep muscles

79

COBRA POSE
(BHUJANGASANA)

① Lie prone on the floor. Bend your elbows, placing your hands flat on the floor beside your chest. Keep your elbows pulled in toward your body. Extend your legs, pressing your pubis, thighs, and tops of your feet into the floor.

② Inhale, and lift your chest off the floor, pushing down with your hands to guide your lift. Keep your pubis pressed against the floor.

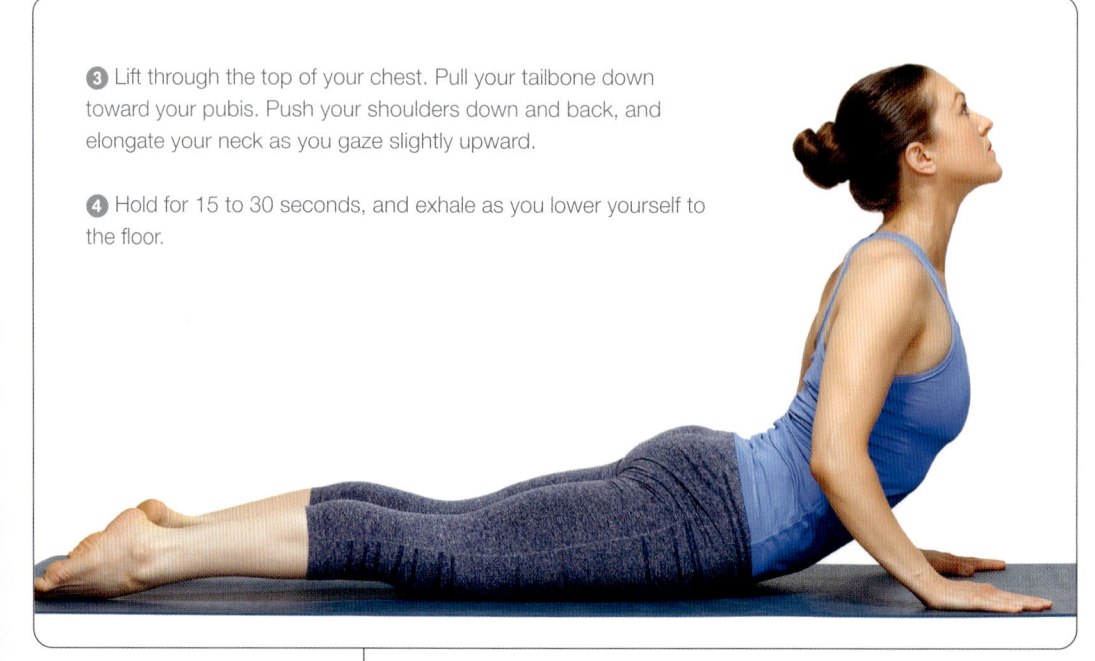

③ Lift through the top of your chest. Pull your tailbone down toward your pubis. Push your shoulders down and back, and elongate your neck as you gaze slightly upward.

④ Hold for 15 to 30 seconds, and exhale as you lower yourself to the floor.

FORWARD BENDS & BACKBENDS

PRONUNCIATION & MEANING
- Bhujangasana (boo-jang-GAHS-anna)
- *bhujang* = snake, serpent; *bhuja* = arm or shoulder; *anga* = limb

BENEFITS
- Strengthens spine and buttocks
- Stretches chest, abdominals, and shoulders

CONTRA-INDICATIONS & CAUTIONS
- Back injury

AVOID
- Tensing your buttocks, which adds pressure on your lower back.
- Splaying your elbows out to the sides.
- Lifting your hips off the floor.

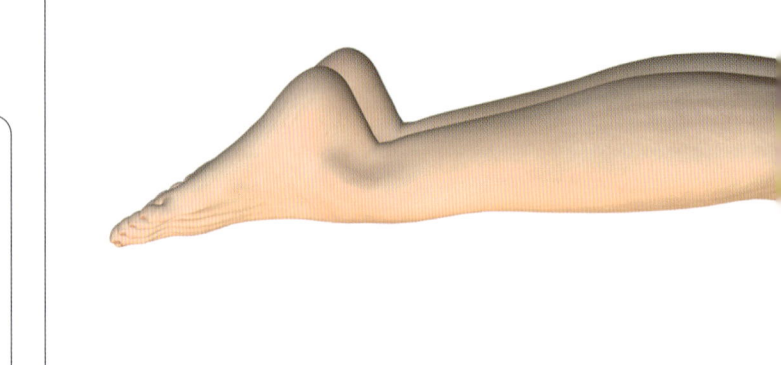

COBRA POSE • FORWARD BENDS & BACKBENDS

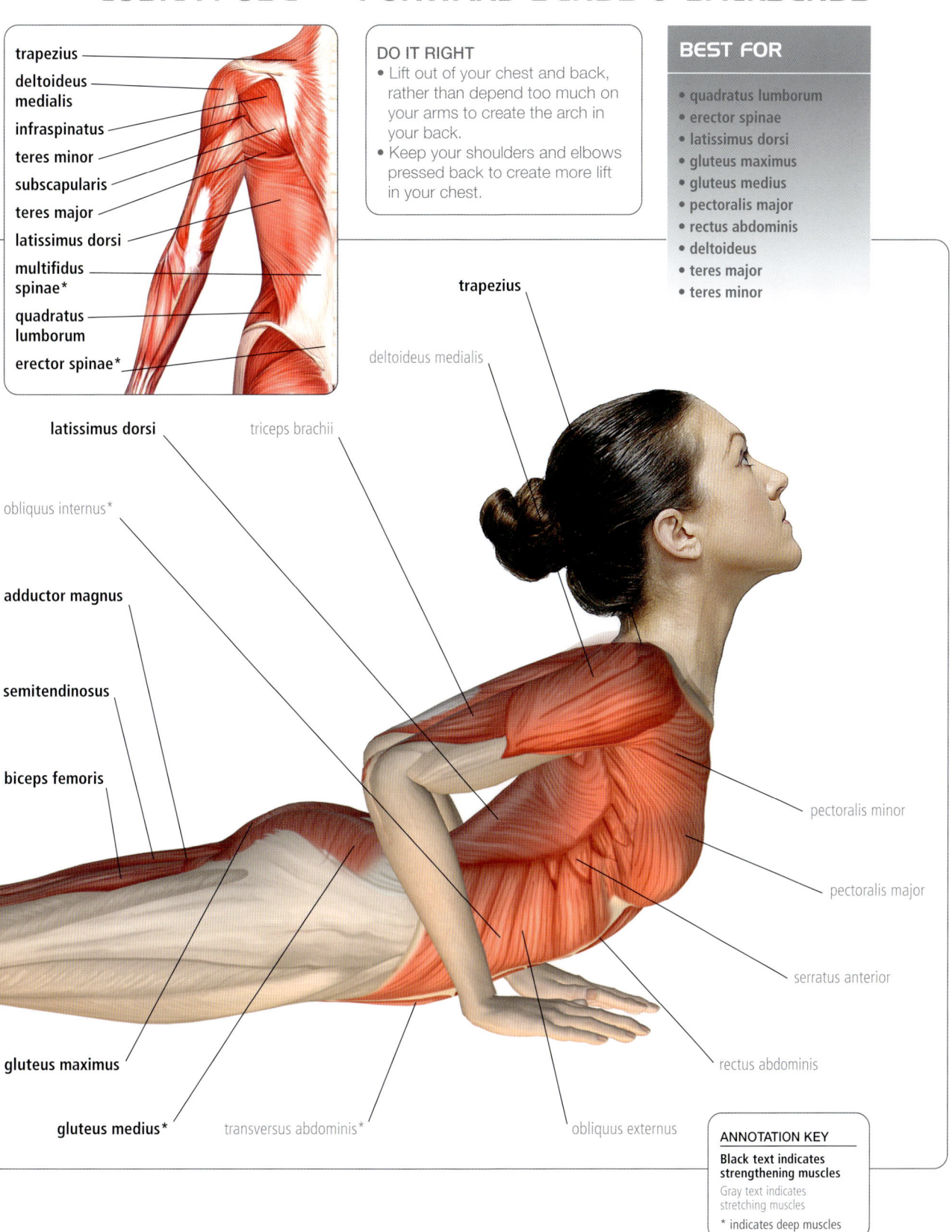

DO IT RIGHT
- Lift out of your chest and back, rather than depend too much on your arms to create the arch in your back.
- Keep your shoulders and elbows pressed back to create more lift in your chest.

BEST FOR
- quadratus lumborum
- erector spinae
- latissimus dorsi
- gluteus maximus
- gluteus medius
- pectoralis major
- rectus abdominis
- deltoideus
- teres major
- teres minor

Labels (inset): trapezius, deltoideus medialis, infraspinatus, teres minor, subscapularis, teres major, latissimus dorsi, multifidus spinae*, quadratus lumborum, erector spinae*

Labels (main figure): latissimus dorsi, obliquus internus*, adductor magnus, semitendinosus, biceps femoris, gluteus maximus, gluteus medius*, transversus abdominis*, trapezius, deltoideus medialis, triceps brachii, pectoralis minor, pectoralis major, serratus anterior, rectus abdominis, obliquus externus

ANNOTATION KEY
Black text indicates strengthening muscles
Gray text indicates stretching muscles
* indicates deep muscles

81

BOW POSE
(DHANURASANA)

FORWARD BENDS & BACKBENDS

① Lie prone on the floor, and place your arms by your sides with your palms facing upward.

② Place your chin on the floor, and exhale as you bend your knees. Reach your arms behind you, and grasp the outside of your ankles with your hands.

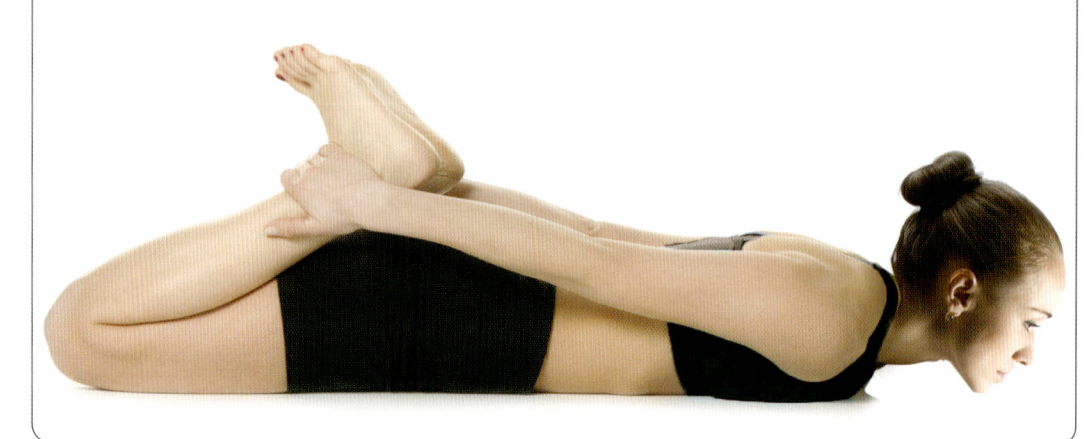

③ Inhale, and lift your chest off the floor. Simultaneously lift your thighs by pulling your ankles up with your hands. Shift your weight onto your abdominals.

④ Keep your head in a neutral position, and make sure that your knees don't separate more than the width of your hips. Tuck your tailbone into your pubis.

⑤ Hold for 20 to 30 seconds. Exhale, and release your ankles, gently returning to the floor.

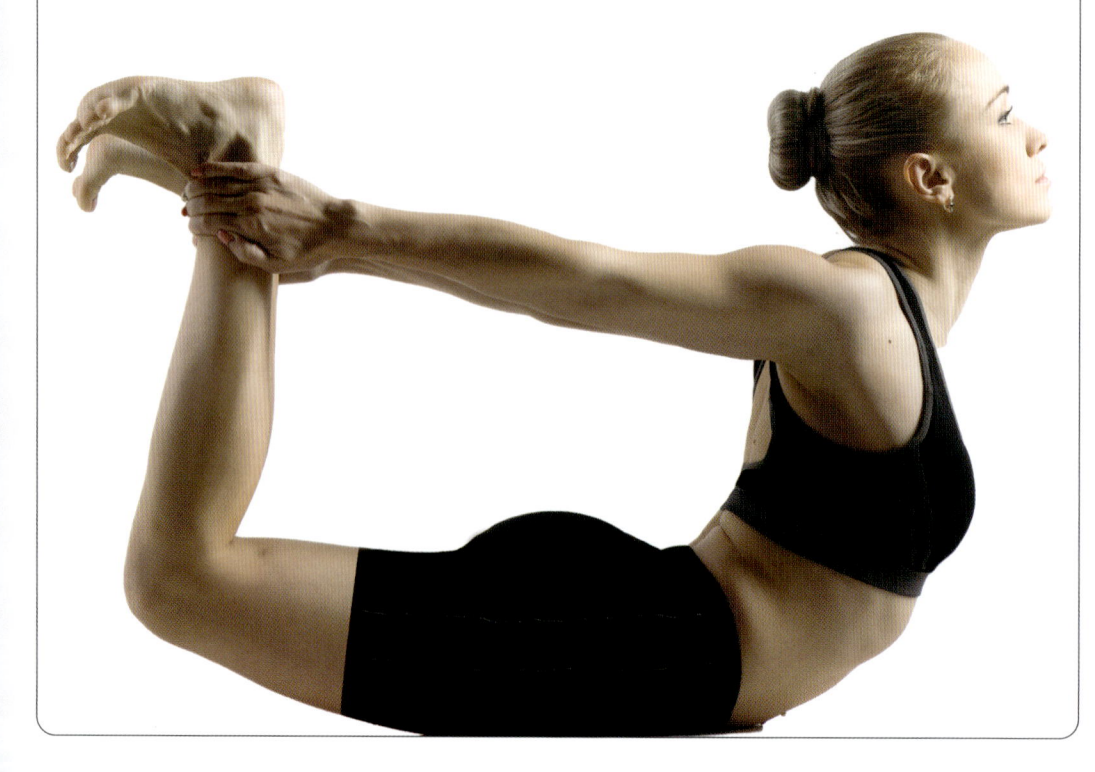

PRONUNCIATION & MEANING
- Dhanurasana (don-your-AHS-anna)
- *dhanu* = bow

BENEFITS
- Strengthens spine
- Stretches chest, abdominals, hip flexors, and quadriceps
- Stimulates digestion

CONTRA-INDICATIONS & CAUTIONS
- Headache
- High or low blood pressure
- Back injury

BOW POSE • FORWARD BENDS & BACKBENDS

DO IT RIGHT
- Keep your knees close together during the duration of the posture, making sure that they don't separate more than the width of your hips.

AVOID
- Holding your breath. Breathing in this pose can be difficult, so make sure to take short, controlled breaths from the back of your torso.
- Rolling back onto your pelvis to support your weight.

BEST FOR
- pectoralis major
- pectoralis minor
- deltoideus
- erector spinae
- gluteus medius
- gluteus maximus
- iliopsoas
- rectus femoris

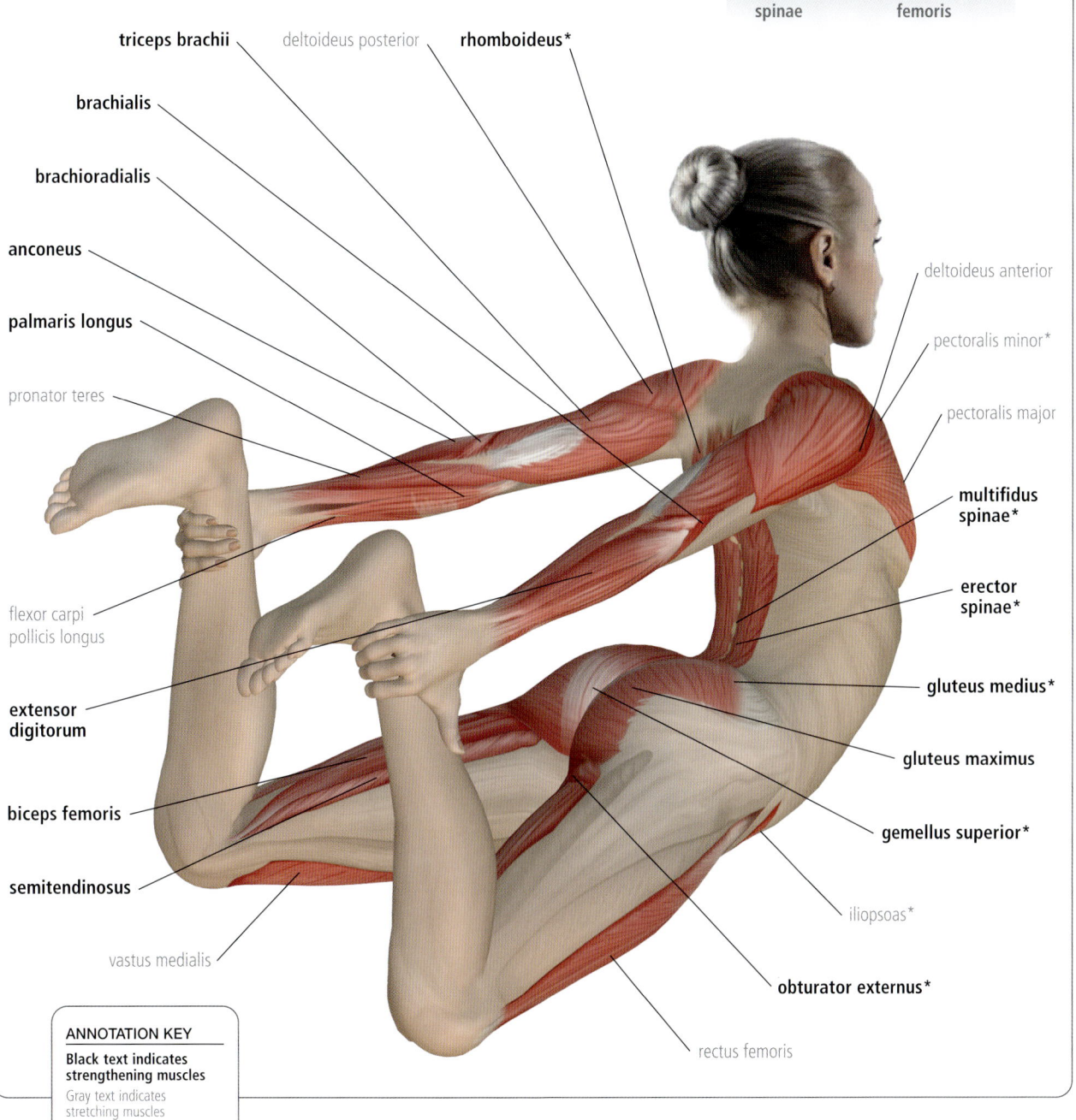

triceps brachii
deltoideus posterior
rhomboideus*
brachialis
brachioradialis
anconeus
palmaris longus
pronator teres
flexor carpi pollicis longus
extensor digitorum
biceps femoris
semitendinosus
vastus medialis

deltoideus anterior
pectoralis minor*
pectoralis major
multifidus spinae*
erector spinae*
gluteus medius*
gluteus maximus
gemellus superior*
iliopsoas*
obturator externus*
rectus femoris

ANNOTATION KEY
Black text indicates strengthening muscles
Gray text indicates stretching muscles
* indicates deep muscles

BRIDGE POSE
(SETU BANDHASANA)

FORWARD BENDS & BACKBENDS

① Lie supine on the floor. Bend your knees and draw you heels close to your buttocks. Place you hands flat on the floor by your sides.

② Exhale, and press down though your feet to lift your buttocks off the floor. With your feet and thighs parallel, push your arms into the floor while extending through your fingertips.

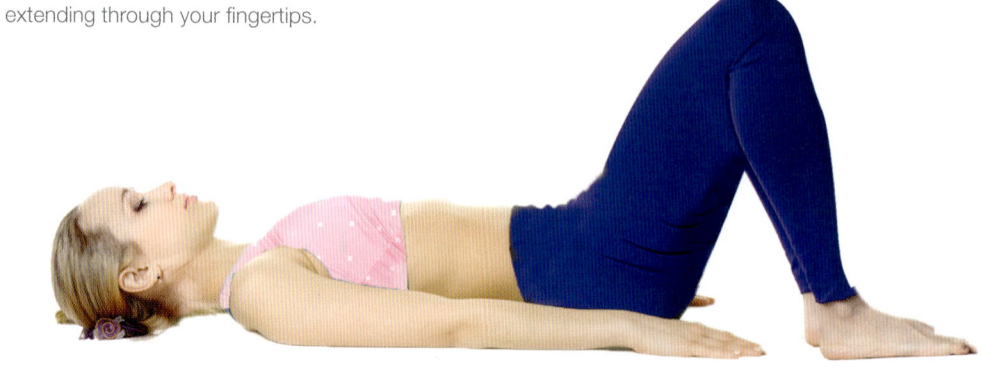

③ Lengthen your neck away from your shoulders. Lift your hips higher so that your torso rises from the floor.

④ Hold for 30 seconds to 1 minute. Exhale as you release your spine onto the floor, one vertebra at a time. Repeat at least one more time.

AVOID
- Tucking your chin in toward your chest.
- Using your buttocks more than your hamstrings to lift your hips.

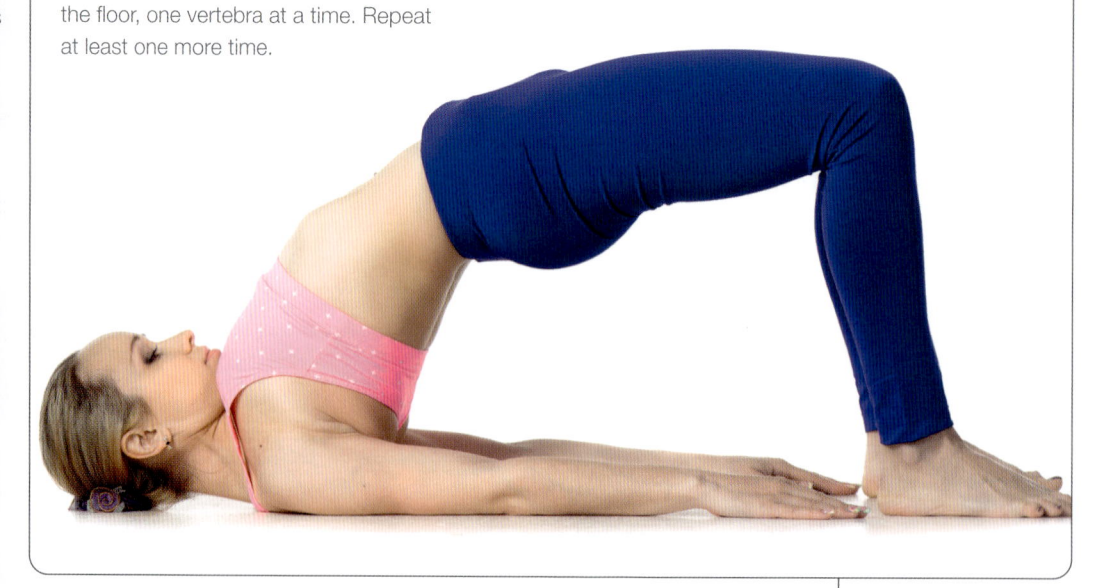

PRONUNCIATION & MEANING
- Setu Bandhasana (SET-too BAHN-dahs-anna)
- *setu* = dam, dike, bridge; *bandha* = lock

BENEFITS
- Strengthens thighs and buttocks
- Stretches chest and spine
- Stimulates digestion
- Stimulates thyroid
- Reduces stress

CONTRA-INDICATIONS & CAUTIONS
- Shoulder injury
- Back injury
- Neck issues

BRIDGE POSE • FORWARD BENDS & BACKBENDS

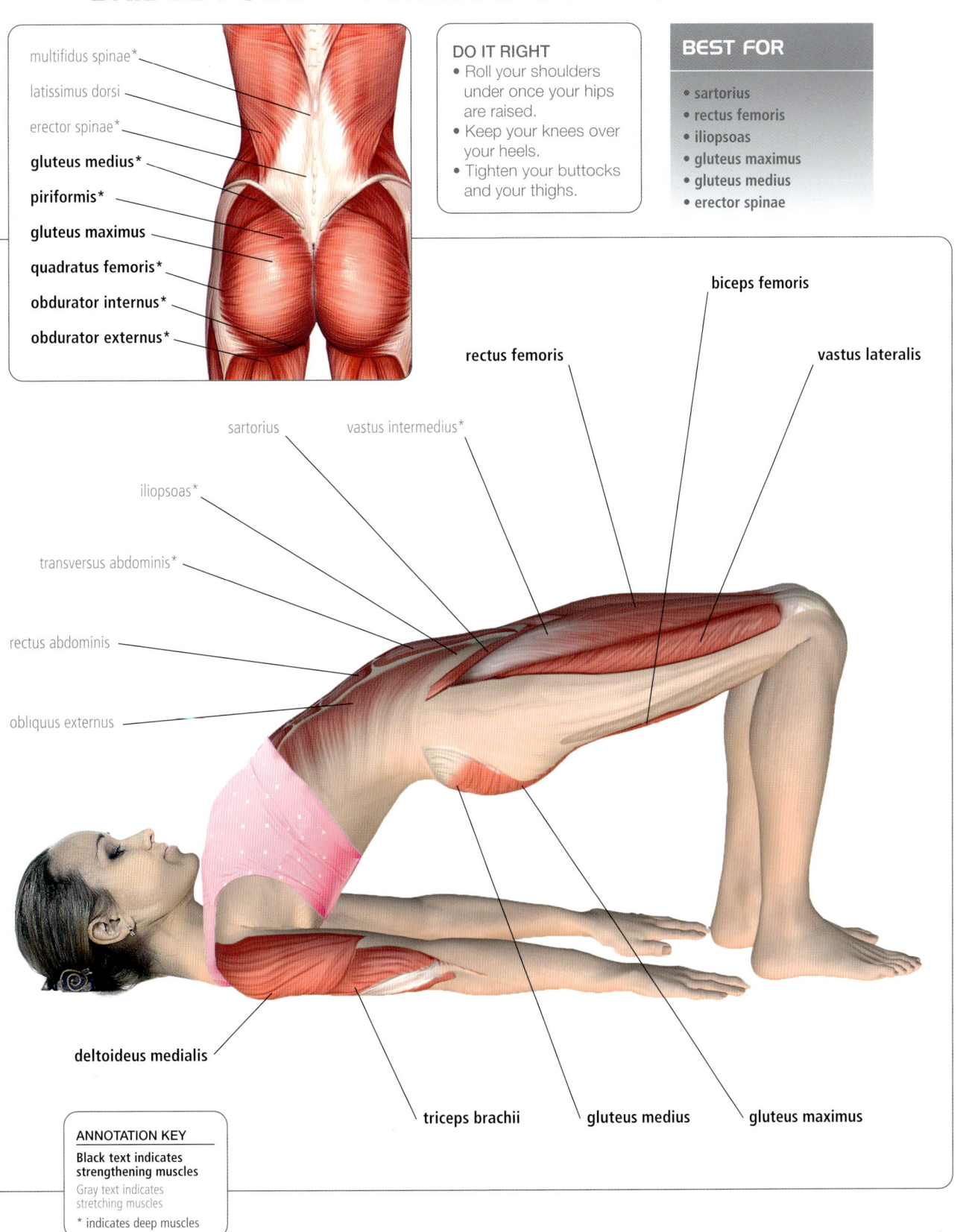

Muscle labels (upper diagram):
- multifidus spinae*
- latissimus dorsi
- erector spinae*
- **gluteus medius***
- **piriformis***
- **gluteus maximus**
- **quadratus femoris***
- **obdurator internus***
- **obdurator externus***

DO IT RIGHT
- Roll your shoulders under once your hips are raised.
- Keep your knees over your heels.
- Tighten your buttocks and your thighs.

BEST FOR
- sartorius
- rectus femoris
- iliopsoas
- gluteus maximus
- gluteus medius
- erector spinae

Muscle labels (lower diagram):
- sartorius
- vastus intermedius*
- **rectus femoris**
- biceps femoris
- vastus lateralis
- iliopsoas*
- transversus abdominis*
- rectus abdominis
- obliquus externus
- **deltoideus medialis**
- triceps brachii
- gluteus medius
- gluteus maximus

ANNOTATION KEY
Black text indicates strengthening muscles
Gray text indicates stretching muscles
* indicates deep muscles

85

CAMEL POSE
(UTRASANA)

FORWARD BENDS & BACKBENDS

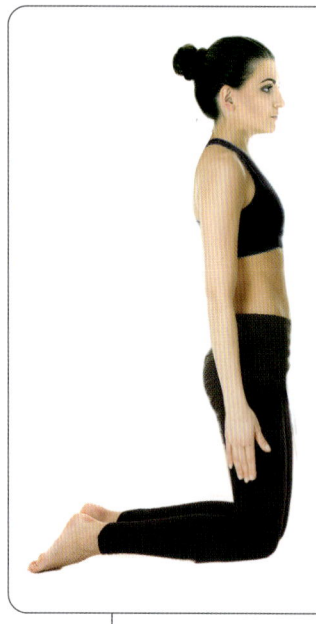

① With your knees one hip-width apart, kneel on the floor with your thighs perpendicular to the floor and your hips open. Tuck your tailbone toward your pubis, and lift up through your spine.

② Place your hands on your lower back with your elbows bent and your fingers pointed toward your buttocks. Lean your shoulders and upper torso backward, opening your chest and pushing forward with your hips.

③ Exhale, and drop back, pressing your pelvis upward and elongating your spine. Pressing your shoulder blades back, lean slightly to your right, and place your right hand on your right heel. Lean slightly to your left, and place your left hand on your left heel. Your fingers should be pointed toward your toes.

④ Push your thighs forward and center your weight in between your knees, lifting your chest into the arch. Drop your head back, and relax your throat.

⑤ Hold for 20 seconds to 1 minute. To come out of the pose, contract your abdominals to lift your chest forward, and slowly bring your hands to your lower back before returning to the starting position.

PRONUNCIATION & MEANING
- Utrasana (oosh-TRAHS-anna)
- *ustra* = camel

BENEFITS
- Strengthens spine
- Stretches thighs, hip flexors, chest, and abdominals
- Stimulates digestion

CONTRA-INDICATIONS & CAUTIONS
- Back injury
- High or low blood pressure
- Headache

AVOID
- Compressing your lower back.
- Rushing into the back bend, which can strain your back.

DO IT RIGHT
- Keep your pelvis pressed forward, and lift up with your abdominals.

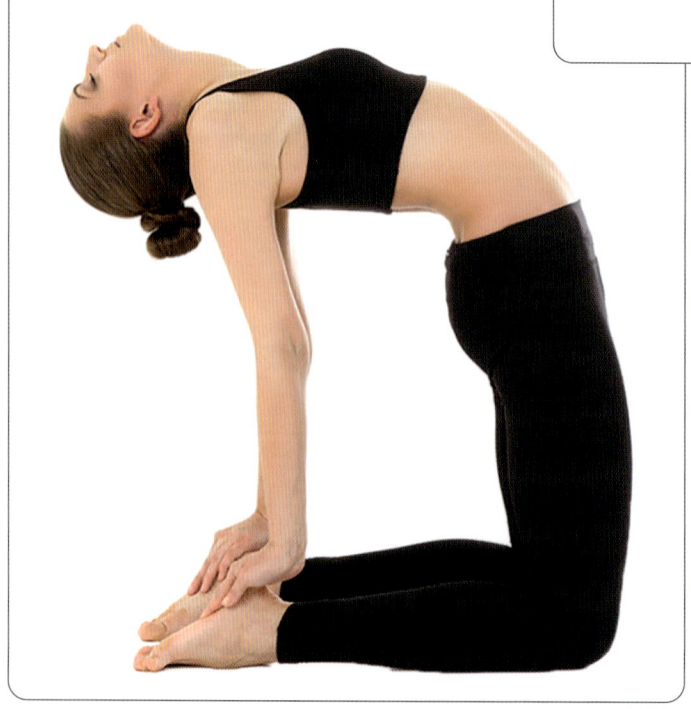

CAMEL POSE • FORWARD BENDS & BACKBENDS

BEST FOR
- pectoralis major
- pectoralis minor
- sternocleidomastoideus
- trapezius
- rectus abdominis
- erector spinae
- gluteus medius
- gluteus maximus
- iliopsoas
- deltoideus anterior
- quadratus lumborum

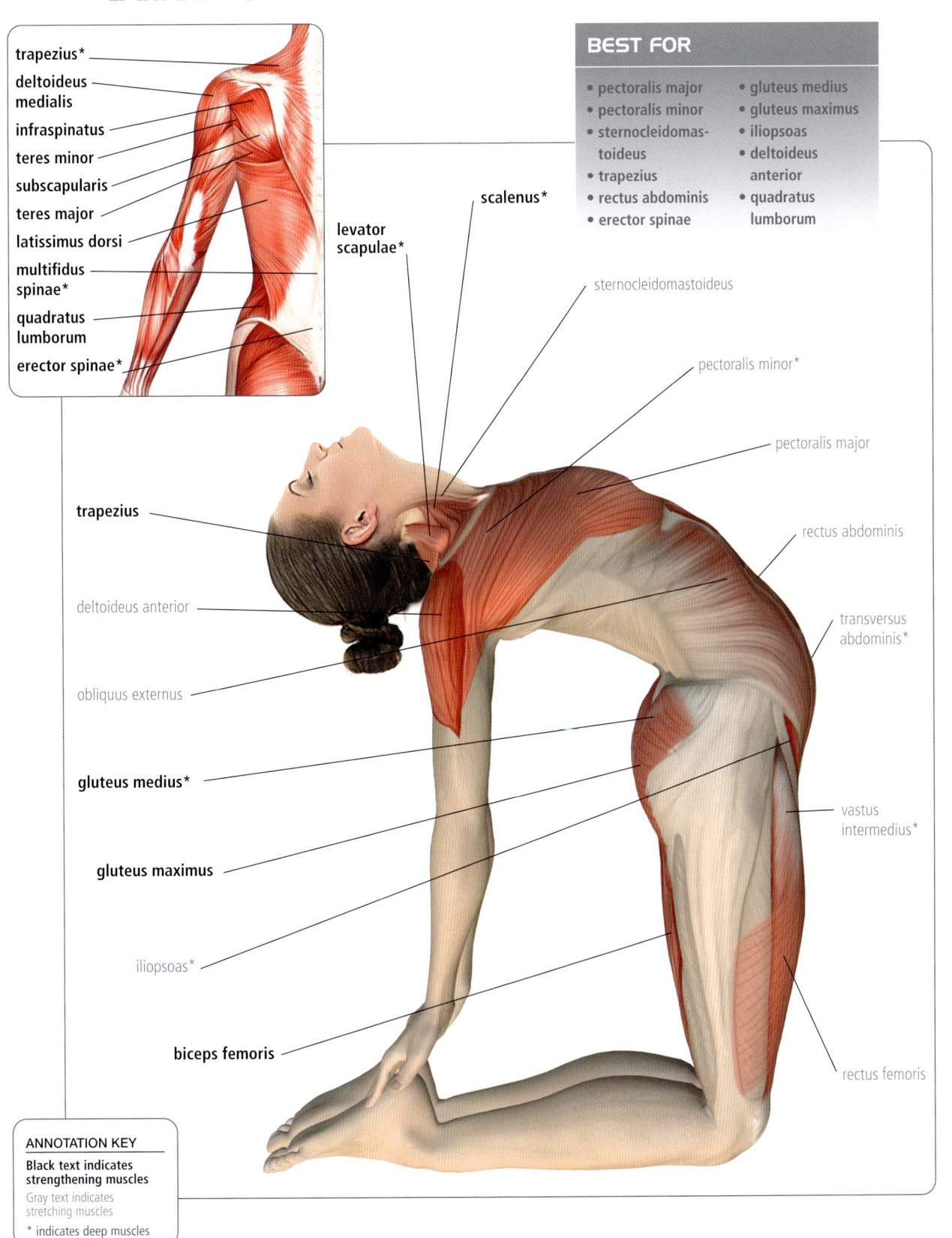

trapezius*
deltoideus medialis
infraspinatus
teres minor
subscapularis
teres major
latissimus dorsi
multifidus spinae*
quadratus lumborum
erector spinae*

levator scapulae*
scalenus*
sternocleidomastoideus
pectoralis minor*
pectoralis major
trapezius
rectus abdominis
deltoideus anterior
transversus abdominis*
obliquus externus
gluteus medius*
vastus intermedius*
gluteus maximus
iliopsoas*
biceps femoris
rectus femoris

ANNOTATION KEY
Black text indicates strengthening muscles
Gray text indicates stretching muscles
* indicates deep muscles

REVERSE TABLETOP POSE
(ARDHA PURVOTTANASANA)

FORWARD BENDS & BACKBENDS

① Begin in Staff Pose (pages 98-99), sitting with your legs straight in front of you. Place your palms flat on the mat at your hips, with your fingers pointing toward your feet.

② Bend your knees and place your feet flat on the mat. Leave some space between your hips and feet, so that when you come up into position, your knees are perpendicular to the floor.

③ Pressing firmly into your hands and feet, inhale and squeeze your buttocks and thighs as you lift your hips up to knee height..

④ Straighten your arms, and check that your thighs and torso are parallel to the floor.

⑤ Your wrists should be directly beneath your shoulders. Draw your shoulder blades together, and open your chest. Keep your neck neutral, or gently begin to drop your head if this feels comfortable. Try to relax your buttocks, and hold the pose only with the strength of your legs

⑥ Hold for the recommended breaths, then release your hips back to the mat, and straighten your legs.

PRONUNCIATION & MEANING
- ARE-dah – PUR-voh-tun-AHS-anna

BENEFITS
- Opens chest
- Stretches quads and hamstrings
- Strengthens glutes and upper back

CONTRA-INDICATIONS & CAUTIONS
- Recent or chronic injury to the knees, hips, arms, back or shoulders.

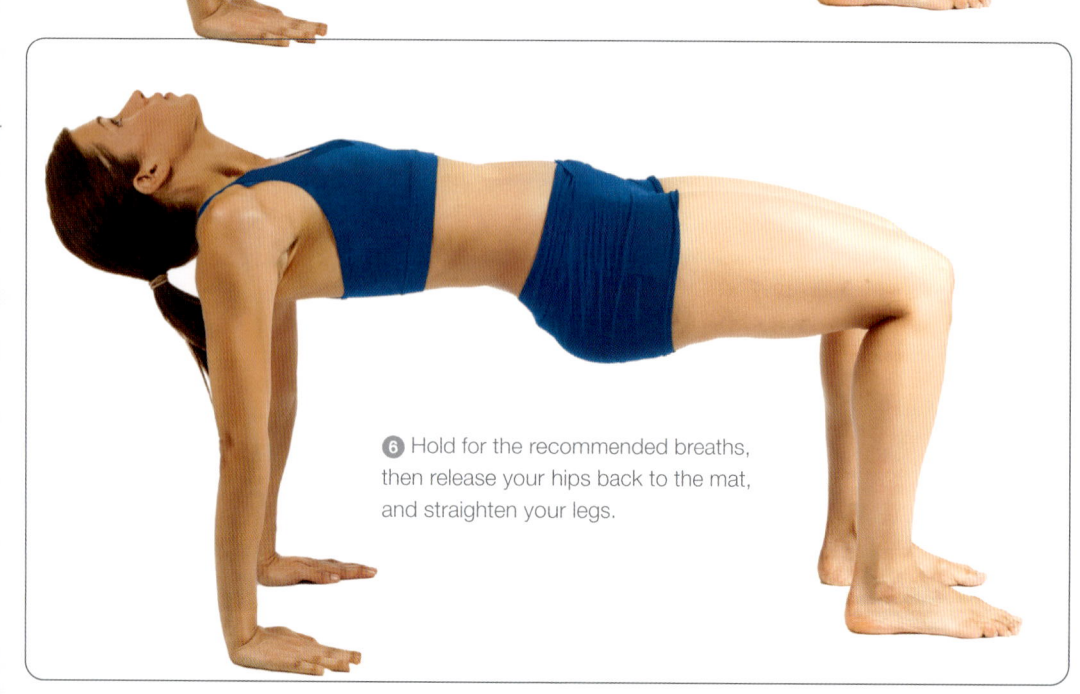

88

REVERSE TABLETOP POSE • FORWARD BENDS & BACKBENDS

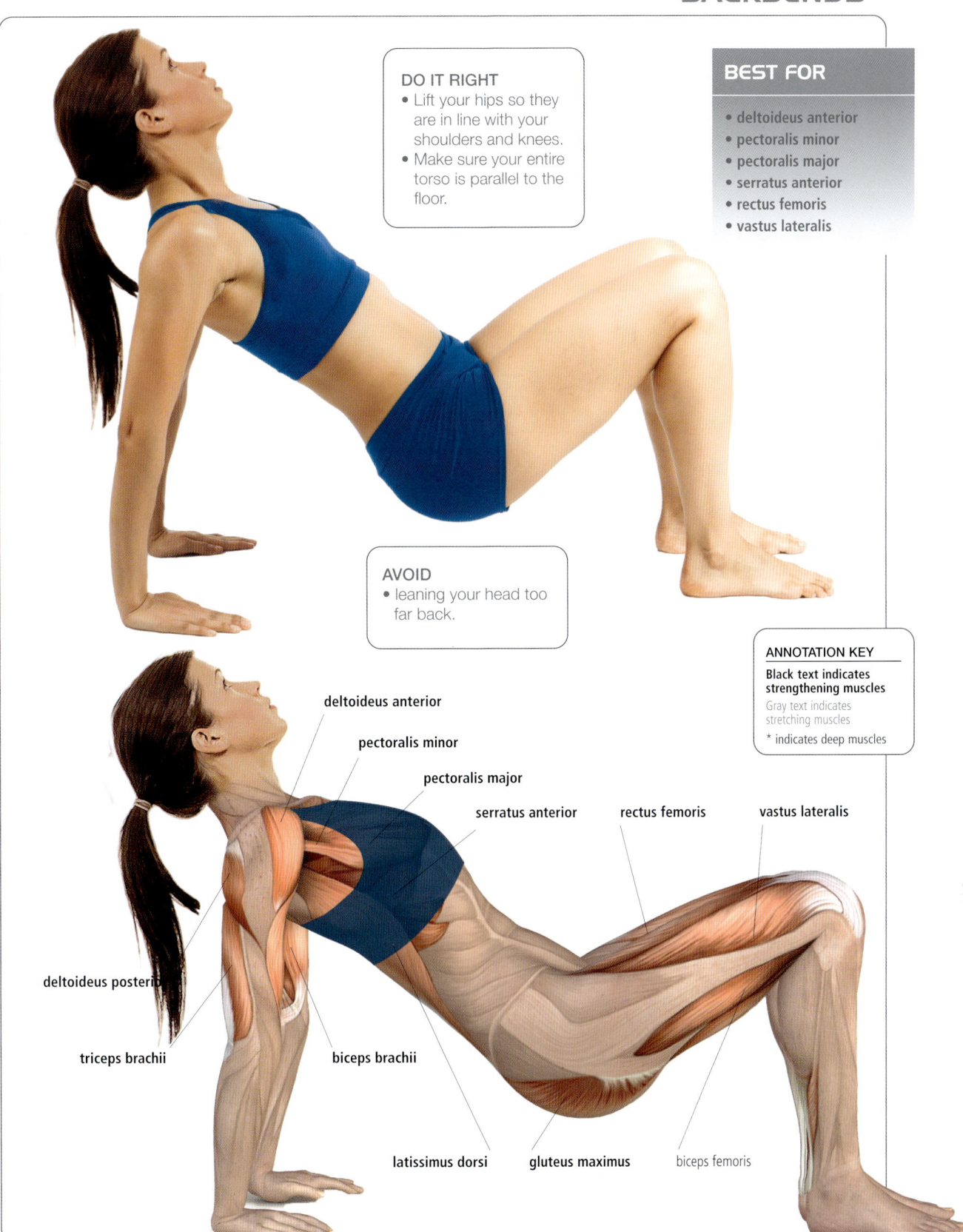

DO IT RIGHT
- Lift your hips so they are in line with your shoulders and knees.
- Make sure your entire torso is parallel to the floor.

BEST FOR
- deltoideus anterior
- pectoralis minor
- pectoralis major
- serratus anterior
- rectus femoris
- vastus lateralis

AVOID
- leaning your head too far back.

ANNOTATION KEY
Black text indicates strengthening muscles
Gray text indicates stretching muscles
* indicates deep muscles

Labels: deltoideus anterior, pectoralis minor, pectoralis major, serratus anterior, rectus femoris, vastus lateralis, deltoideus posterior, triceps brachii, biceps brachii, latissimus dorsi, gluteus maximus, biceps femoris

89

FISH POSE
(MATSYASANA)

① Lie supine on the floor with your arms by your sides. Push down into your heels to lift your hips, and place your hands beneath your buttocks, with your palms facing down.

AVOID
- Pushing your weight onto your head and neck.
- Lifting your hips as you push up into the arch.

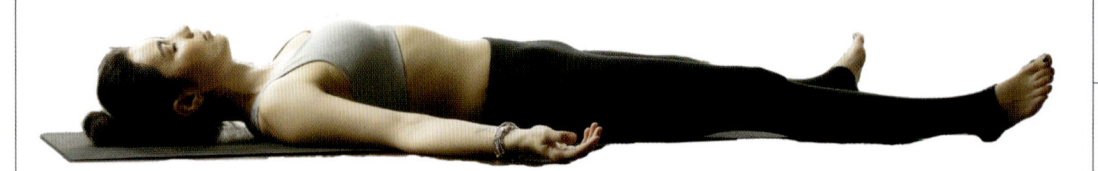

② Rest your buttocks on the tops of your hands, and elongate your legs. Inhale, and press down with your forearms, slightly bending your elbows. Lift up with your chest and head off the floor, creating an arch in your upper back.

③ Tilt your head back, and place it on the floor. Keep the majority of your weight on your elbows.

④ Hold for 15 to 30 seconds.

DO IT RIGHT
- Keep your elbows and forearms pulled in toward your torso throughout the pose.
- Perform this pose with your legs straight, bent, or in Full Lotus (Padmasana, see page 109).

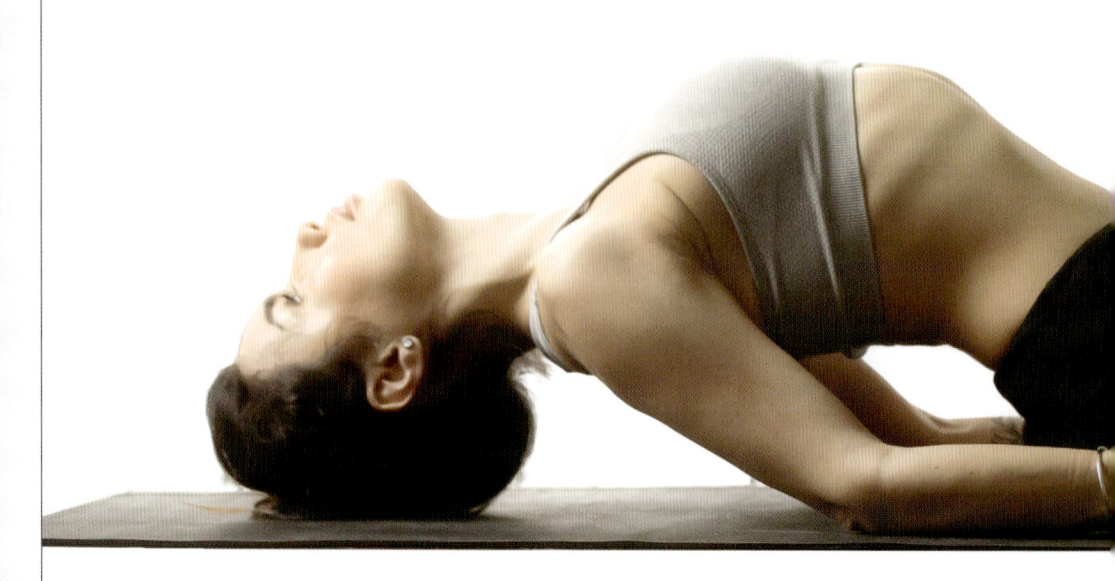

FORWARD BENDS & BACKBENDS

PRONUNCIATION & MEANING
- Matsyasana (mot-see-AHS-anna)
- *matsya* = fish

BENEFITS
- Stretches chest and abdominals
- Strengthens neck, shoulders, and spine
- Improves posture

CONTRA-INDICATIONS & CAUTIONS
- Back injury
- High or low blood pressure
- Headache

FISH POSE • FORWARD BENDS & BACKBENDS

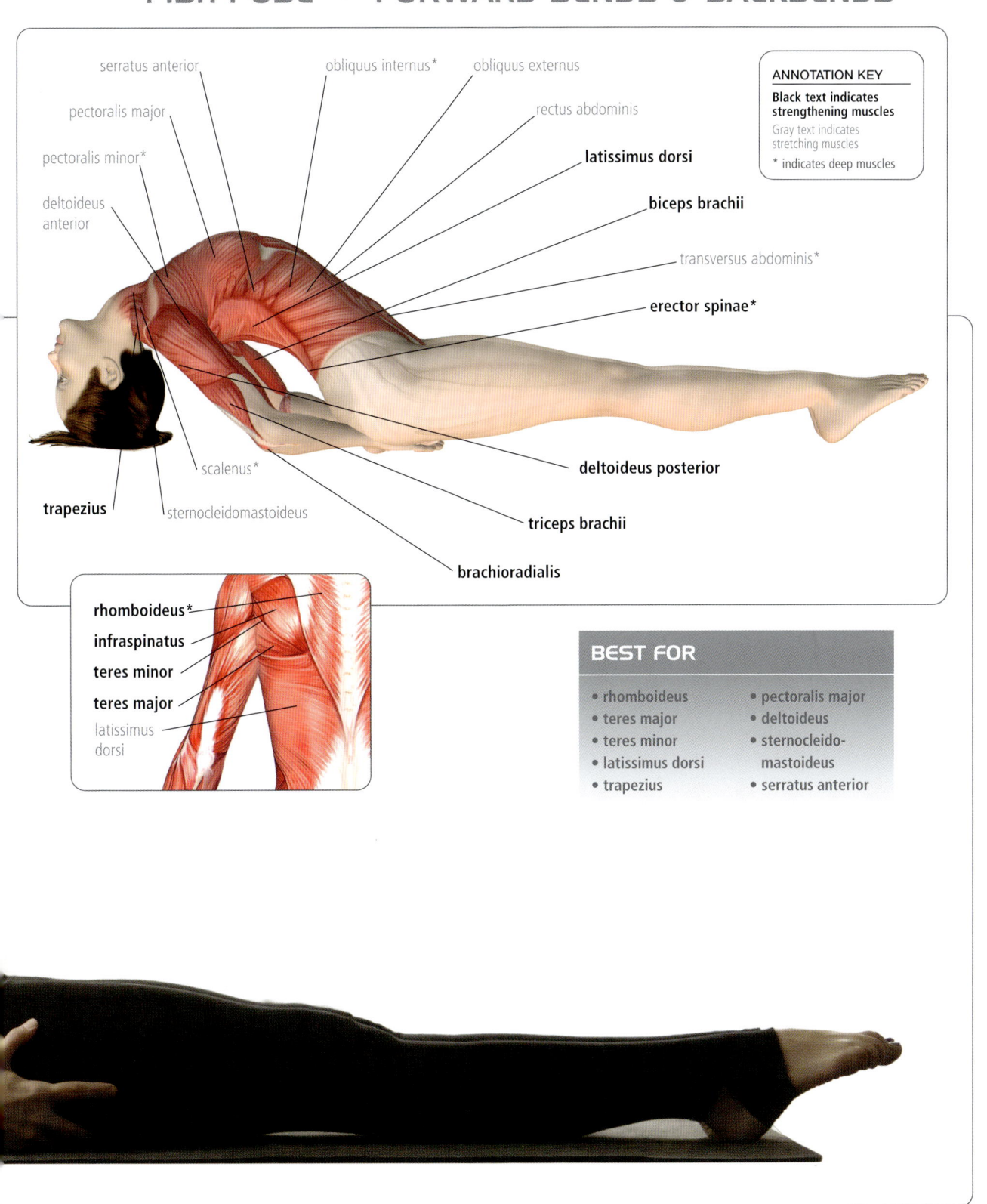

serratus anterior
obliquus internus*
obliquus externus
pectoralis major
rectus abdominis
pectoralis minor*
latissimus dorsi
deltoideus anterior
biceps brachii
transversus abdominis*
erector spinae*
scalenus*
sternocleidomastoideus
trapezius
deltoideus posterior
triceps brachii
brachioradialis

ANNOTATION KEY
Black text indicates strengthening muscles
Gray text indicates stretching muscles
* indicates deep muscles

rhomboideus*
infraspinatus
teres minor
teres major
latissimus dorsi

BEST FOR

- rhomboideus
- teres major
- teres minor
- latissimus dorsi
- trapezius
- pectoralis major
- deltoideus
- sternocleido-mastoideus
- serratus anterior

HALF-FROG POSE
(ARDHA BHEKASANA)

FORWARD BENDS & BACKBENDS

① Lie prone on the floor with your legs fully extended. Bend your elbows, placing your hands flat on the floor on either side of your chest. Keep your elbows pulled in toward your body.

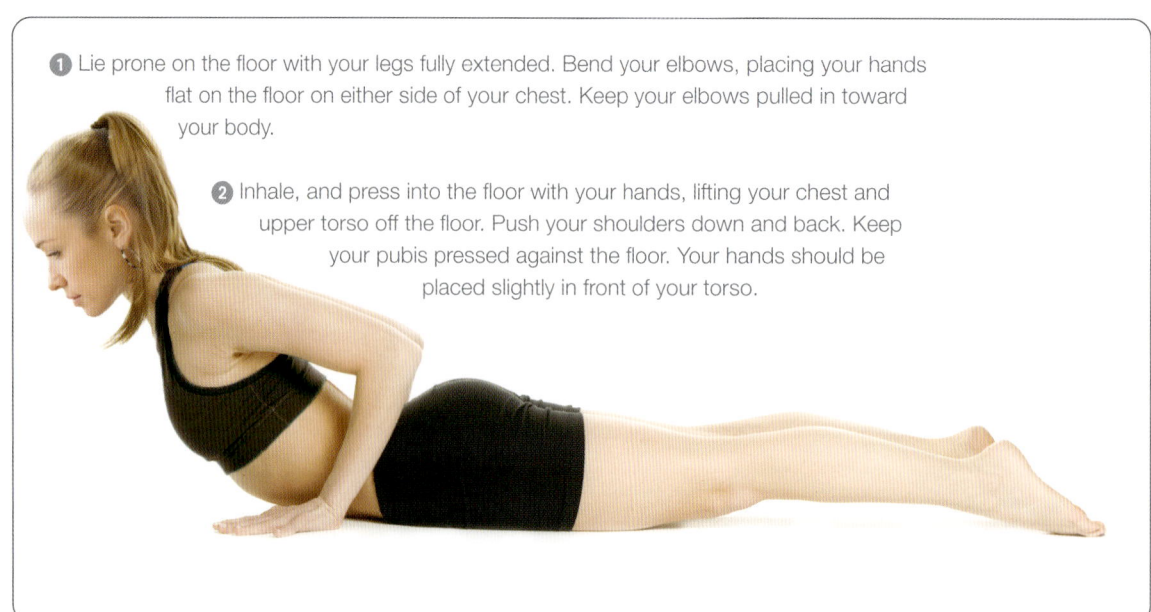

② Inhale, and press into the floor with your hands, lifting your chest and upper torso off the floor. Push your shoulders down and back. Keep your pubis pressed against the floor. Your hands should be placed slightly in front of your torso.

PRONUNCIATION & MEANING
- Ardha Bhekasana (are-dah BEK-has-anna)
- *ardha* = half; *bheka* = frog

BENEFITS
- Strengthens spine and shoulders
- Stretches chest, abdominals, hip flexors, quadriceps, and ankles

CONTRA-INDICATIONS & CAUTIONS
- High or low blood pressure
- Back injury
- Shoulder injury

③ Bend your left knee, drawing your left heel toward your left buttock. Shift your weight onto your right hand, and reach behind you with your left hand to grasp the inside of your left foot. Continue to lift your chest and push down with your right shoulder.

④ Bend your left elbow up toward the ceiling, and rotate your hand so that it rests on top of your foot with your fingers facing forward. Exhale, and press down on your foot with your left hand to stretch it toward your left buttock.

⑤ Without separating your legs more than one hip-width apart, deepen the stretch by moving your left foot slightly to the outside of your left thigh, aiming the sole of your foot toward the floor.

⑥ Hold for 30 seconds to 2 minutes. Repeat on the opposite side.

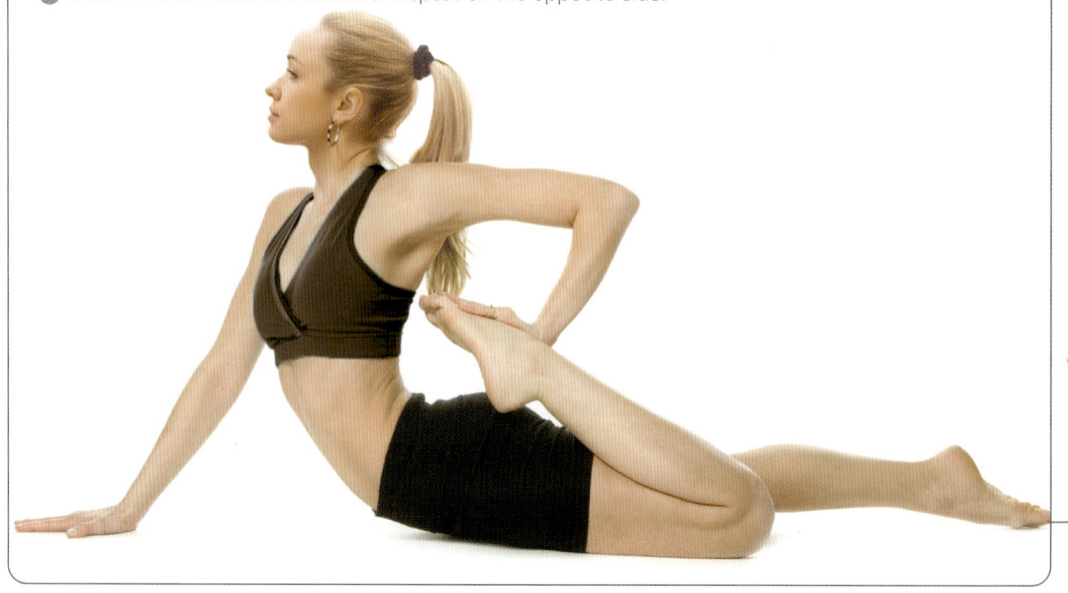

HALF-FROG POSE • FORWARD BENDS & BACKBENDS

DO IT RIGHT
- Keep your hips and shoulders squared forward.
- If you have trouble supporting yourself on your hand, lower yourself onto your forearm and elbow.

AVOID
- Pushing so hard on your foot that it causes discomfort in your knee.
- Sinking into your supporting shoulder.

BEST FOR
- latissimus dorsi
- quadratus lumborum
- erector spinae
- pectoralis major
- deltoideus medialis
- rectus abdominis
- transversus
- abdominis
- iliopsoas
- vastus intermedius
- rectus femoris
- sartorius
- tibialis anterior
- extensor hallucis

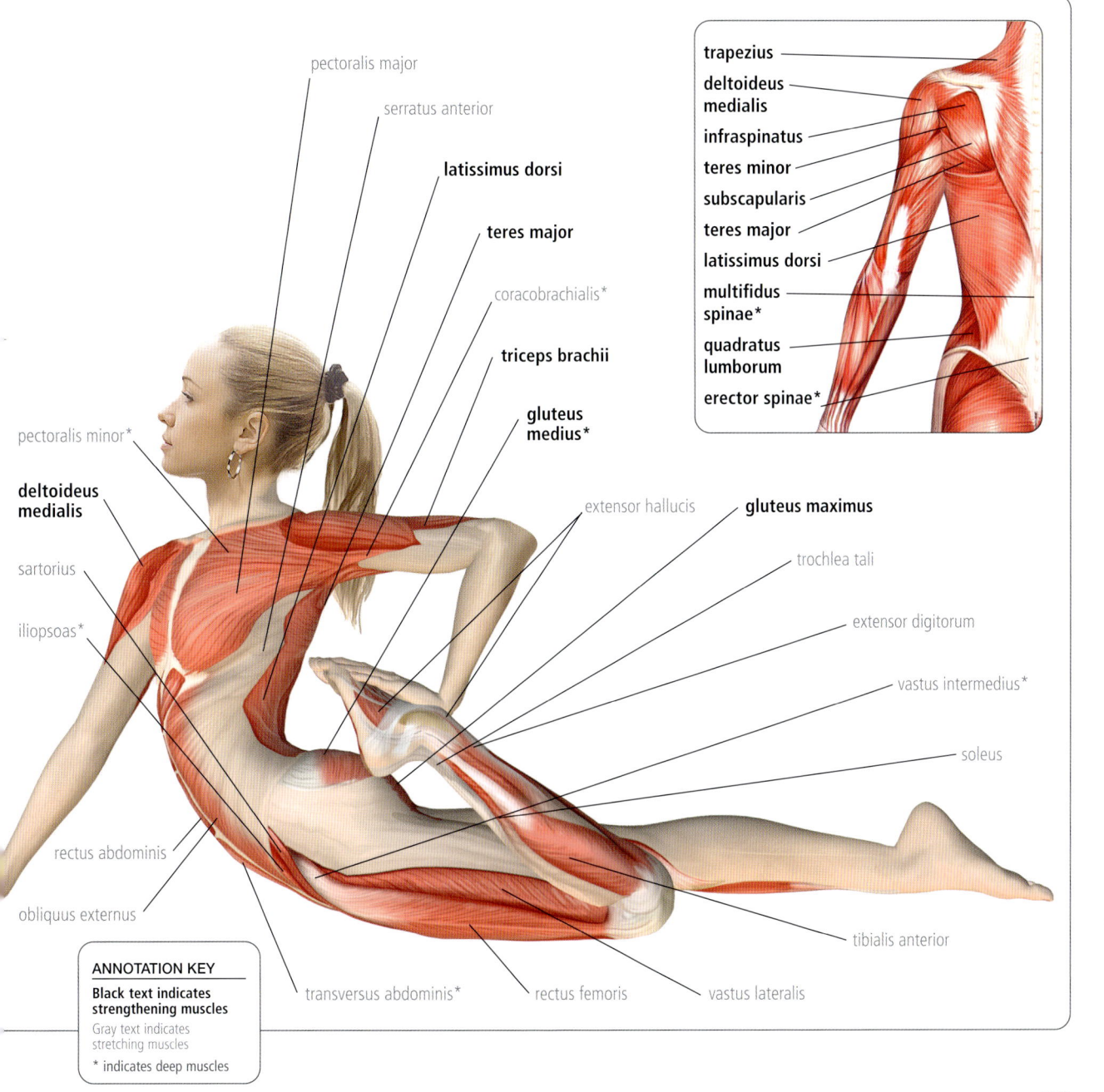

Labels (main figure)
- pectoralis major
- serratus anterior
- **latissimus dorsi**
- **teres major**
- coracobrachialis*
- **triceps brachii**
- gluteus medius*
- extensor hallucis
- **gluteus maximus**
- trochlea tali
- extensor digitorum
- vastus intermedius*
- soleus
- tibialis anterior
- vastus lateralis
- rectus femoris
- transversus abdominis*
- obliquus externus
- rectus abdominis
- iliopsoas*
- sartorius
- **deltoideus medialis**
- pectoralis minor*

Labels (inset)
- trapezius
- deltoideus medialis
- infraspinatus
- teres minor
- subscapularis
- teres major
- latissimus dorsi
- multifidus spinae*
- quadratus lumborum
- erector spinae*

ANNOTATION KEY
Black text indicates strengthening muscles
Gray text indicates stretching muscles
* indicates deep muscles

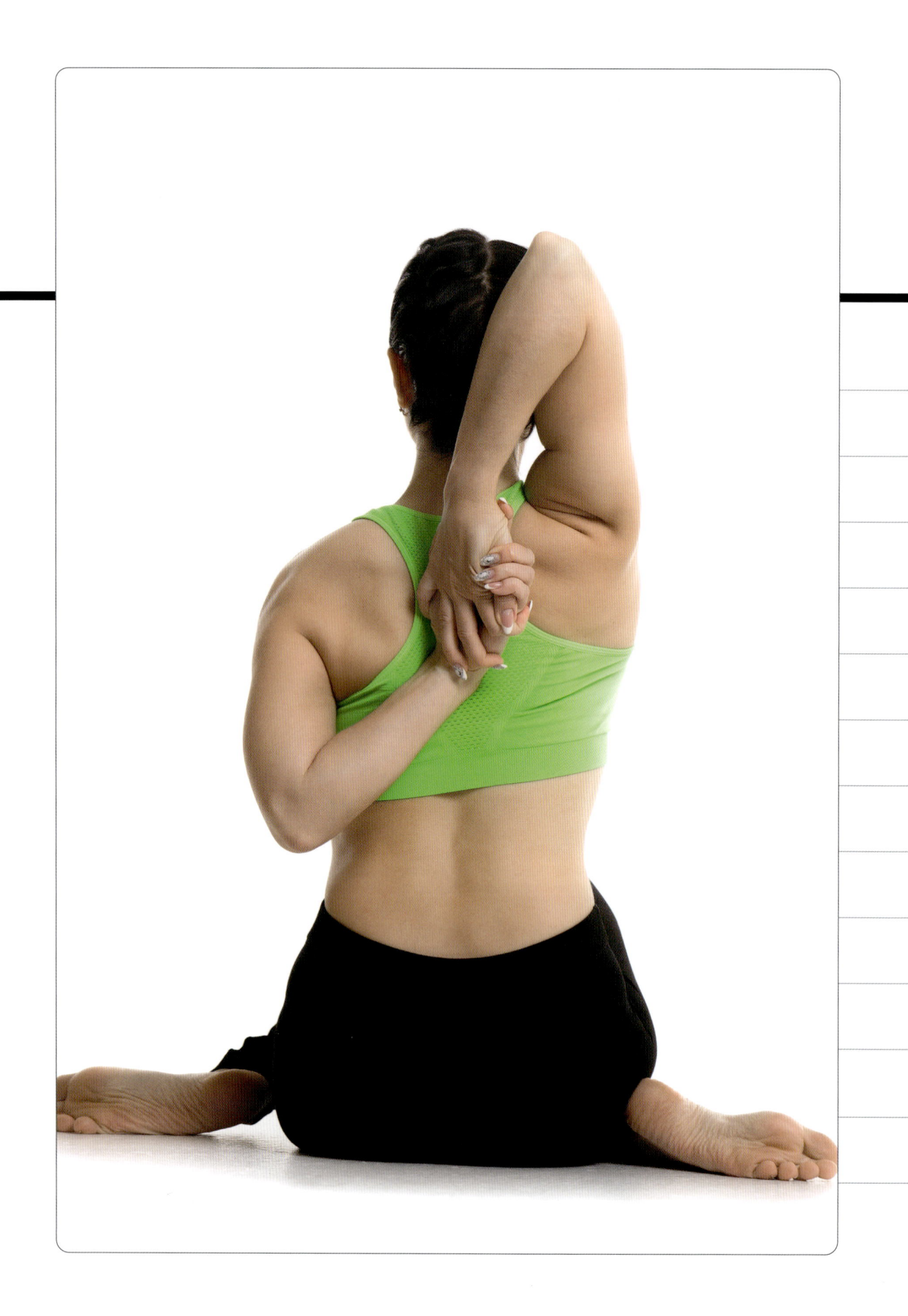

SEATED POSES AND TWISTS

Seated and twisting poses invigorate the body and alleviate tension caused by poor posture and back pain. These poses are among the most stable, allowing you to concentrate on your breathing and form and worry less about balance. When you align your spine correctly and ground yourself in seated poses, you can unlock long-standing tension in your hips, groin, pelvis, and lower back.

Twisting poses cause your muscles to contract and stretch on alternate sides of your body. These actions benefit your internal organs and circulatory system, as well as greatly improving your overall flexibility. As you engage in a twist, your organs compress and then relax when you release, flushing out internal toxins. Keeping your spine extended during a twist is vital to maximize spinal rotation.

EASY POSE
(SUKHASANA)

SEATED POSES AND TWISTS

① Sit on the floor with your legs extended in front of you.

② Bend your knees, and cross your shins inward, sliding your left foot beneath your right knee and your right foot beneath your left knee, forming a gap between your feet and your groins. Relax your knees toward the floor.

③ Draw your sit bones to the floor, and lift up through your spine. Maintain a neutral position from your pelvis to your shoulders. Open your chest, and relax your shoulders.

④ Place the backs of your hands on your knees, forming an "O" with your thumb and index finger. Breathe slowly and evenly.

⑤ Hold for as long as you wish. Be sure to also practice the pose with your opposite leg in front.

AVOID
- Pulling your feet in toward your groins.
- Arching your lower back beyond its neutral spinal position.

PRONUNCIATION & MEANING
- Sukhasana (sook-AHS-anna)
- *sukh* = joy, comfort

BENEFITS
- Opens hips
- Strengthens spine
- Relieves stress

CONTRA-INDICATIONS & CAUTIONS
- Knee injury
- Hip injury

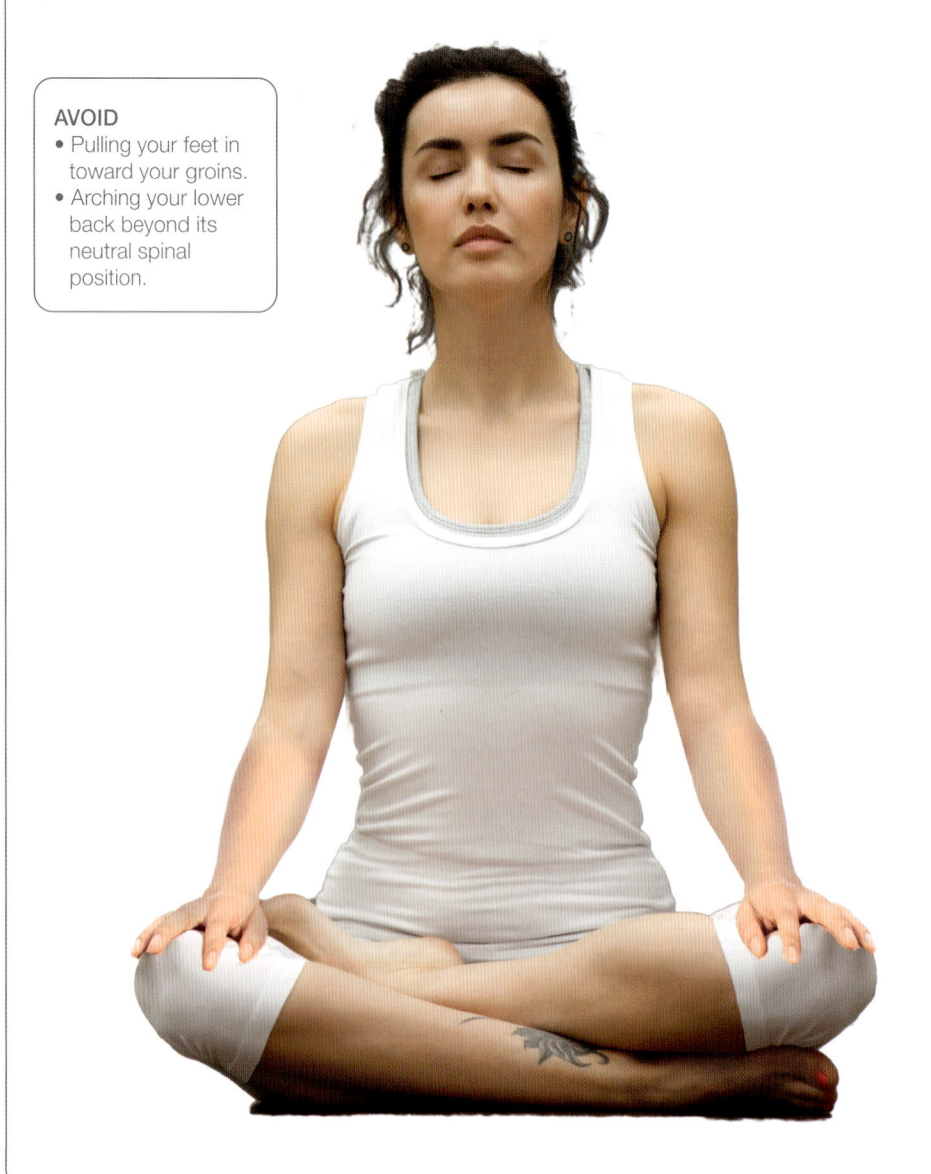

EASY POSE • SEATED POSES AND TWISTS

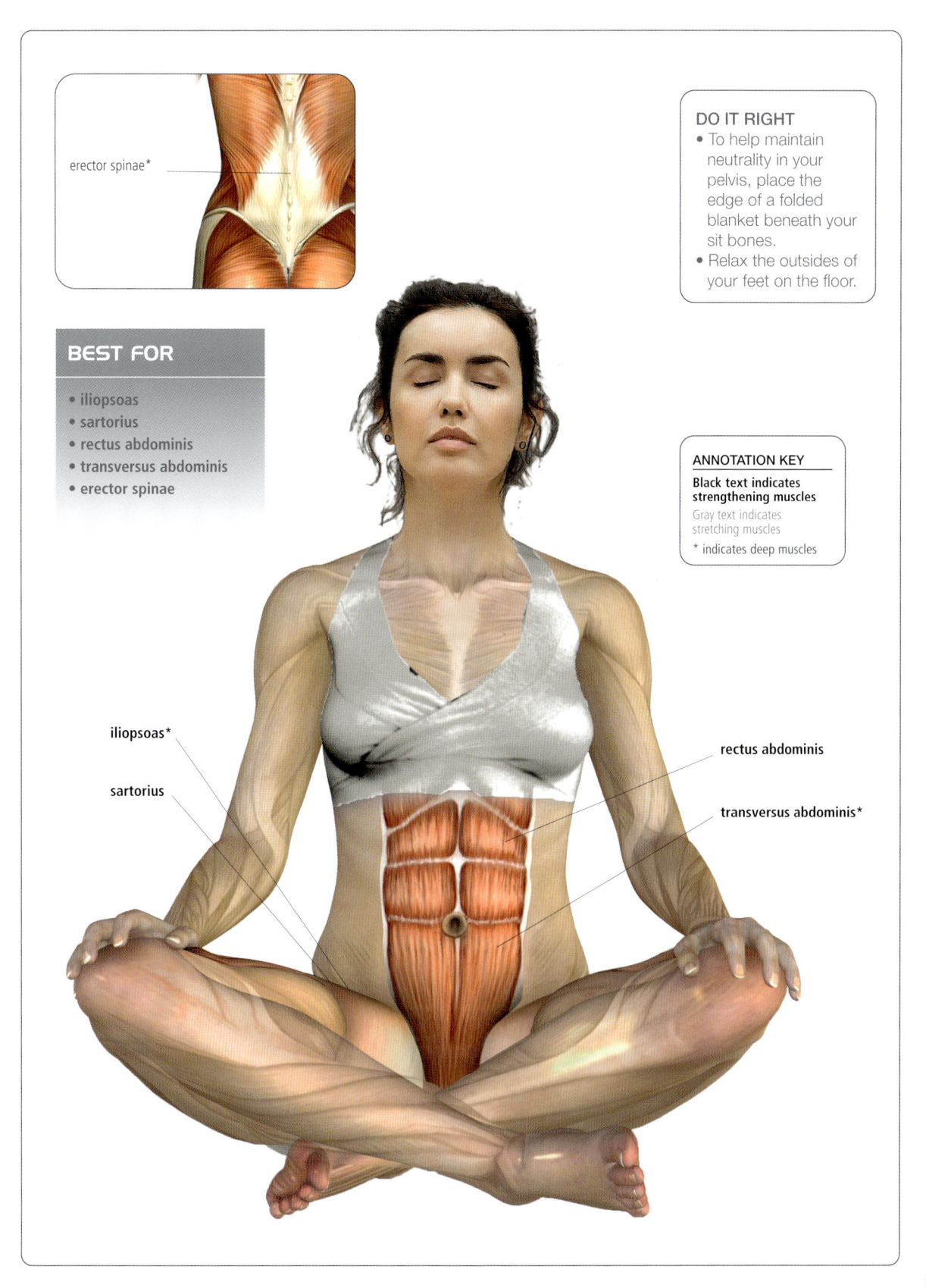

erector spinae*

DO IT RIGHT
- To help maintain neutrality in your pelvis, place the edge of a folded blanket beneath your sit bones.
- Relax the outsides of your feet on the floor.

BEST FOR
- iliopsoas
- sartorius
- rectus abdominis
- transversus abdominis
- erector spinae

ANNOTATION KEY
Black text indicates strengthening muscles
Gray text indicates stretching muscles
* indicates deep muscles

iliopsoas*

sartorius

rectus abdominis

transversus abdominis*

97

STAFF POSE
(DANDASANA)

SEATED POSES AND TWISTS

DO IT RIGHT
- Keep your legs firm and active.
- Draw your shoulder blades together.
- If you find that your lower back is rounding and your pelvis tucks under when your legs are straight, try sitting on a block or blanket.

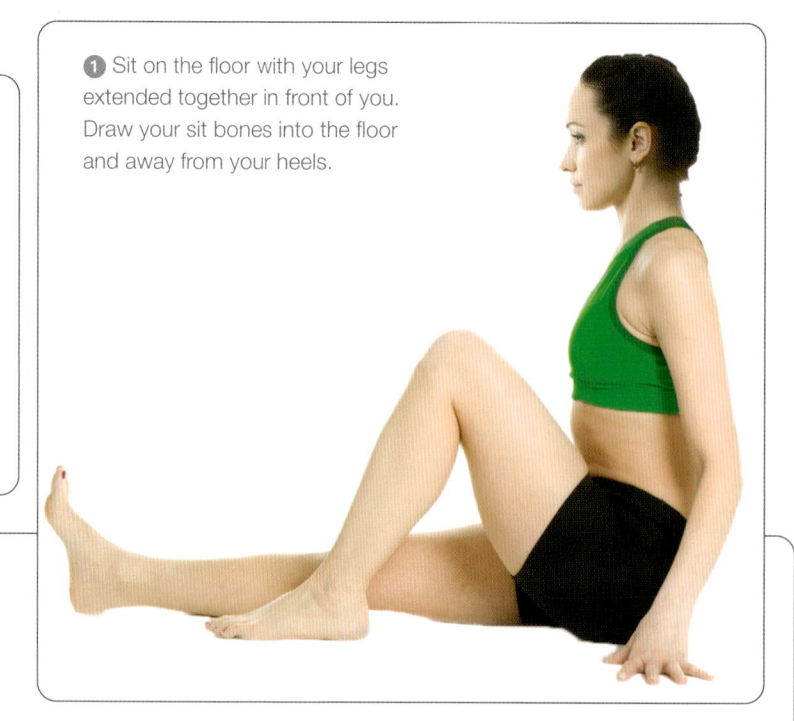

❶ Sit on the floor with your legs extended together in front of you. Draw your sit bones into the floor and away from your heels.

❷ Contract the muscles in your legs, pressing them against the floor. Place the palms of your hands on the floor beside your hips, and lift up through your spine. Flex your feet.

❸ Lift your chest, and gaze forward, tucking your chin slightly downward. Relax your shoulders, and pull your abdominals in toward your spine.

❹ Hold for 1 minute or more.

PRONUNCIATION & MEANING
- Dandasana (Dand-AHS-anna)
- 'Danda' means staff or stick, and 'asana' means pose.

BENEFITS
- Improves posture
- Stretches legs
- Strengthens spine

CONTRA-INDICATIONS & CAUTIONS
- Lower-back pain
- Tight hamstrings

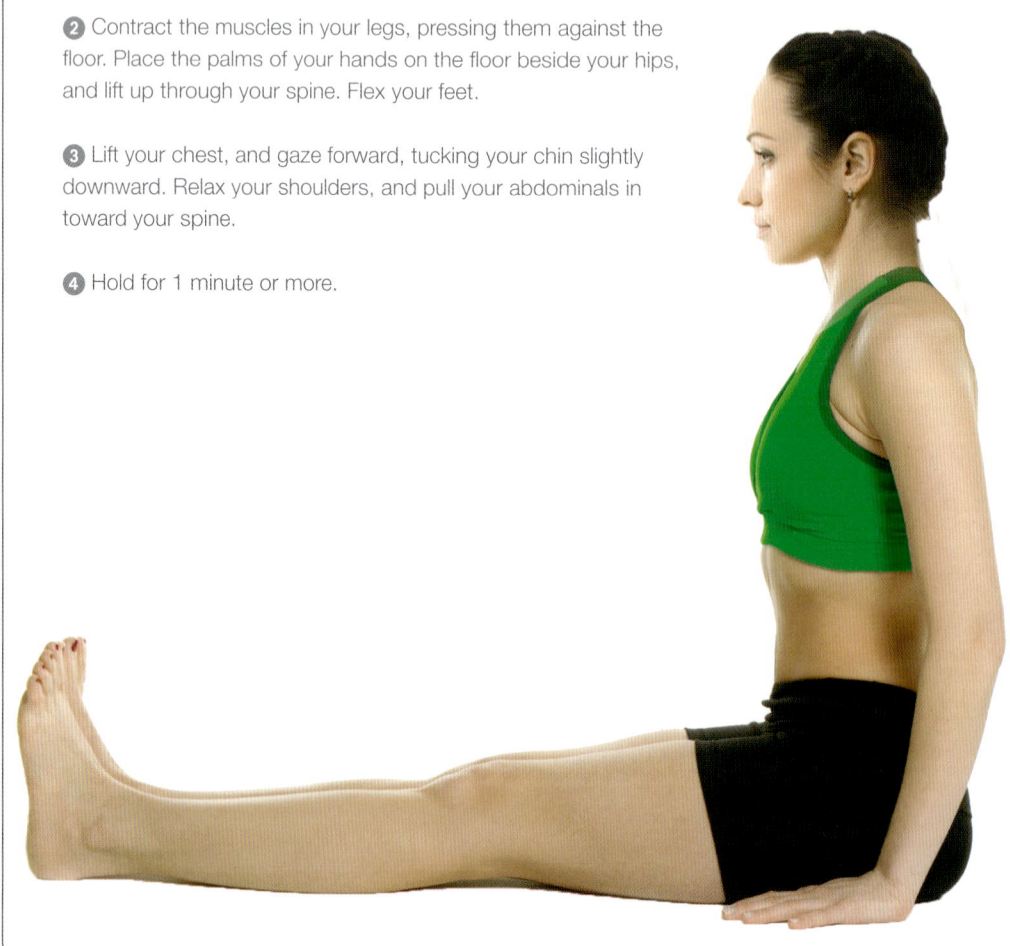

98

STAFF POSE • SEATED POSES AND TWISTS

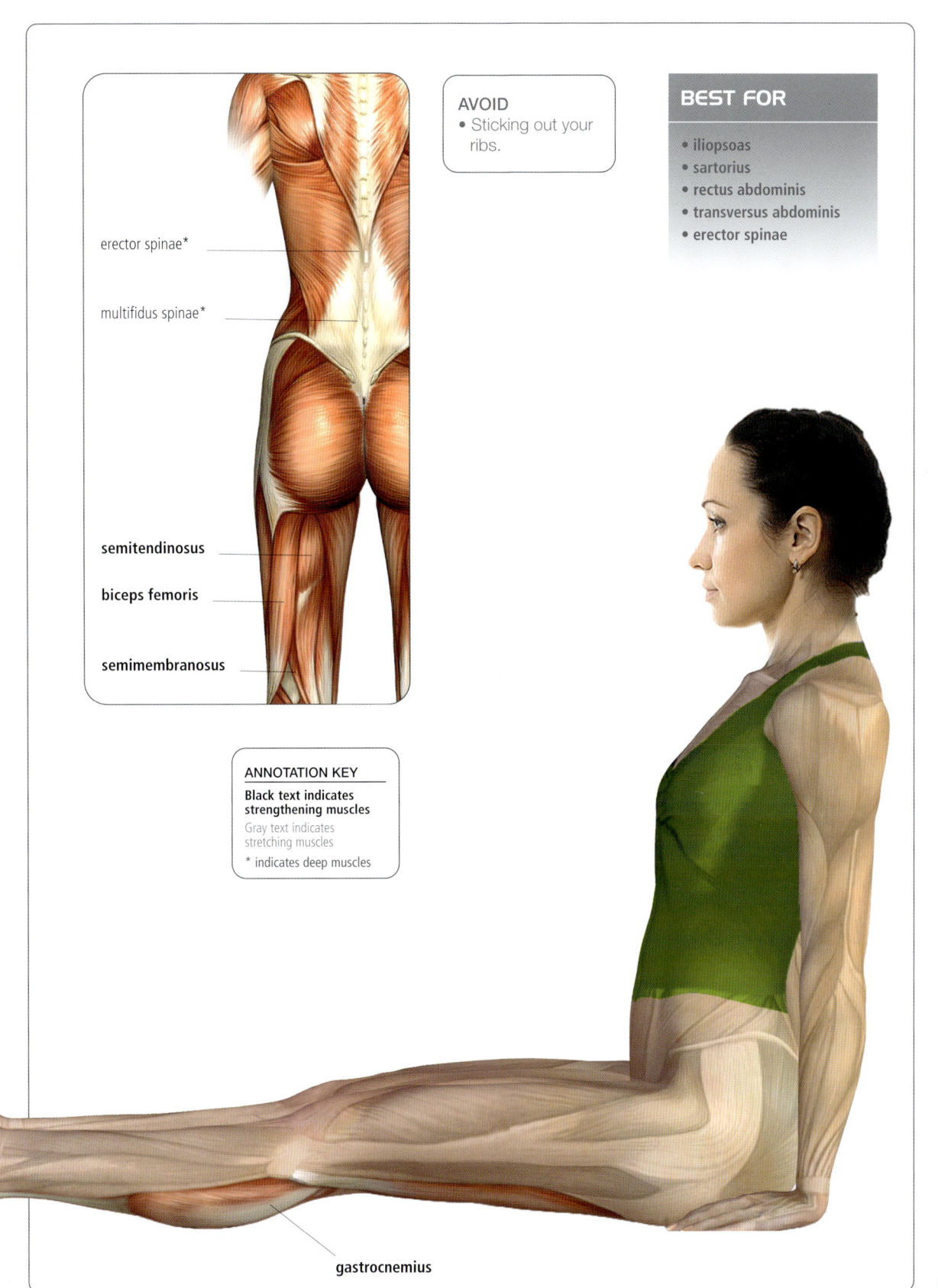

AVOID
- Sticking out your ribs.

BEST FOR
- iliopsoas
- sartorius
- rectus abdominis
- transversus abdominis
- erector spinae

erector spinae*

multifidus spinae*

semitendinosus

biceps femoris

semimembranosus

ANNOTATION KEY

Black text indicates strengthening muscles

Gray text indicates stretching muscles

* indicates deep muscles

gastrocnemius

SEATED POSES AND TWISTS

BOUND ANGLE POSE
(BADDHA KONASANA)

1. Sit with your legs extended in front of you. Sit up tall with your shoulders relaxed.

2. Bring your knees toward your chest with your feet flat on the floor.

3. Exhale, and open hips, drawing your thighs to the floor. Use your hands to press your feet together, and keep the outsides of your feet on the floor.

4. Draw your torso upward, and focus on keeping the spine in the neutral position. Your weight should be balanced evenly on your sit bones. Allow your hips to open farther and your thighs to drop to the floor.

5. Hold for 1 to 5 minutes.

AVOID
- Pushing your knees down with your hands.
- Rounding your back.

DO IT RIGHT
- Lift upward from your spine, and keep your chest and shoulders pressed open, creating a straight line from your sit bones to your shoulders.
- If your groins and inner thighs are very tight, place a folded blanket beneath your buttocks for elevation.
- If you are comfortable in the pose and want to deepen the stretch, bend forward, leading with your chest.

BEST FOR
- iliopsoas
- tensor fasciae latae
- adductor magnus
- adductor longus
- iliacus

PRONUNCIATION & MEANING
- Baddha Konasana (BAH-dah cone-AHS-anna)
- *baddha* = bound; *kona* = angle
- Also called Tailor Pose

BENEFITS
- Stretches inner thighs, groins, and knees
- Provides relief from menstrual discomfort

CONTRA-INDICATIONS & CAUTIONS
- Knee injury
- Groin injury

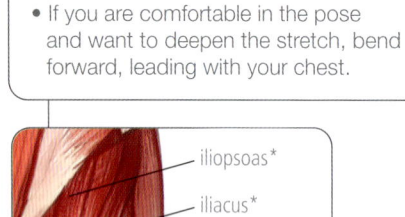

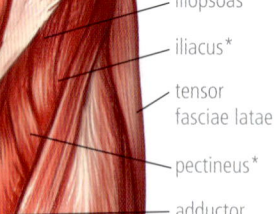

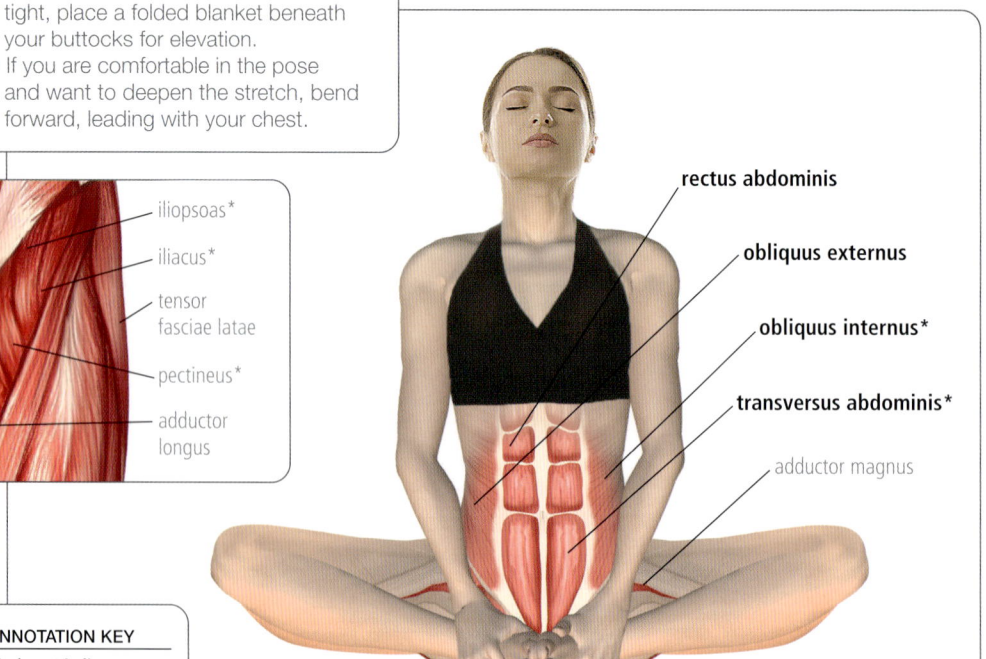

Muscles labeled:
- iliopsoas*
- iliacus*
- tensor fasciae latae
- pectineus*
- adductor longus
- rectus abdominis
- obliquus externus
- obliquus internus*
- transversus abdominis*
- adductor magnus

ANNOTATION KEY
Black text indicates strengthening muscles
Gray text indicates stretching muscles
* indicates deep muscles

100

BOUND ANGLE POSE WITH FORWARD BEND
(BADDHA KONASANA UTTANASANA)

SEATED POSES AND TWISTS

① Sit up tall on your mat, with the soles of your feet pressed together.

② Place your forearms or elbows on your inner thighs, and grab your feet and toes with your hands.

③ Draw your heels closer, keeping your heels a comfortable distance from your core.

④ Fold your upper body forward until you feel a stretch in your groin.

⑤ Hold for the recommended breaths, and then slowly roll up.

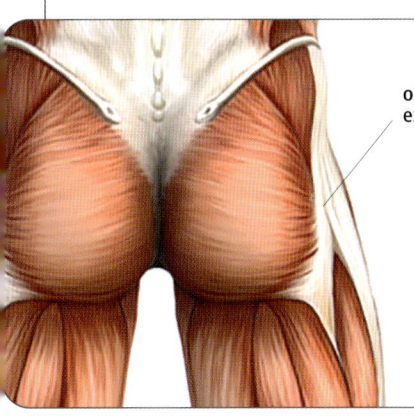

obturator externus*

DO IT RIGHT
- Make sure you exhale as you drop your chest toward the floor.

AVOID
- Slouching or rocking backward off your hip bones; instead, you should feel them anchored on the floor.
- Holding your breath.

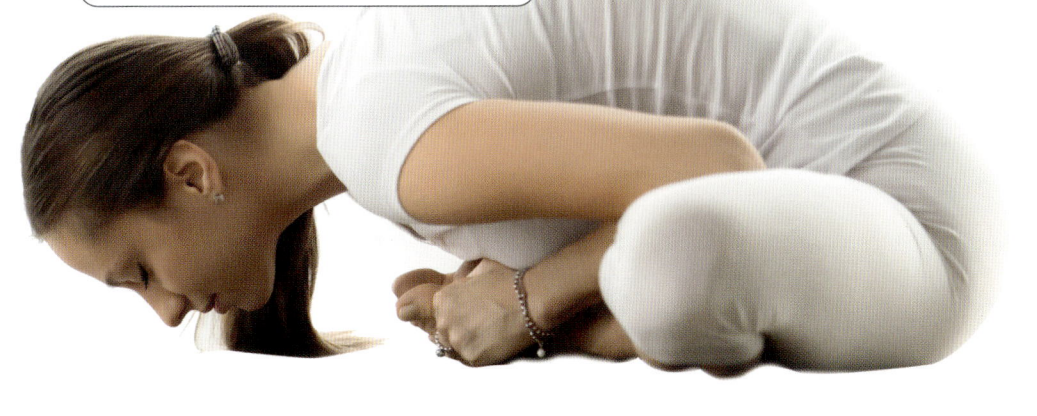

PRONUNCIATION & MEANING
- Baddha Konasana (BAH-dah cone-AHS-anna)
- *baddha* = bound; *kona* = angle
- Also called Tailor Pose

BENEFITS
- Stretches inner thighs, groins, and knees
- Provides relief from menstrual discomfort

CONTRA-INDICATIONS & CAUTIONS
- Knee injury
- Groin injury

SEATED POSES AND TWISTS

FIRE LOG POSE
(AGNISTAMBHASANA)

① Sit in Easy Pose (pages 96-97)) with your torso lifted tall.

② Place your right ankle on top of your left knee. Your right foot should rest on the outside of your left knee.

③ Slide your left ankle below your right knee, so that your shins are stacked one on top of the other. Flex both of your feet.

④ Lift up in your spine through your torso to sit tall on your sit bones. Exhale, and allow your hips to stretch open.

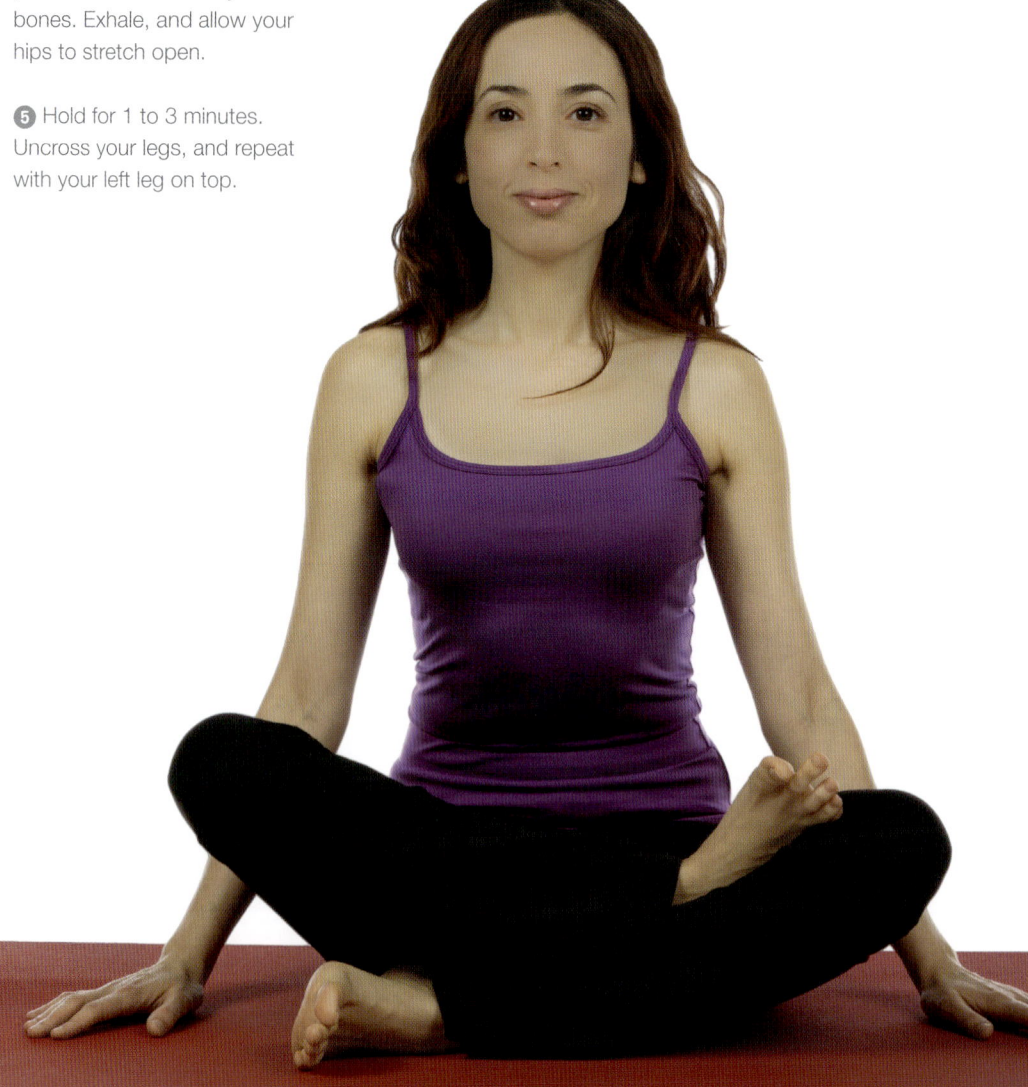

⑤ Hold for 1 to 3 minutes. Uncross your legs, and repeat with your left leg on top.

BEST FOR
- iliopsoas
- iliacus
- adductor magnus
- adductor longus
- tensor fasciae latae
- pectineus
- vastus lateralis
- iliacus
- vastus medialis
- gracilis
- sartorius

PRONUNCIATION & MEANING
- Agnistambhasana (AHG-nih stom-BAHS-anna)
- *agni* = fire; *stambha* = pillar

BENEFITS
- Stretches hips and groins

CONTRA-INDICATIONS & CAUTIONS
- Knee injury
- Groin injury

FIRE LOG POSE • SEATED POSES AND TWISTS

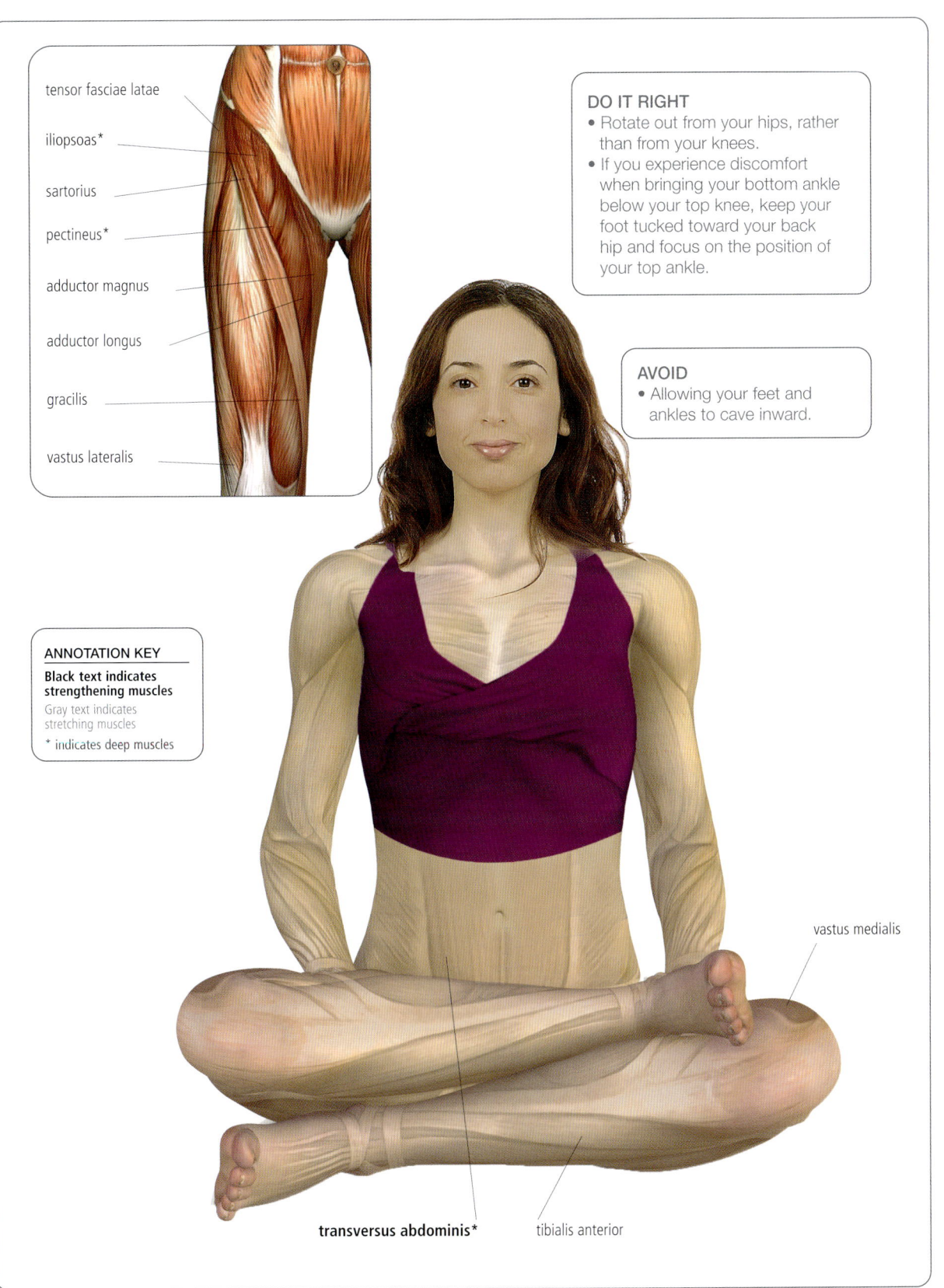

- tensor fasciae latae
- iliopsoas*
- sartorius
- pectineus*
- adductor magnus
- adductor longus
- gracilis
- vastus lateralis

DO IT RIGHT
- Rotate out from your hips, rather than from your knees.
- If you experience discomfort when bringing your bottom ankle below your top knee, keep your foot tucked toward your back hip and focus on the position of your top ankle.

AVOID
- Allowing your feet and ankles to cave inward.

ANNOTATION KEY

Black text indicates strengthening muscles

Gray text indicates stretching muscles

* indicates deep muscles

vastus medialis

transversus abdominis*   tibialis anterior

103

COW-FACE POSE
(GOMUKHASANA)

① Sit in Fire Log Pose (pages 102-03), with your right leg stacked on top of your left.

② Slide your left ankle to the left and your right ankle to the right so that your knees are stacked on top of each other. Your heels should angle toward your hips at approximately the same distance from your hips.

③ Lift up from your spine, sitting with equal weight on your sit bones. Inhale, and reach your right hand to the side, parallel to the floor.

④ Bend your elbow, and rotate your shoulder downward so that the palm of your hand faces behind you. Reach behind your back, palm still up, and draw your elbow into your right side. Continue to rotate your shoulder downward as you reach upward with your hand until your forearm is parallel to your spine. Your right hand should rest in between your shoulder blades.

⑤ With your next inhalation, reach your left arm up toward the ceiling with your palm facing the back wall. Exhale, and bend your elbow, reaching your left hand down the center of your back.

⑥ Hook your hands together behind your back. Lift your chest, and pull your abdominals in toward your spine.

⑦ Hold for approximately 1 minute. Repeat with your left leg stacked on top of your right, and your right elbow pointed toward the ceiling.

DO IT RIGHT
- Allow gravity to stretch your hips open.
- Make sure that whichever leg is on top, the opposite elbow is pointed toward the ceiling.
- If you cannot hook your hands behind your back, try using a strap to help you pull your hands closer together.

AVOID
- Lifting either of your sit bones off the floor.

SEATED POSES AND TWISTS

PRONUNCIATION & MEANING
- Gomukhasana (go-moo-KAHS-anna)
- *go* = cow; *mukha* = face

BENEFITS
- Stretches hips, thighs, shoulders, and triceps

CONTRA-INDICATIONS & CAUTIONS
- Shoulder injury

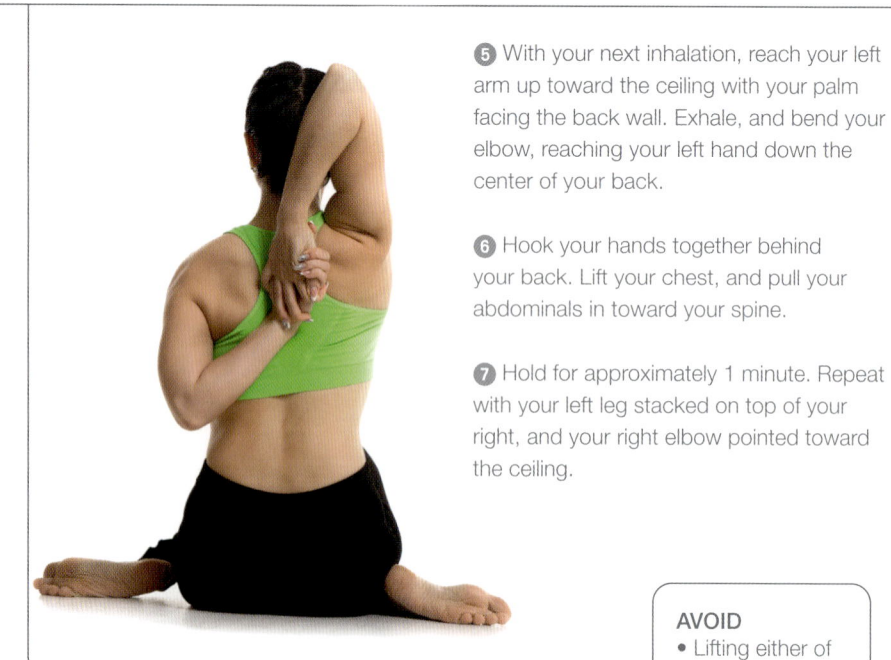

COW-FACE POSE • SEATED POSES AND TWISTS

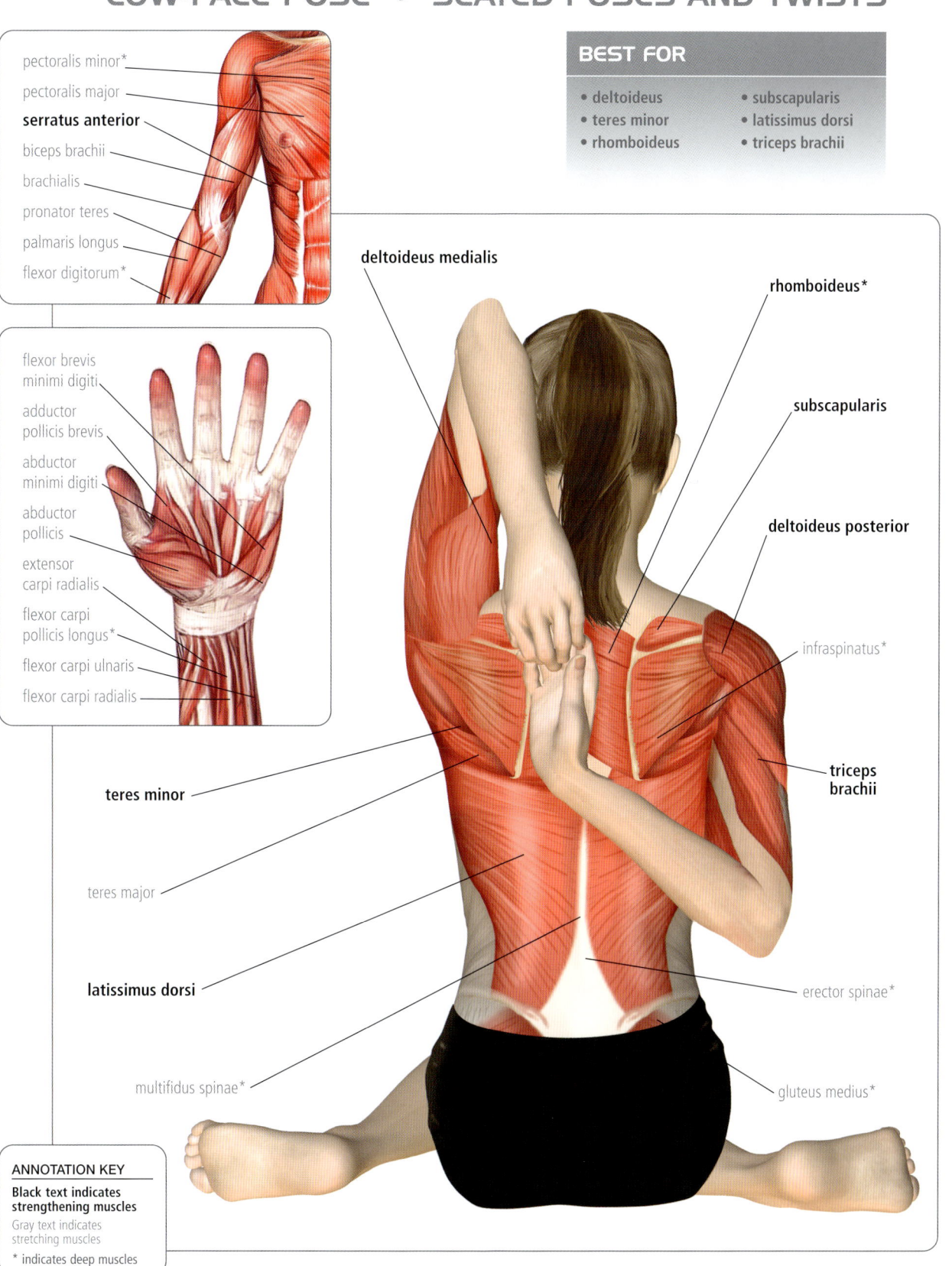

BEST FOR

- deltoideus
- teres minor
- rhomboideus
- subscapularis
- latissimus dorsi
- triceps brachii

pectoralis minor*
pectoralis major
serratus anterior
biceps brachii
brachialis
pronator teres
palmaris longus
flexor digitorum*

flexor brevis minimi digiti
adductor pollicis brevis
abductor minimi digiti
abductor pollicis
extensor carpi radialis
flexor carpi pollicis longus*
flexor carpi ulnaris
flexor carpi radialis

deltoideus medialis
rhomboideus*
subscapularis
deltoideus posterior
infraspinatus*
triceps brachii
teres minor
teres major
latissimus dorsi
erector spinae*
multifidus spinae*
gluteus medius*

ANNOTATION KEY
Black text indicates strengthening muscles
Gray text indicates stretching muscles
* indicates deep muscles

SEATED POSES AND TWISTS

HALF LOTUS POSE
(ARDHA PADMASANA)

① Sit in Staff Pose (pages 98-99). Lift up through your spine.

② Bend your right knee and open it to the side. Allow your hip to open, and lower your right thigh to the floor.

BEST FOR
- rectus abdominis
- transversus abdominis
- tibialis anterior
- sartorius
- rectus femoris

AVOID
- Overextending your outer ankle.

③ Lean forward slightly, and grab your right shin with your hands. Place your right foot on top of your left thigh, with your heel nestled against your groin. Make sure that the rotation is coming from your hips.

④ Carefully position your left foot beneath your right thigh. Draw your knees closer together. Push into the floor with your groins, as you keep both sit bones on the floor.

⑤ Extend upward through your spine, and place the backs of your hands on each knee, forming an "O" with your index finger and your thumb.

⑥ Hold for 5 seconds to 1 minute. Repeat with your left leg on top.

PRONUNCIATION & MEANING
- Ardha Padmasana (are-dah pod-MAHS-anna)
- *ardha* = half; *padma* = lotus

BENEFITS
- Stretches hips, thighs, and knees, and ankles
- Works the abdominals to stimulate digestion

CONTRA-INDICATIONS & CAUTIONS
- Knee injury

DO IT RIGHT
- Hold the position for the same length of time on both sides.

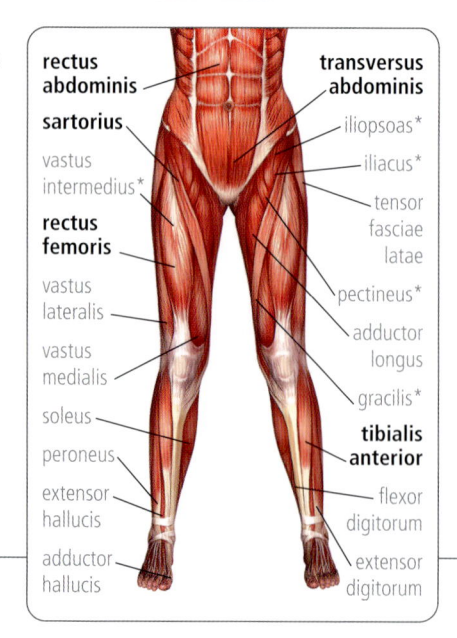

Muscles labeled: rectus abdominis, transversus abdominis, sartorius, iliopsoas*, vastus intermedius*, iliacus*, rectus femoris, tensor fasciae latae, vastus lateralis, pectineus*, vastus medialis, adductor longus, soleus, gracilis*, peroneus, tibialis anterior, extensor hallucis, flexor digitorum, adductor hallucis, extensor digitorum

106

FULL LOTUS POSE
(PADMASANA)

SEATED POSES AND TWISTS

① Begin in Half Lotus ((pages 106)), with your right leg on top of your left.

② Extend your left leg from below your right hip. With the knee bent, grab your left shin with your hands. Lean back slightly as you bring your left shin on top of your right, and place your left foot on top of your right thigh. Nestle your left heel against your right groin.

③ Push into the floor with your groins and rotate your hips open to press your thighs to the floor. Be sure to keep both sit bones on the floor.

④ Extend upward through your spine and place the backs of your hands on each knee, forming an "O" with your index finger and your thumb.

⑤ Hold for 5 seconds to 1 minute. Repeat with your right leg on top.

BEST FOR
- rectus abdominis
- transversus abdominis
- tibialis anterior

DO IT RIGHT
- If you have trouble keeping your spine in a straight, neutral position, place a folded blanked beneath your hips to elevate your hips above your knees.

AVOID
- Straining your knees. If you experience discomfort in this position, practice the Half Lotus Pose (Ardha Padmasana, see page 108) or the Bound Angle Pose (Baddha Konasana, see page 104) until your hips are flexible enough to practice the Full Lotus.

Annotations:
- obliquus externus
- obliquus internus*
- rectus abdominis
- transversus abdominis*
- tibialis anterior

ANNOTATION KEY
Black text indicates strengthening muscles
Gray text indicates stretching muscles
* indicates deep muscles

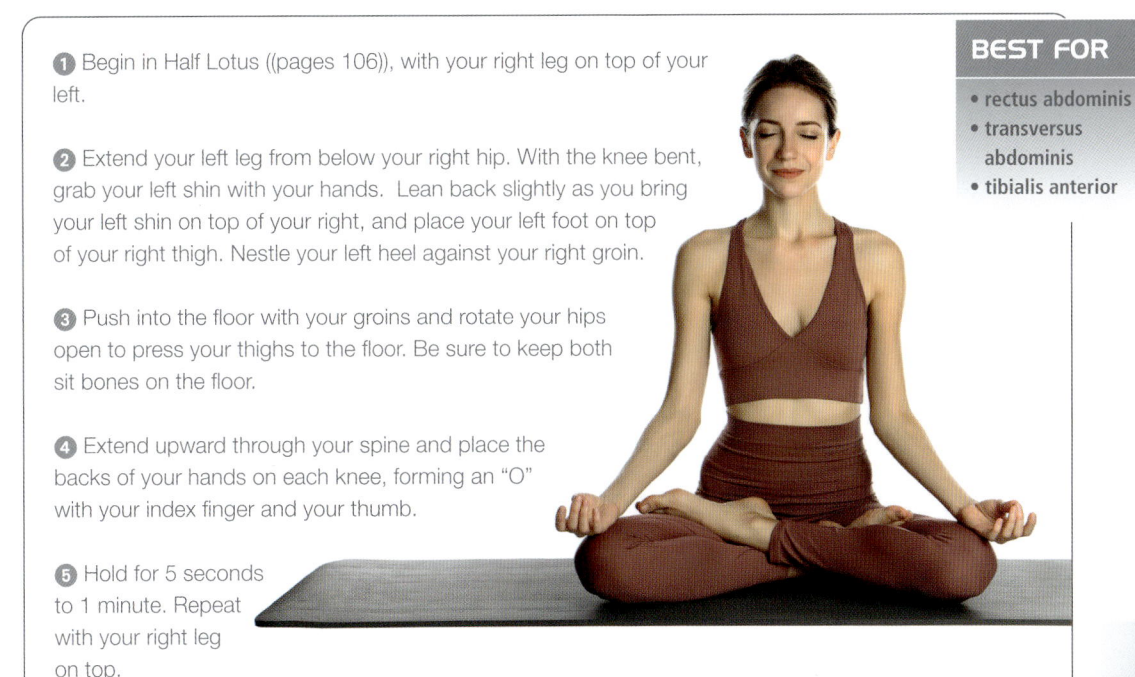

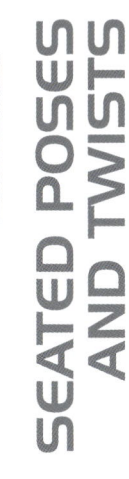

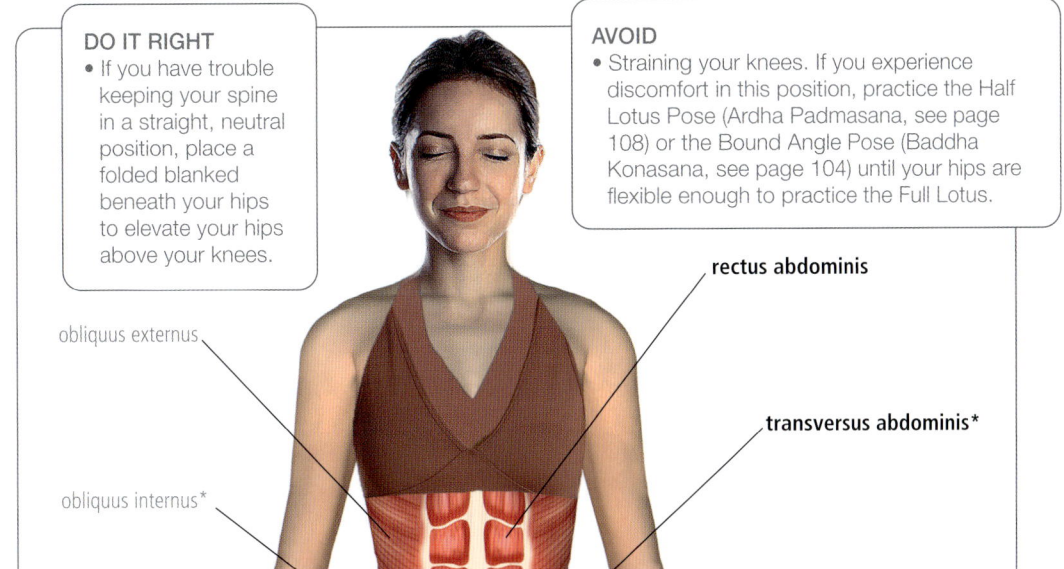

PRONUNCIATION & MEANING
- Padmasana (pod-MAHS-anna)
- padma = lotus

LEVEL
- Advanced

BENEFITS
- Stretches hips, thighs, and knees, and ankles
- Stimulates digestion
- Calms the brain for meditation

CONTRA-INDICATIONS & CAUTIONS
- Knee injury
- Hip injury
- Ankle injury

107

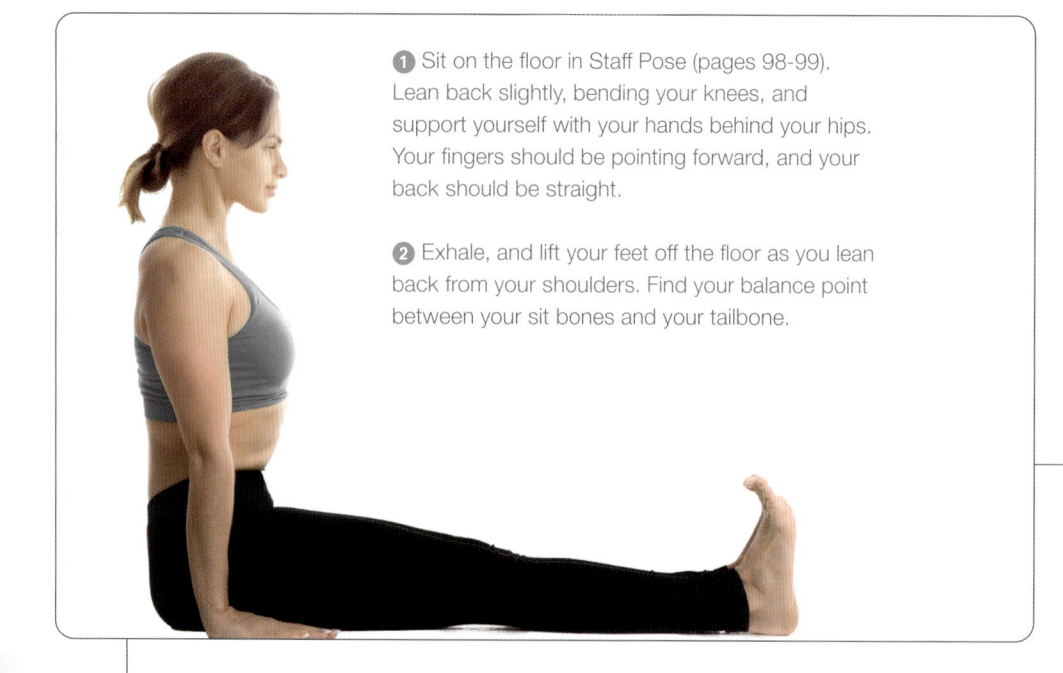

SEATED POSES AND TWISTS

BOAT POSE
(PARIPURNA NAVASANA)

① Sit on the floor in Staff Pose (pages 98-99). Lean back slightly, bending your knees, and support yourself with your hands behind your hips. Your fingers should be pointing forward, and your back should be straight.

② Exhale, and lift your feet off the floor as you lean back from your shoulders. Find your balance point between your sit bones and your tailbone.

③ Slowly straighten your legs in front of you so that they form a 45-degree angle with your torso. Point your toes. Lift your arms to your sides, parallel to the floor.

④ Pull your abdominals in toward your spine as they work to keep your balance. Stretch your arms forward through your fingertips, and elongate the back of your neck.

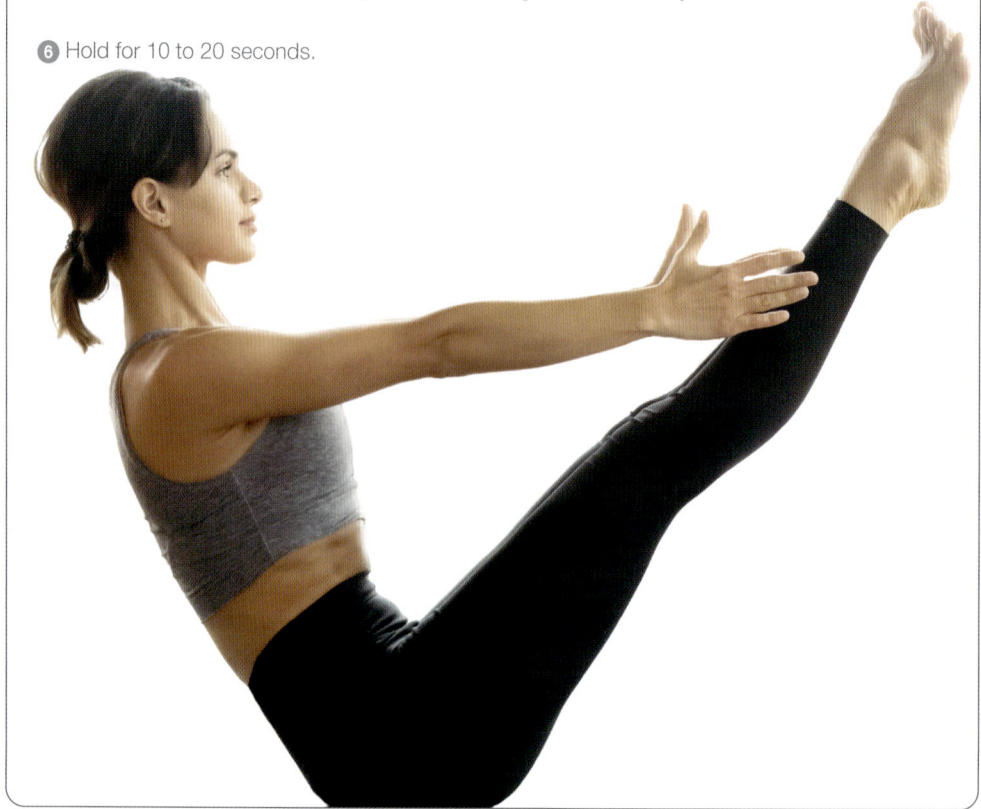

⑤ Hold for 10 to 20 seconds.

PRONUNCIATION & MEANING
- Paripurna Navasana (par-ee-POOR-nah nah-VAHS-anna)
- *paripurna* = full, entire, complete; *nava* = boat

BENEFITS
- Strengthens abdominals, hip flexors, spine, and thighs
- Stretches hamstrings
- Stimulates digestion
- Alleviates thyroid problems

CONTRA-INDICATIONS & CAUTIONS
- Neck injury
- Headache
- Lower back pain

108

BOAT POSE • SEATED POSES AND TWISTS

BEST FOR
- rectus abdominis
- obliquus internus
- obliquus externus
- iliopsoas
- transversus abdominis
- vastus intermedius
- rectus femoris
- iliacus
- erector spinae

DO IT RIGHT
- Keep your neck elongated and relaxed, minimizing the tension in your upper spine.
- If you are unable to straighten your legs, balance with your knees bent.

AVOID
- Rounding your spine, causing you to sink into your lower back.

sternocleidomastoideus
brachialis
triceps brachii
rectus abdominis
rectus femoris
transversus abdominis*
vastus lateralis
biceps femoris
vastus intermedius*

obliquus externus
obliquus internus*
erector spinae*
iliopsoas*
iliacus*

ANNOTATION KEY
Black text indicates strengthening muscles
Gray text indicates stretching muscles
* indicates deep muscles

109

BHARADVAJA'S TWIST
(BHARADVAJASANA I)

SEATED POSES AND TWISTS

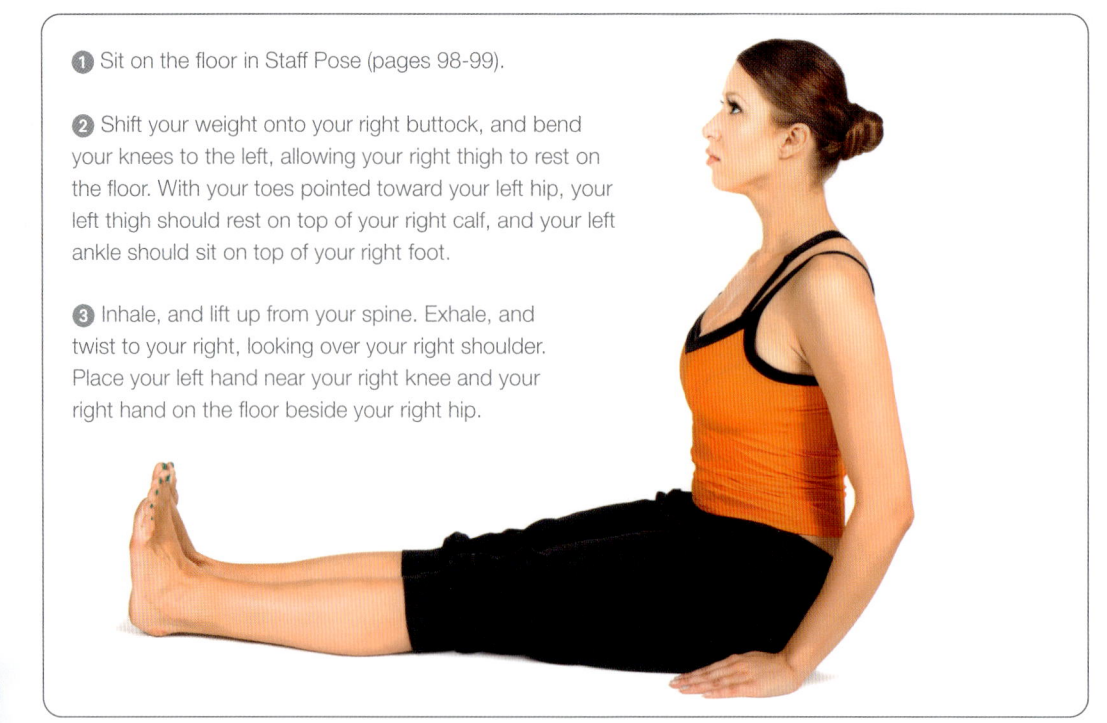

❶ Sit on the floor in Staff Pose (pages 98-99).

❷ Shift your weight onto your right buttock, and bend your knees to the left, allowing your right thigh to rest on the floor. With your toes pointed toward your left hip, your left thigh should rest on top of your right calf, and your left ankle should sit on top of your right foot.

❸ Inhale, and lift up from your spine. Exhale, and twist to your right, looking over your right shoulder. Place your left hand near your right knee and your right hand on the floor beside your right hip.

❹ With each exhale, deepen the twist while keeping your torso upright and your shoulders pressed back. If possible, bend your right elbow, and reach across your back. Hook your right hand beneath the bend in your left elbow.

❺ Hold for 30 seconds to 1 minute. Repeat on the opposite side.

PRONUNCIATION & MEANING
- Bharadvajasana I (bah-ROD-va-JAHS-anna)
- Bharadvaja = the name of a great Hindu sage

BENEFITS
- Stretches spine, shoulders, and hips
- Stimulates digestion
- Relieves stress

CONTRA-INDICATIONS & CAUTIONS
- Low or high blood pressure
- Diarrhea

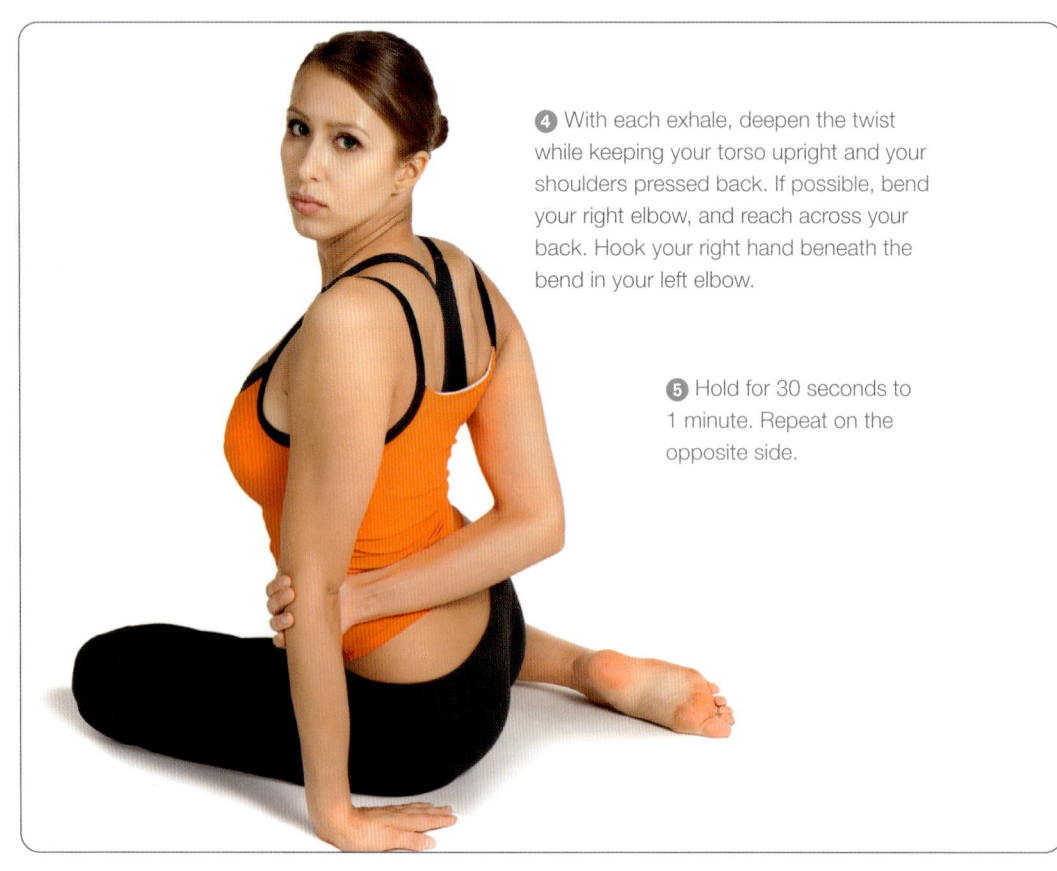

BHARADVAJA'S TWIST • SEATED POSES AND TWISTS

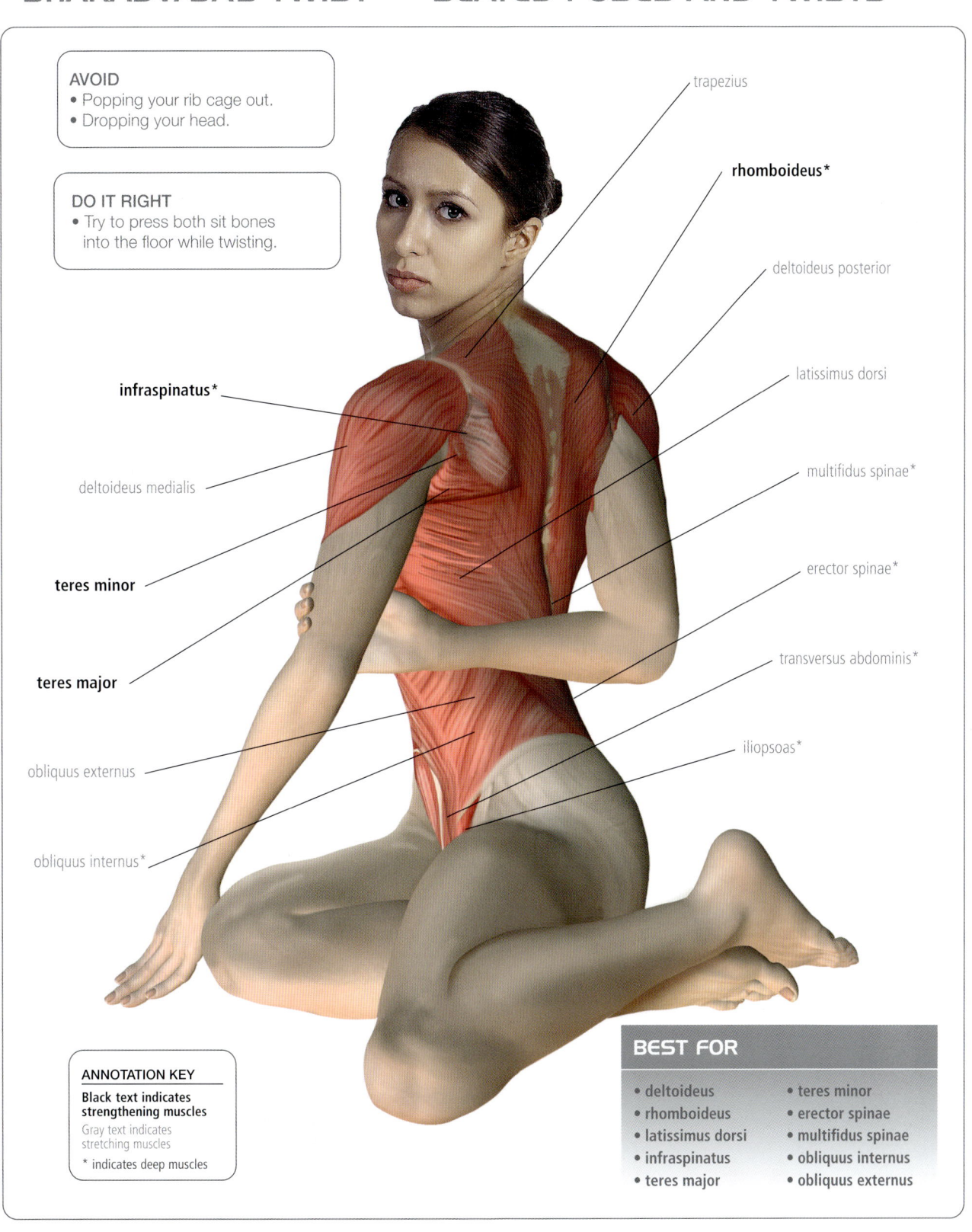

AVOID
- Popping your rib cage out.
- Dropping your head.

DO IT RIGHT
- Try to press both sit bones into the floor while twisting.

trapezius

rhomboideus*

deltoideus posterior

infraspinatus*

latissimus dorsi

deltoideus medialis

multifidus spinae*

teres minor

erector spinae*

teres major

transversus abdominis*

iliopsoas*

obliquus externus

obliquus internus*

ANNOTATION KEY
Black text indicates strengthening muscles
Gray text indicates stretching muscles
* indicates deep muscles

BEST FOR
- deltoideus
- rhomboideus
- latissimus dorsi
- infraspinatus
- teres major
- teres minor
- erector spinae
- multifidus spinae
- obliquus internus
- obliquus externus

MARICHI'S POSE
(MARICHYASANA)

SEATED POSES AND TWISTS

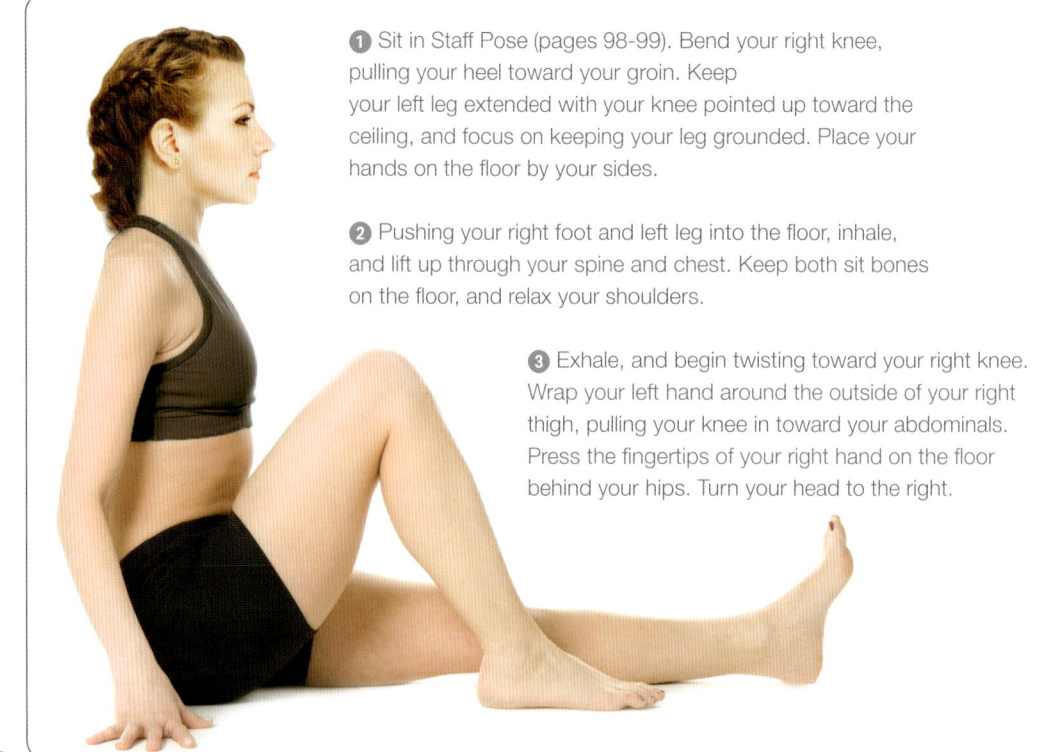

① Sit in Staff Pose (pages 98-99). Bend your right knee, pulling your heel toward your groin. Keep your left leg extended with your knee pointed up toward the ceiling, and focus on keeping your leg grounded. Place your hands on the floor by your sides.

② Pushing your right foot and left leg into the floor, inhale, and lift up through your spine and chest. Keep both sit bones on the floor, and relax your shoulders.

③ Exhale, and begin twisting toward your right knee. Wrap your left hand around the outside of your right thigh, pulling your knee in toward your abdominals. Press the fingertips of your right hand on the floor behind your hips. Turn your head to the right.

④ Twist deeper with each exhalation. If possible, place your left elbow on the outside of your right knee. Lean back slightly, leading with your upper torso. This will help you twist your entire spine.

⑤ Hold for 30 seconds to 1 minute. Gently untwist as you exhale, and repeat with your left leg bent and your right elbow over your left knee.

PRONUNCIATION & MEANING
- Marichyasana III (mar-ee-chee-AHS-anna)
- *marichi* = ray of light; or name of the Hindu seer credited with intuiting the divine law of the universe, or *dharma*
- Also called the Sage's Pose

BENEFITS
- Stimulates digestion
- Strengthens and stretches spine
- Removes toxins from internal organs

CONTRA-INDICATIONS & CAUTIONS
- High or low blood pressure
- Back injury

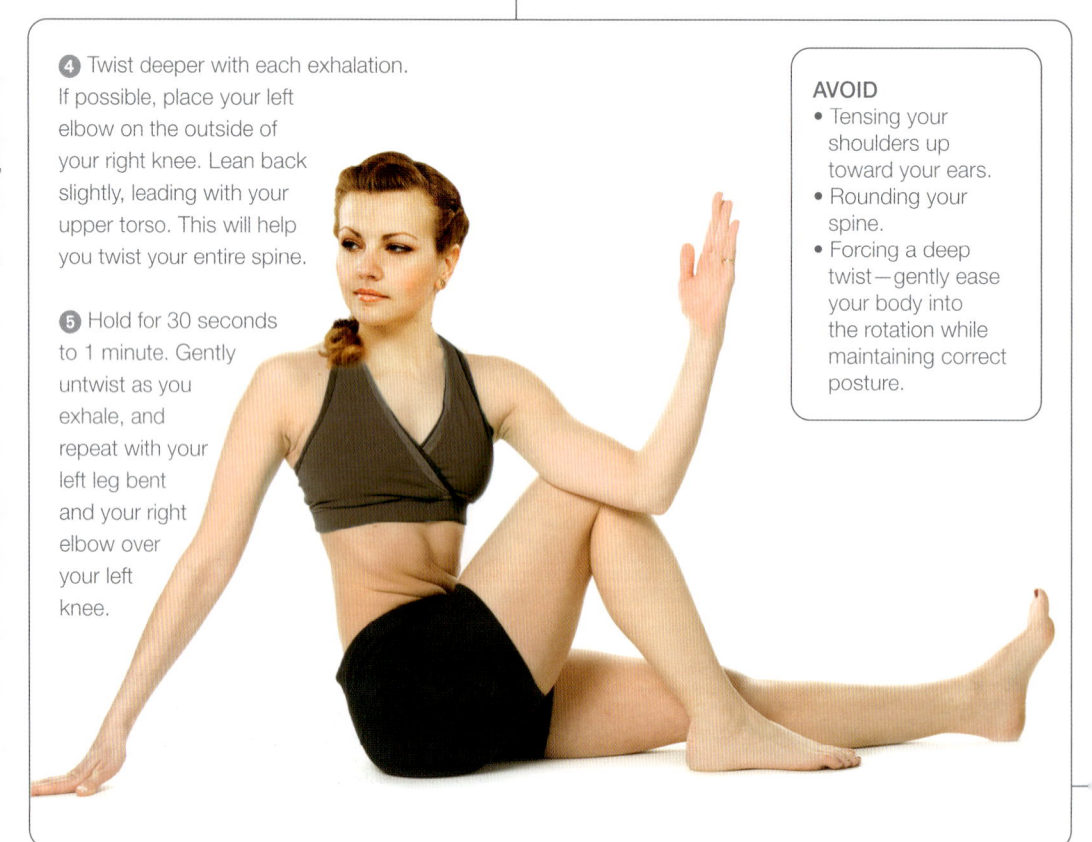

AVOID
- Tensing your shoulders up toward your ears.
- Rounding your spine.
- Forcing a deep twist—gently ease your body into the rotation while maintaining correct posture.

MARICHI'S POSE • SEATED POSES AND TWISTS

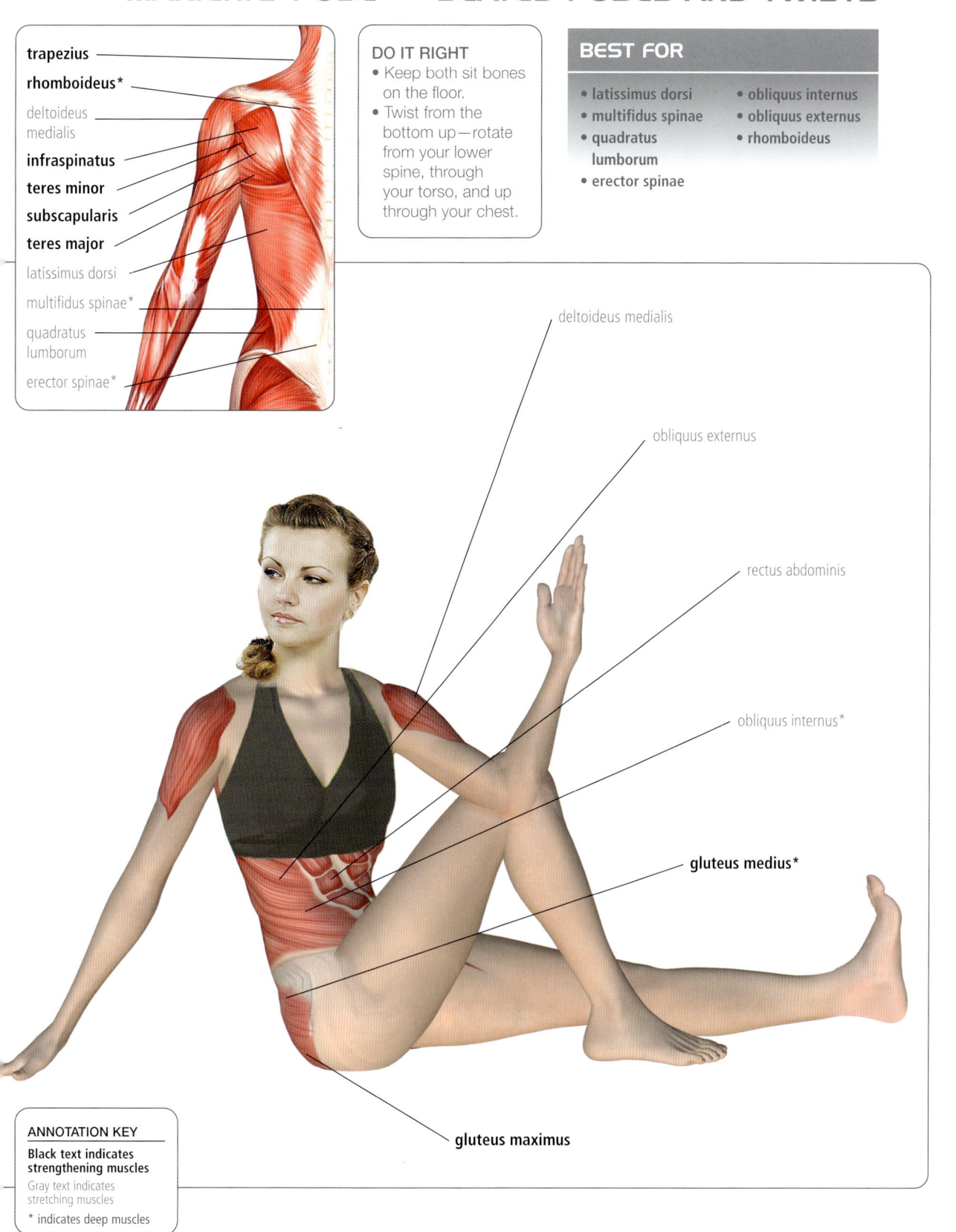

- **trapezius**
- **rhomboideus***
- deltoideus medialis
- **infraspinatus**
- **teres minor**
- **subscapularis**
- **teres major**
- latissimus dorsi
- multifidus spinae*
- quadratus lumborum
- erector spinae*

DO IT RIGHT
- Keep both sit bones on the floor.
- Twist from the bottom up—rotate from your lower spine, through your torso, and up through your chest.

BEST FOR
- latissimus dorsi
- multifidus spinae
- quadratus lumborum
- erector spinae
- obliquus internus
- obliquus externus
- rhomboideus

- deltoideus medialis
- obliquus externus
- rectus abdominis
- obliquus internus*
- **gluteus medius***
- **gluteus maximus**

ANNOTATION KEY
Black text indicates strengthening muscles
Gray text indicates stretching muscles
* indicates deep muscles

HALF LORD OF THE FISHES
(ARDHA MATSYENDRASANA)

SEATED POSES AND TWISTS

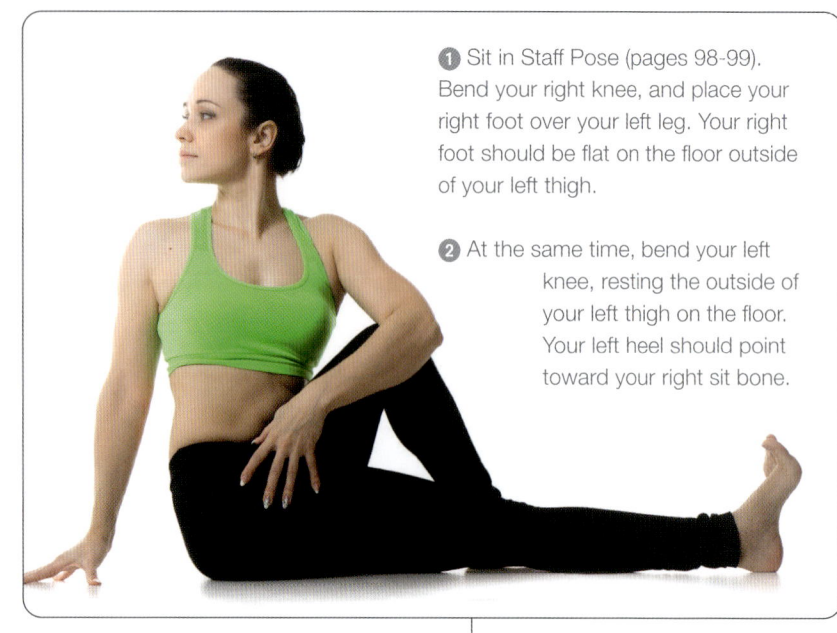

① Sit in Staff Pose (pages 98-99). Bend your right knee, and place your right foot over your left leg. Your right foot should be flat on the floor outside of your left thigh.

② At the same time, bend your left knee, resting the outside of your left thigh on the floor. Your left heel should point toward your right sit bone.

③ Inhale, and lift up through your spine and chest while keeping your shoulders relaxed. Exhale, and begin twisting to your right. Place your left elbow on the outside of your right knee. Press your right hand on the floor behind your hips. Turn your head to the right.

④ Twist deeper with each exhalation. Lean back slightly, leading with your upper torso. Using your left arm, pull your right thigh closer toward your abdominals. Continue to lengthen your spine from the bottom up, pulling your tailbone down toward the floor. Use your right hand to guide your rotation deeper.

⑤ Hold for 30 seconds to 1 minute. Gently untwist as you exhale, and repeat with your left leg over your right thigh.

AVOID
- Tensing your shoulders up toward your ears.
- Rounding your spine.
- Lifting the foot of your raised leg off the ground.

DO IT RIGHT
- Try to pull the thigh of your raised leg and your torso as close together as possible without collapsing your spine.
- Pull your back shoulder toward the back wall as you twist through your entire spine.

PRONUNCIATION & MEANING
- Ardha Matsyendrasana (ARD-ha MOTS-yen-DRAHS-anna)
- *ardha* = half; *matsya* = fish; *indra* = ruler, lord

BENEFITS
- Stimulates digestion
- Stretches hips, spine, and shoulders
- Relieves backache and menstrual discomfort

CONTRA-INDICATIONS & CAUTIONS
- Back injury

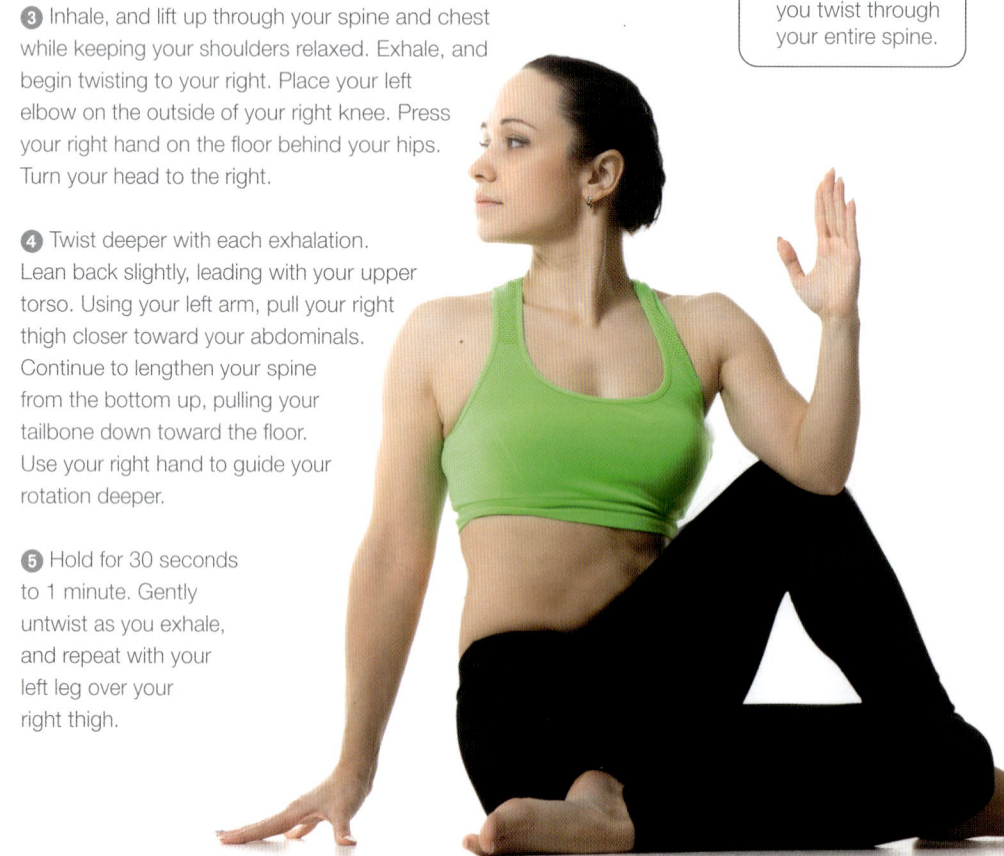

HALF LORD OF THE FISHES • SEATED POSES AND TWISTS

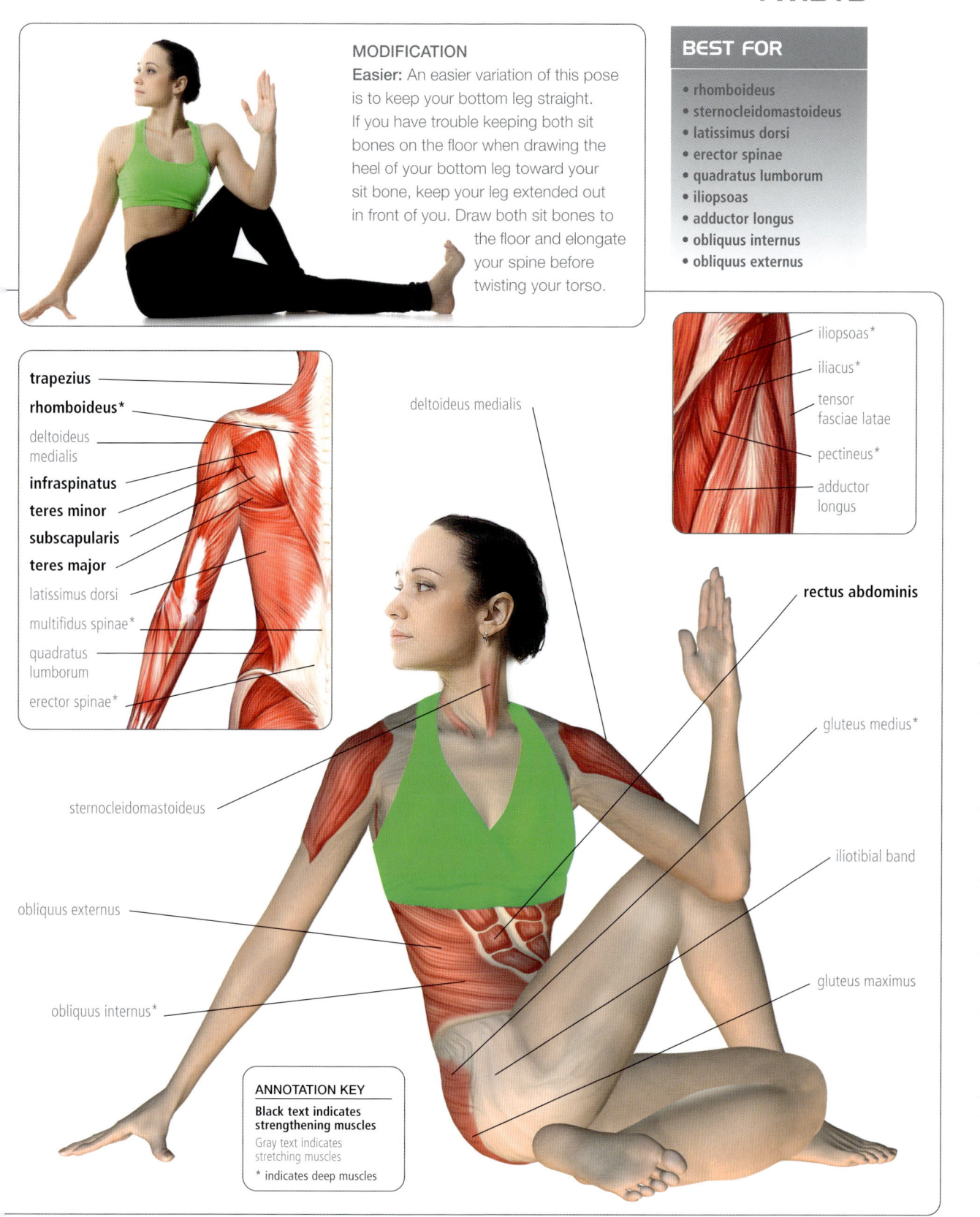

MODIFICATION
Easier: An easier variation of this pose is to keep your bottom leg straight. If you have trouble keeping both sit bones on the floor when drawing the heel of your bottom leg toward your sit bone, keep your leg extended out in front of you. Draw both sit bones to the floor and elongate your spine before twisting your torso.

BEST FOR
- rhomboideus
- sternocleidomastoideus
- latissimus dorsi
- erector spinae
- quadratus lumborum
- iliopsoas
- adductor longus
- obliquus internus
- obliquus externus

trapezius
rhomboideus*
deltoideus medialis
infraspinatus
teres minor
subscapularis
teres major
latissimus dorsi
multifidus spinae*
quadratus lumborum
erector spinae*

sternocleidomastoideus

obliquus externus

obliquus internus*

deltoideus medialis

iliopsoas*
iliacus*
tensor fasciae latae
pectineus*
adductor longus

rectus abdominis
gluteus medius*
iliotibial band
gluteus maximus

ANNOTATION KEY
Black text indicates strengthening muscles
Gray text indicates stretching muscles
* indicates deep muscles

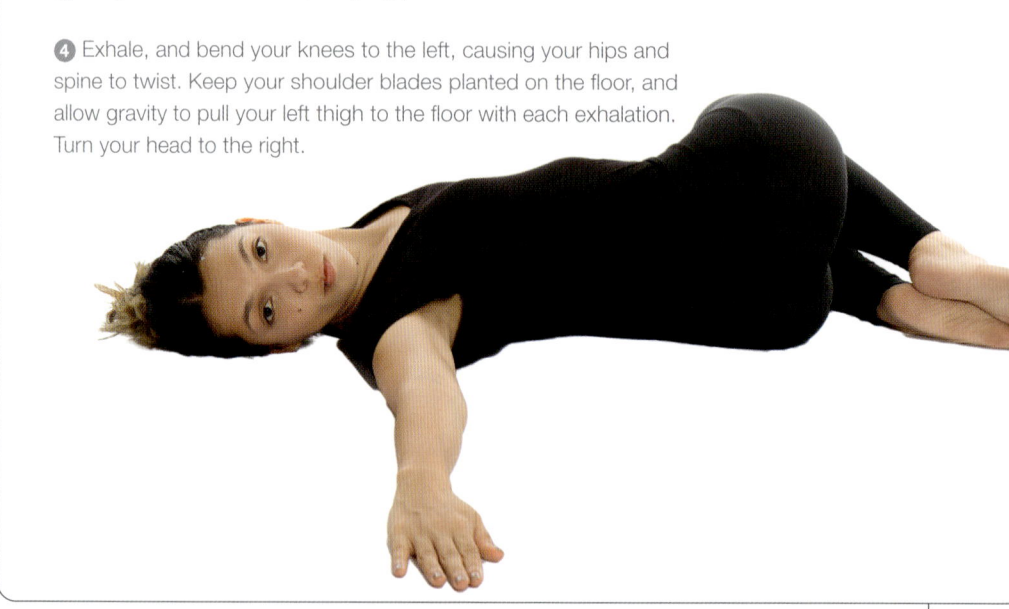

RECLINING TWIST

SEATED POSES AND TWISTS

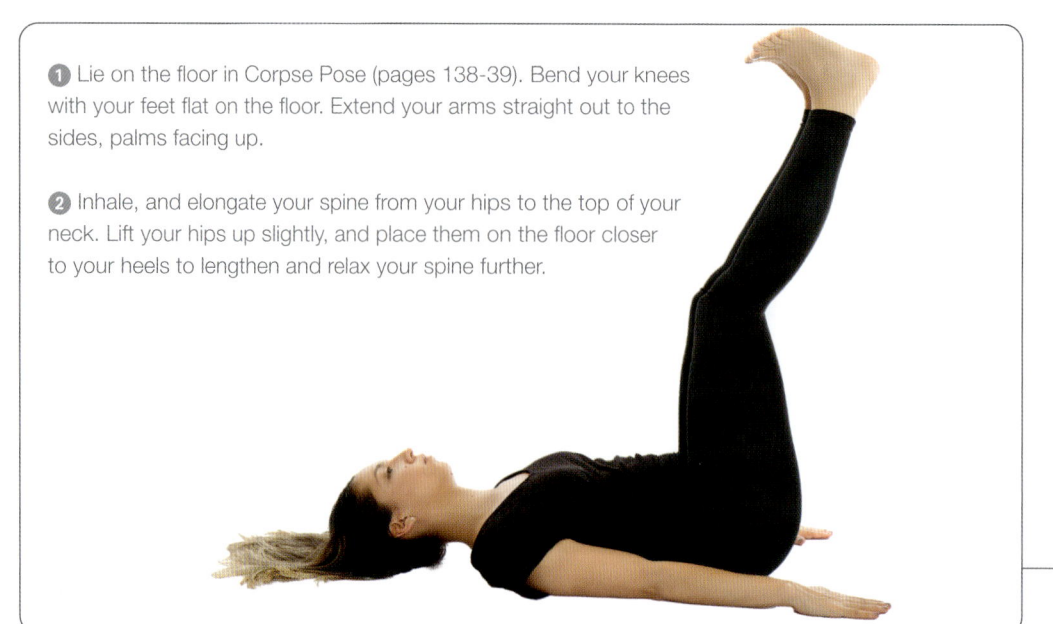

① Lie on the floor in Corpse Pose (pages 138-39). Bend your knees with your feet flat on the floor. Extend your arms straight out to the sides, palms facing up.

② Inhale, and elongate your spine from your hips to the top of your neck. Lift your hips up slightly, and place them on the floor closer to your heels to lengthen and relax your spine further.

PRONUNCIATION & MEANING
- There is no agreed-upon Sanskrit name for this pose.

BENEFITS
- Releases spinal tension
- Loosens hips
- Tones abdominals

CONTRA-INDICATIONS & CAUTIONS
- Shoulder issues

③ Lift your feet off the floor, keeping your knees bent.

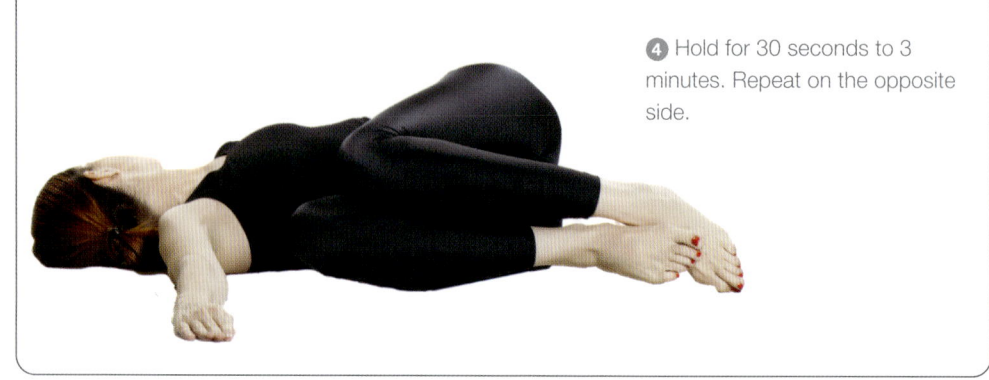

④ Exhale, and bend your knees to the left, causing your hips and spine to twist. Keep your shoulder blades planted on the floor, and allow gravity to pull your left thigh to the floor with each exhalation. Turn your head to the right.

④ Hold for 30 seconds to 3 minutes. Repeat on the opposite side.

RECLINING TWIST • SEATED POSES AND TWISTS

DO IT RIGHT
- Keep your chest open.
- If you struggle to bring your knees to the floor, place a folded blanket beneath them.
- Experiment with turning your head to both sides. This will change the sensation of the stretch.
- Relax—don't push—into the stretch.

AVOID
- Tensing your shoulders up to your ears.
- Allowing your shoulder blades to lift off the floor. If your shoulder comes up, bend the arm of the lifted shoulder, and place your hand beneath your ribs for support.

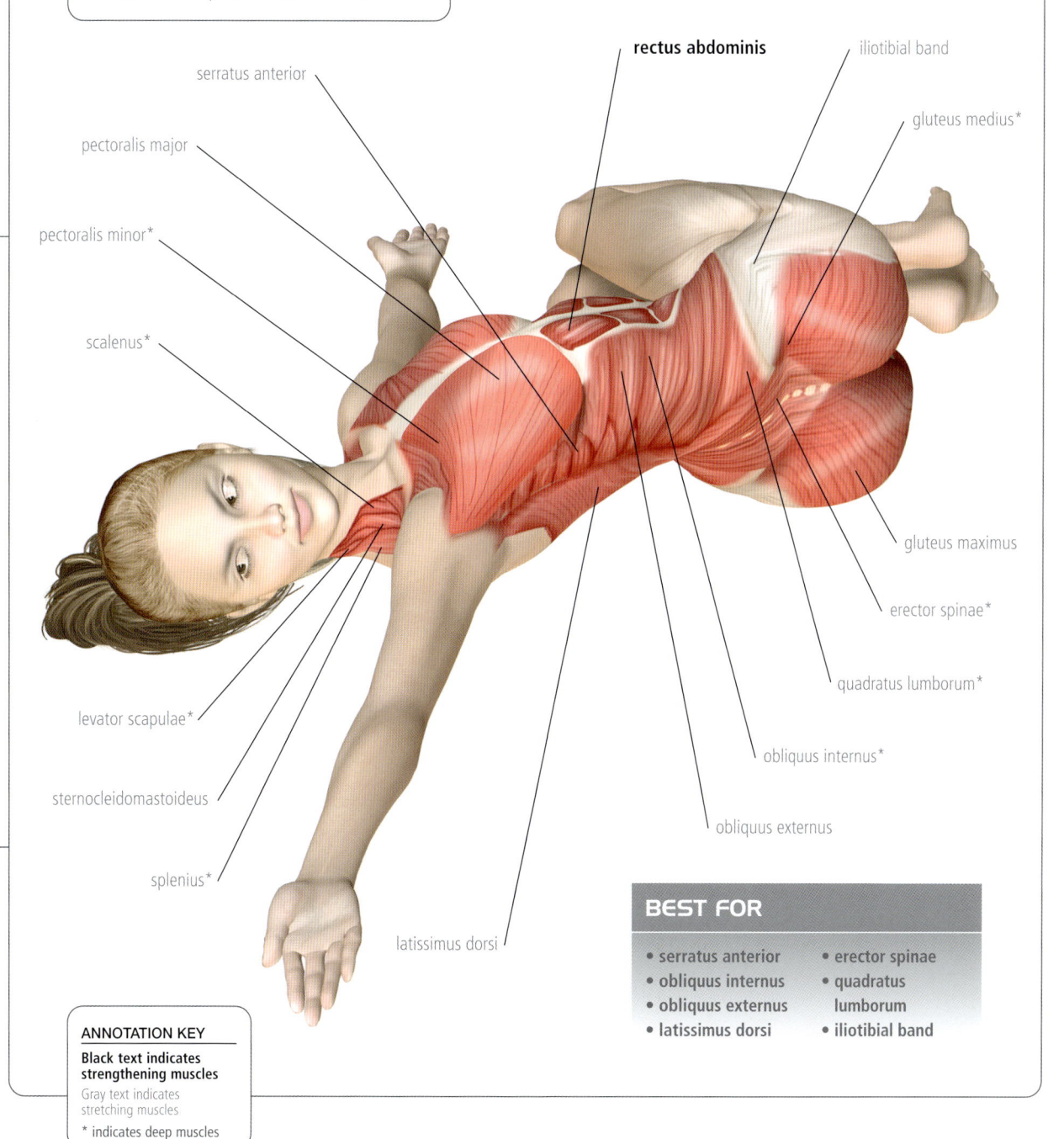

serratus anterior
pectoralis major
pectoralis minor*
scalenus*
levator scapulae*
sternocleidomastoideus
splenius*
latissimus dorsi

rectus abdominis
iliotibial band
gluteus medius*
gluteus maximus
erector spinae*
quadratus lumborum*
obliquus internus*
obliquus externus

BEST FOR
- serratus anterior
- obliquus internus
- obliquus externus
- latissimus dorsi
- erector spinae
- quadratus lumborum
- iliotibial band

ANNOTATION KEY
Black text indicates strengthening muscles
Gray text indicates stretching muscles
* indicates deep muscles

117

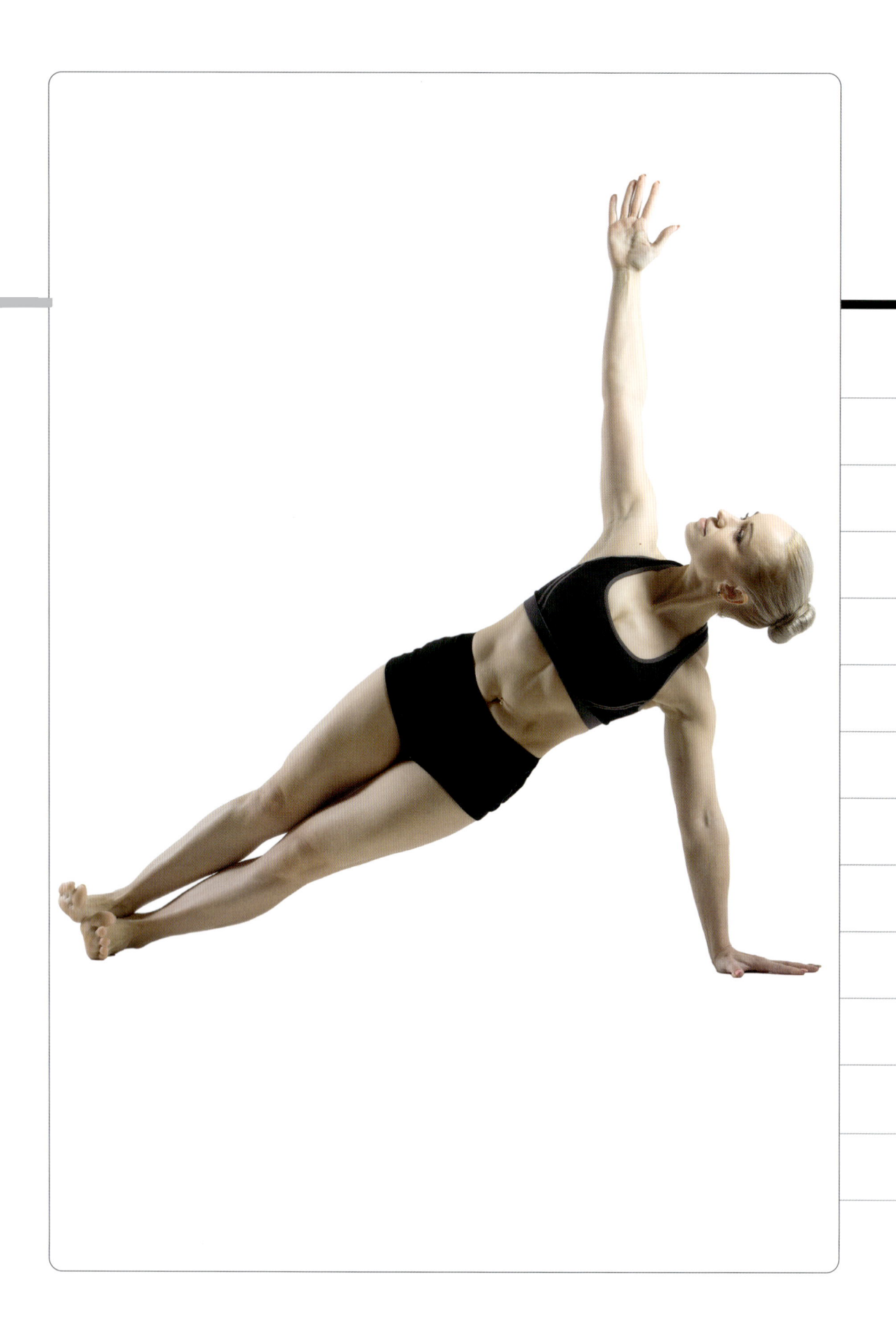

ARM SUPPORTS & INVERSIONS

Bone density and upper body strength both tend to decline as you age. You can help counteract the deterioration of bone and muscle in your arms by practicing arm supports; these postures can help prevent the development of osteoporosis while strengthening your arms, shoulders, chest, and abdominals. A certain amount of flexibility is necessary for arm supports, particularly in the spine and hips.

Inversions reverse the effects of gravity on your body by moving your head below your heart. The cardiovascular, lymphatic, nervous, and endocrine systems all benefit from inversions because they improve blood flow and help to develop healthier tissues. When starting out with inversions, focus on holding the positions for brief periods of time while being gentle on your neck and spine.

UPWARD PLANK POSE
(PURVOTTANASANA)

ARM SUPPORTS & INVERSIONS

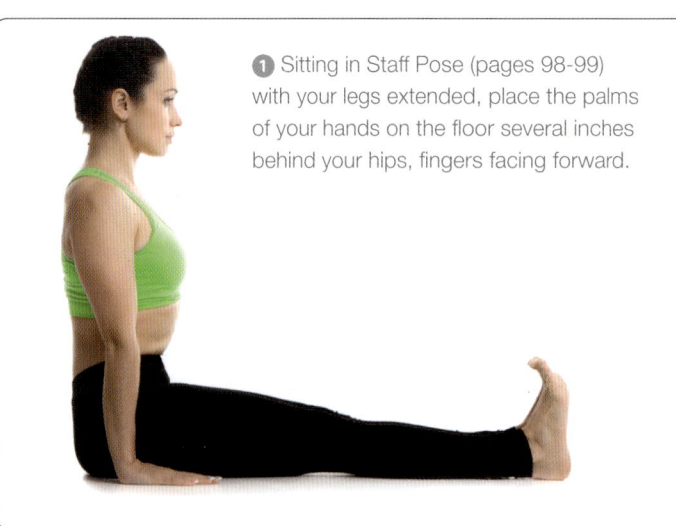

❶ Sitting in Staff Pose (pages 98-99) with your legs extended, place the palms of your hands on the floor several inches behind your hips, fingers facing forward.

DO IT RIGHT
- Use your hamstrings and shoulders to open your hips and chest, rather than overextend your back. If your hamstrings are too weak, keep your legs bent while holding the lift in your hips.
- Breathe steadily, using the breath to deepen the extension in your upper back.

❷ Draw your knees toward your chest. Place your feet on the floor with your heels about 12 inches away from your buttocks, and turn your big toes slightly inward.

❸ Exhale, pressing down with your hands and feet and lifting your hips until your back and thighs are parallel to the floor. Your shoulders should be directly above your wrists.

PRONUNCIATION & MEANING
- Purvottanasana (POOR-vo-tan-AHS-ahna)
- *purva* = front, east; *ut* = intense; *tan* = extend, stretch

BENEFITS
- Strengthens the spine, arms, and hamstrings
- Extends the hips and chest

CONTRA-INDICATIONS & CAUTIONS
- Neck injury
- Wrist injury

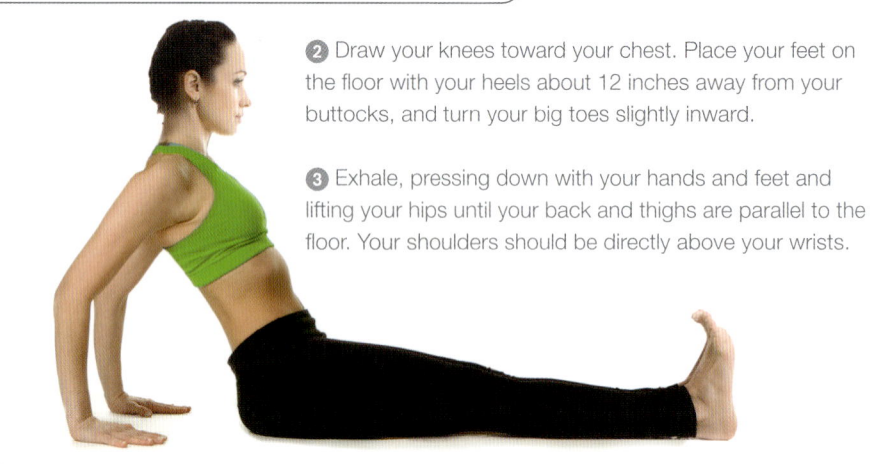

❹ Without lowering your hips, straighten your legs one at a time.

❺ Lifting your chest and bringing your shoulder blades together, push your hips higher, creating a slight arch in your back. Do not squeeze your buttocks to create the lift.

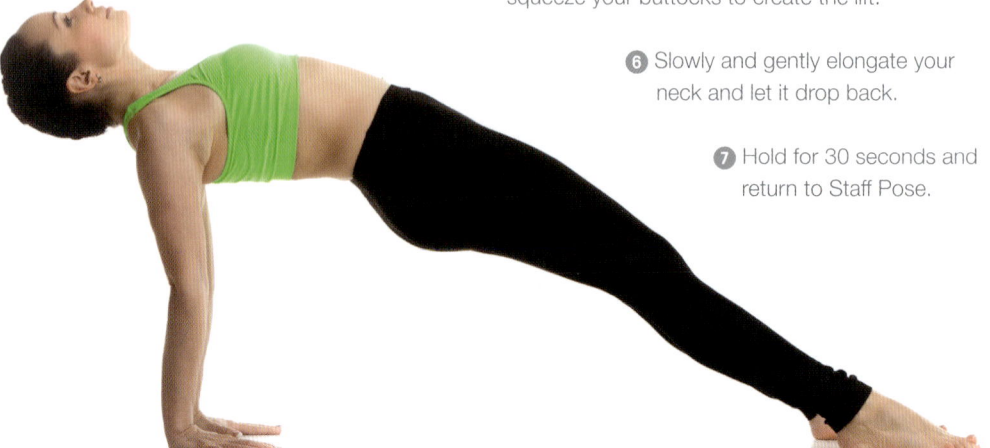

❻ Slowly and gently elongate your neck and let it drop back.

❼ Hold for 30 seconds and return to Staff Pose.

120

UPWARD PLANK POSE • ARM SUPPORTS & INVERSIONS

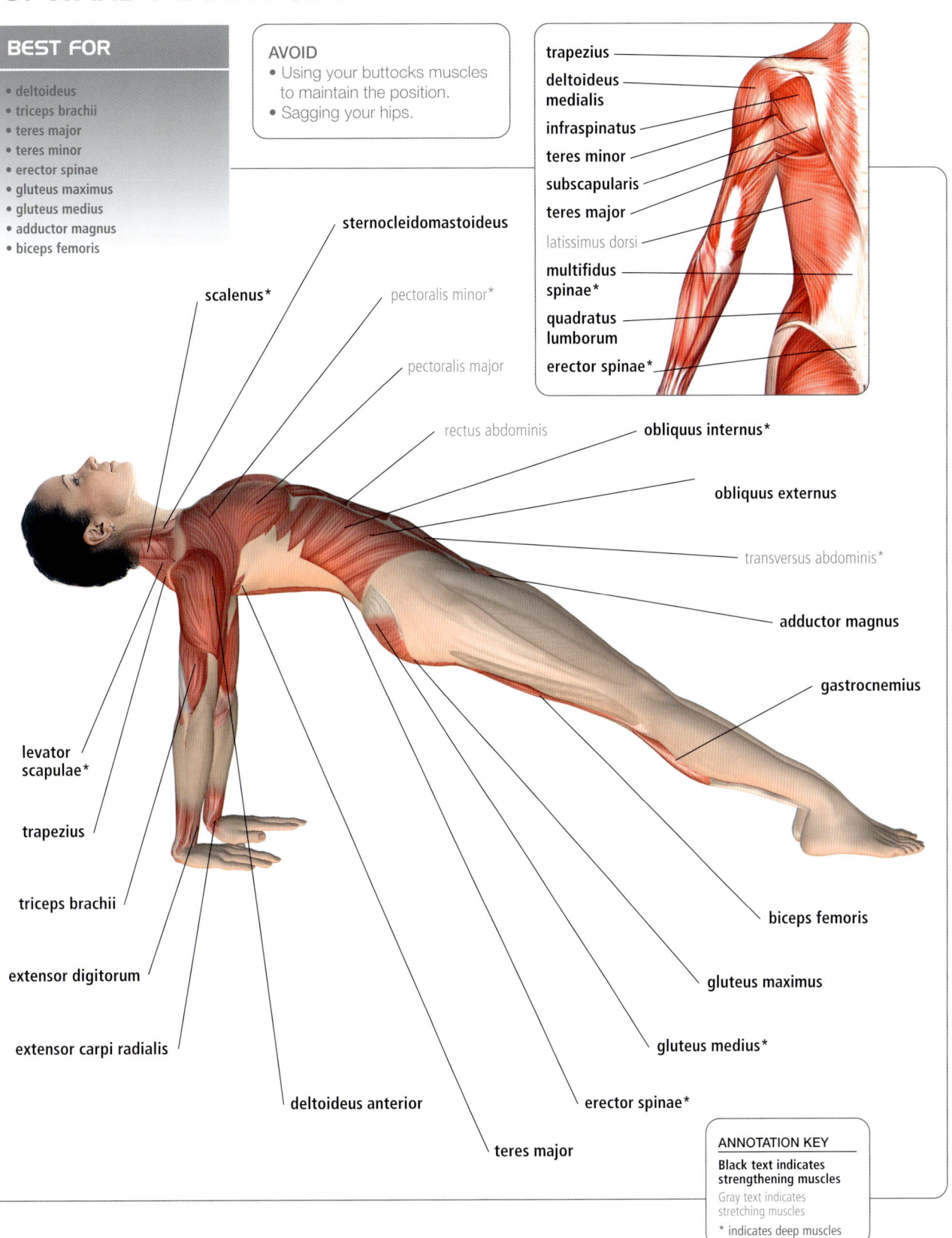

BEST FOR
- deltoideus
- triceps brachii
- teres major
- teres minor
- erector spinae
- gluteus maximus
- gluteus medius
- adductor magnus
- biceps femoris

AVOID
- Using your buttocks muscles to maintain the position.
- Sagging your hips.

trapezius
deltoideus medialis
infraspinatus
teres minor
subscapularis
teres major
latissimus dorsi
multifidus spinae*
quadratus lumborum
erector spinae*

sternocleidomastoideus
scalenus*
pectoralis minor*
pectoralis major
rectus abdominis
obliquus internus*
obliquus externus
transversus abdominis*
adductor magnus
gastrocnemius

levator scapulae*
trapezius
triceps brachii
extensor digitorum
extensor carpi radialis
deltoideus anterior
teres major
erector spinae*
gluteus medius*
gluteus maximus
biceps femoris

ANNOTATION KEY

Black text indicates strengthening muscles
Gray text indicates stretching muscles
* indicates deep muscles

PLANK POSE TO

ARM SUPPORTS & INVERSIONS

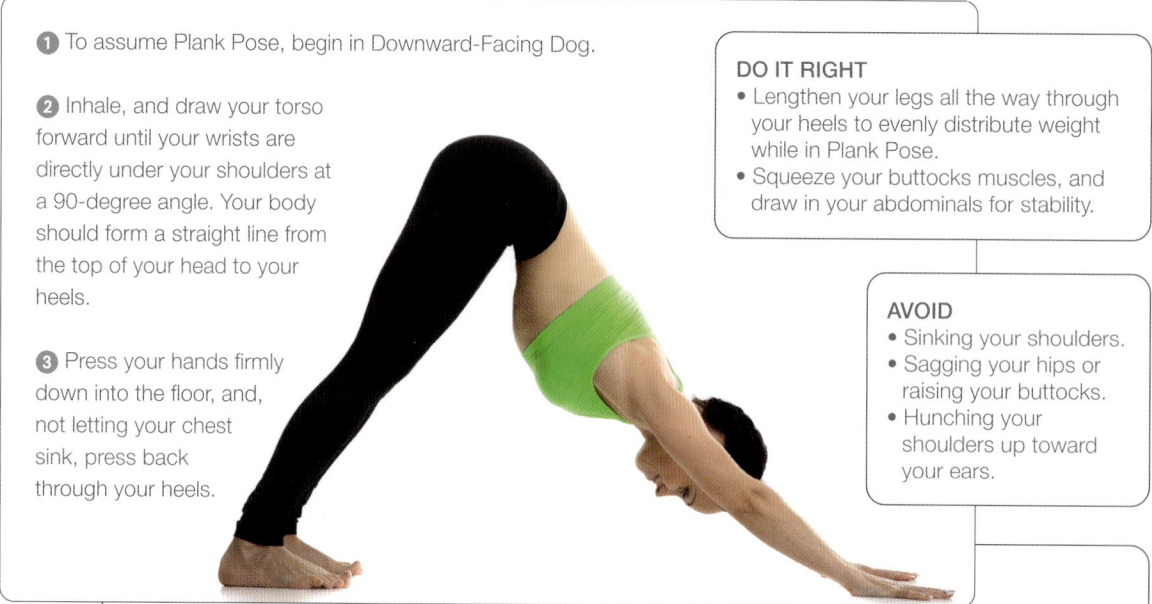

① To assume Plank Pose, begin in Downward-Facing Dog.

② Inhale, and draw your torso forward until your wrists are directly under your shoulders at a 90-degree angle. Your body should form a straight line from the top of your head to your heels.

③ Press your hands firmly down into the floor, and, not letting your chest sink, press back through your heels.

DO IT RIGHT
- Lengthen your legs all the way through your heels to evenly distribute weight while in Plank Pose.
- Squeeze your buttocks muscles, and draw in your abdominals for stability.

AVOID
- Sinking your shoulders.
- Sagging your hips or raising your buttocks.
- Hunching your shoulders up toward your ears.

PRONUNCIATION & MEANING
- There is no agreed-upon Sanskrit name for the Plank Pose.
- Chaturanga Dandasana (chaht-tour-ANG-ah don-DAHS-anna)
- *chatur* = four; *anga* = limb; *danda* = staff, stick

BENEFITS
- Strengthens and tones arms and abdominals
- Strengthens wrists

CONTRA-INDICATIONS & CAUTIONS
- Shoulder issues
- Wrist injury
- Lower-back injury

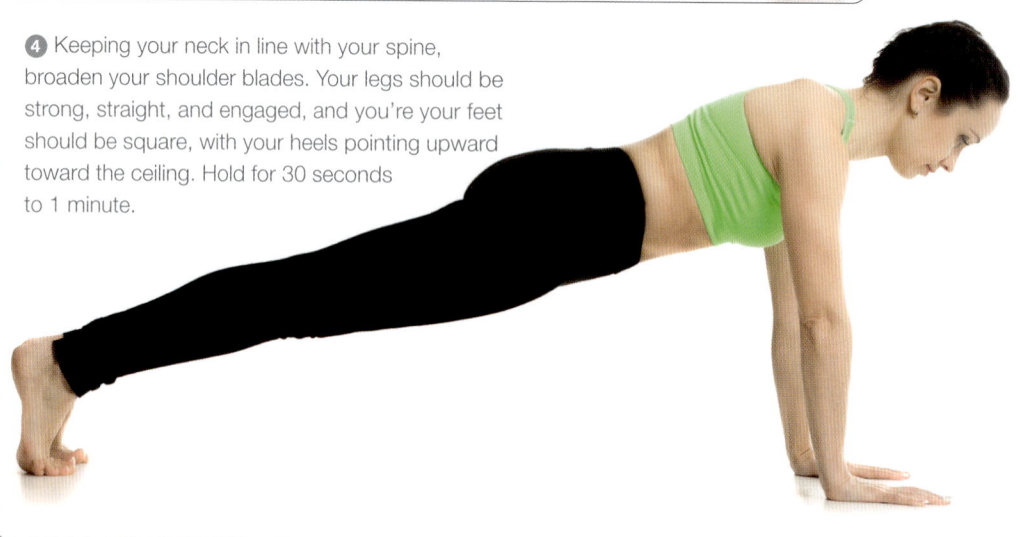

④ Keeping your neck in line with your spine, broaden your shoulder blades. Your legs should be strong, straight, and engaged, and you're your feet should be square, with your heels pointing upward toward the ceiling. Hold for 30 seconds to 1 minute.

⑤ From Plank Pose, open your chest, and broaden your shoulder blades while tucking in your tailbone.

⑥ Exhale, and with your legs turned slightly inward, lower yourself to the floor until your upper arms are parallel to your spine.

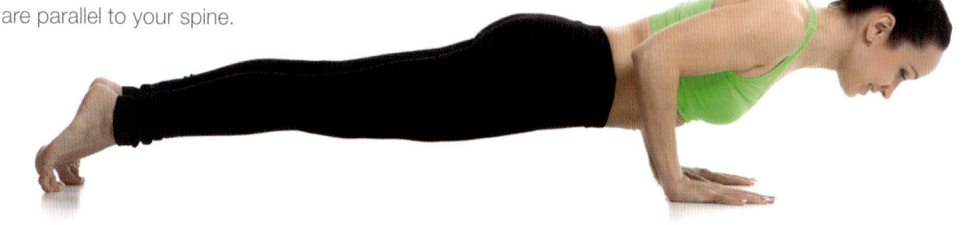

FOUR-LIMBED STAFF POSE
(CHATURANGA DANDASANA)

7 Tuck your tailbone under, and draw your abdominals in toward your spine to maintain the straight line from your shoulders to your heels. Keep your elbows in by your sides. Lift your head and look forward.

8 Hold for 10 to 30 seconds.

BEST FOR
- rectus abdominis
- triceps brachii
- subscapularis
- supraspinatus
- infraspinatus
- teres major
- pectoralis major
- pectoralis minor

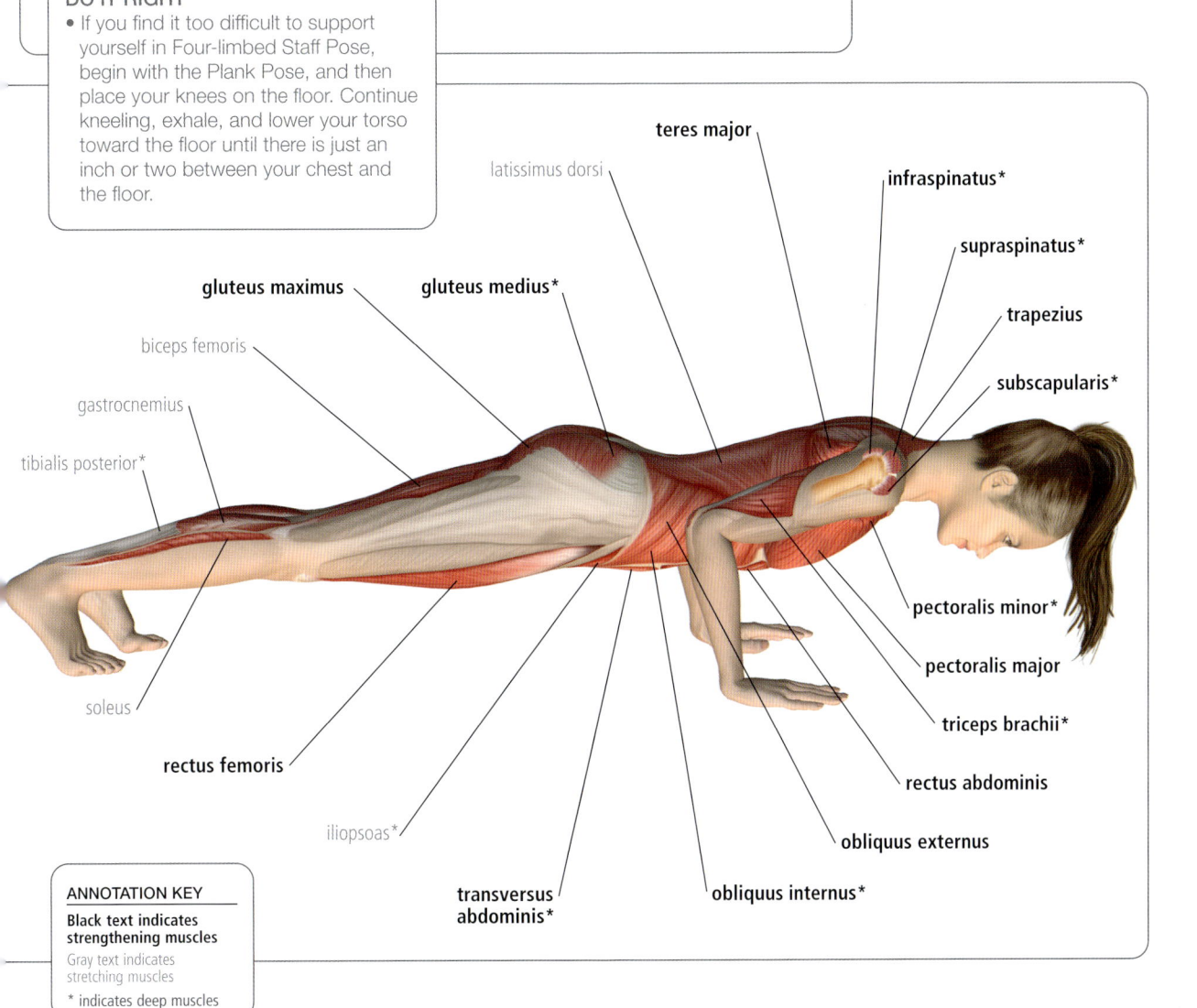

DO IT RIGHT
- If you find it too difficult to support yourself in Four-limbed Staff Pose, begin with the Plank Pose, and then place your knees on the floor. Continue kneeling, exhale, and lower your torso toward the floor until there is just an inch or two between your chest and the floor.

ANNOTATION KEY
Black text indicates strengthening muscles
Gray text indicates stretching muscles
* indicates deep muscles

SIDE PLANK POSE
(VASISTHASANA)

ARM SUPPORTS & INVERSIONS

① Begin in Plank Pose (see page 122). Your arms should be straight with your wrists aligned under the shoulder. To prepare for the Side Plank Pose, you may want your hands slightly in front of your shoulders to push into the support.

DO IT RIGHT
- Elongate your limbs as much as possible, stretching through your legs into the floor and reaching your top arm high to the ceiling.
- Your feet should be stacked and flexed as if they were side by side in standing position.

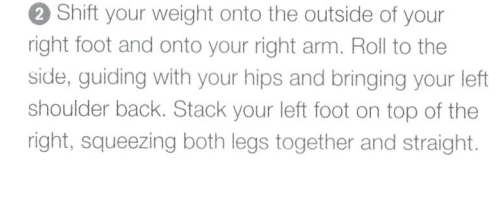

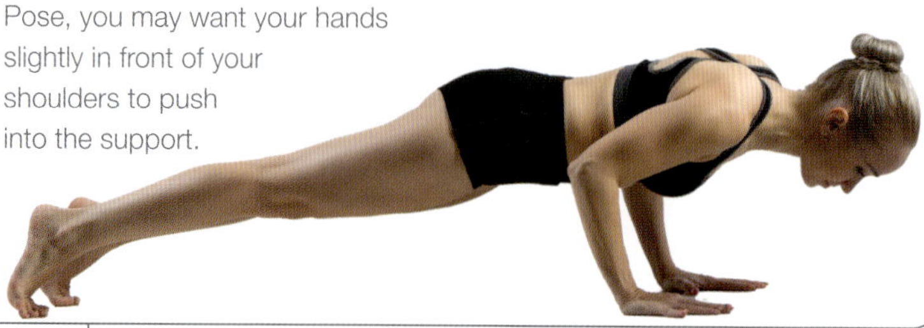

② Shift your weight onto the outside of your right foot and onto your right arm. Roll to the side, guiding with your hips and bringing your left shoulder back. Stack your left foot on top of the right, squeezing both legs together and straight.

③ Exhale, bring the left arm up to the ceiling, and elongate your body, making a straight line from your head to your heels. Gaze up at your fingertips as you continue to push through your shoulder into the floor, maintaining a strong balance.

④ Breathe, and hold the posture for 15 to 30 seconds. Return to Plank Pose or Downward-Facing Dog (Adho Mukha Svanasana, see page 24), and repeat on the left side.

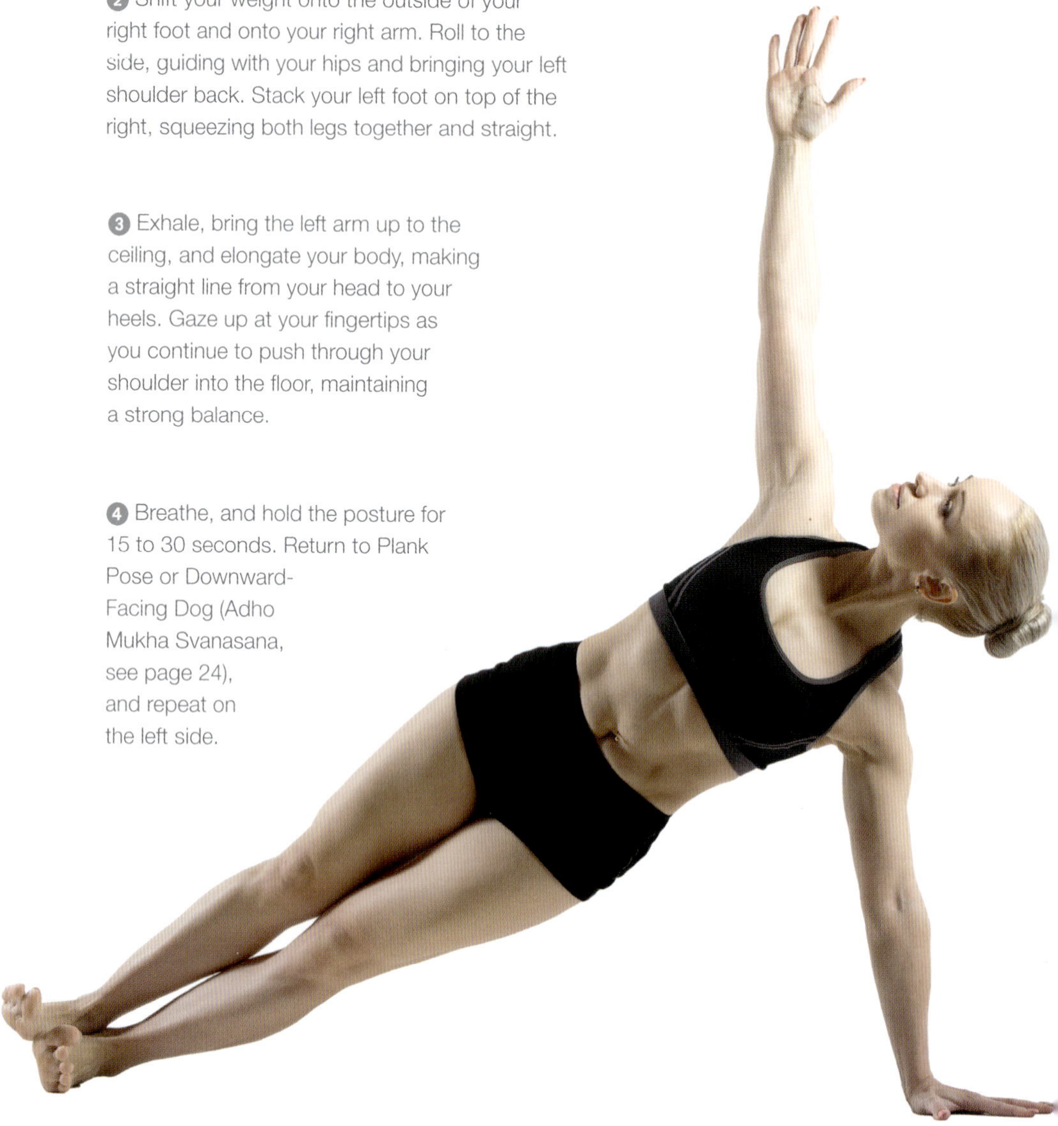

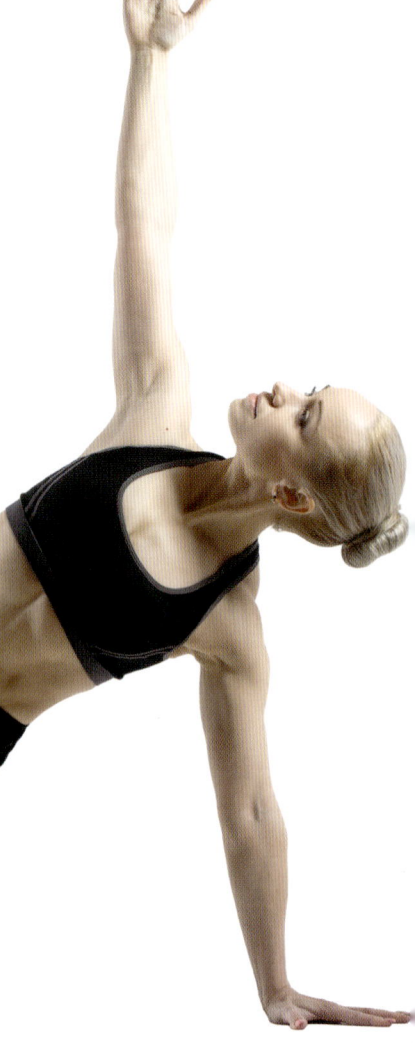

PRONUNCIATION & MEANING
- Vasisthasana (vah-sish-TAHS-anna)
- *vasistha* = most excellent, best, richest

BENEFITS
- Strengthens wrists, arms, legs, and abdominals
- Improves balance

CONTRA-INDICATIONS & CAUTIONS
- Shoulder issues
- Wrist injury
- Elbow injury

124

SIDE PLANK POSE • ARM SUPPORTS & INVERSIONS

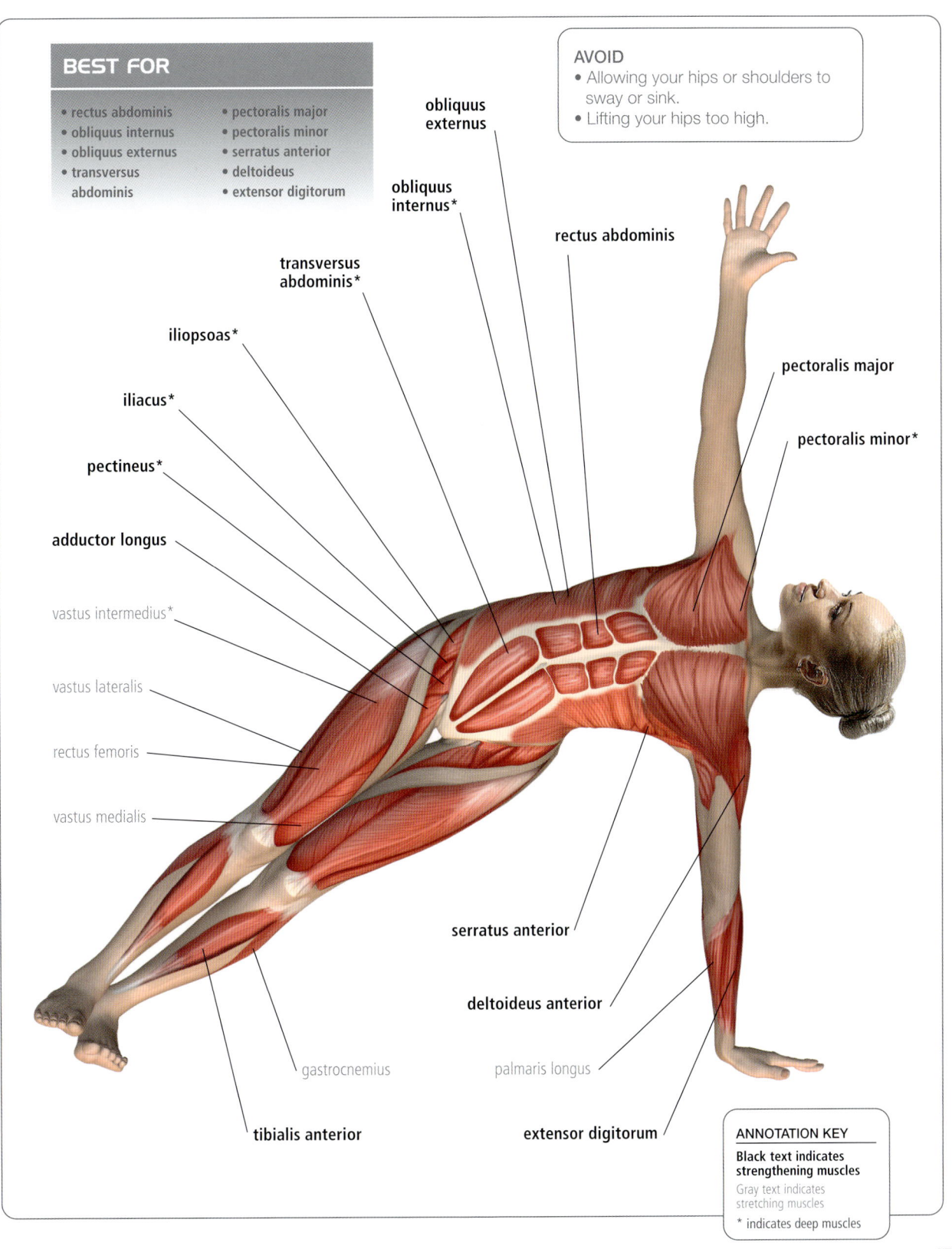

BEST FOR
- rectus abdominis
- obliquus internus
- obliquus externus
- transversus abdominis
- pectoralis major
- pectoralis minor
- serratus anterior
- deltoideus
- extensor digitorum

AVOID
- Allowing your hips or shoulders to sway or sink.
- Lifting your hips too high.

obliquus externus

obliquus internus*

rectus abdominis

transversus abdominis*

iliopsoas*

iliacus*

pectineus*

adductor longus

vastus intermedius*

vastus lateralis

rectus femoris

vastus medialis

pectoralis major

pectoralis minor*

serratus anterior

deltoideus anterior

gastrocnemius

palmaris longus

tibialis anterior

extensor digitorum

ANNOTATION KEY
Black text indicates strengthening muscles
Gray text indicates stretching muscles
* indicates deep muscles

125

BACKBENDS

LOCUST POSE
(SALABHASANA)

1 Lie prone on the floor with your arms resting by your sides and the palms of your hands facing downward. Turn your legs in toward each other so that your knees point directly into the floor.

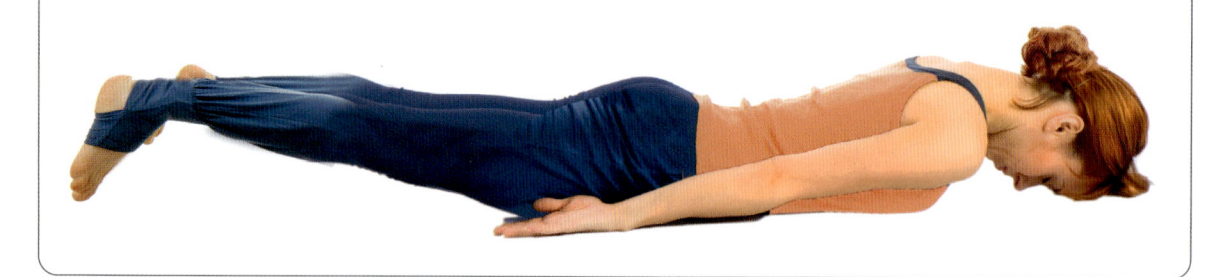

2 Squeezing your buttocks, inhale, and lift up your head, chest, arms and legs simultaneously. Extend your arms and legs behind you, with your arms parallel to the floor. Lift up as high as possible, with your pelvis and lower abdominals stabilizing your body on the floor. Keep your head in neutral position.

3 Hold for 30 seconds to 1 minute. Repeat 1 to 2 times.

AVOID
- Bending your knees.
- Holding your breath.

DO IT RIGHT
- Elongate the back of your neck.
- Open your chest to extend the arch through your entire spine.

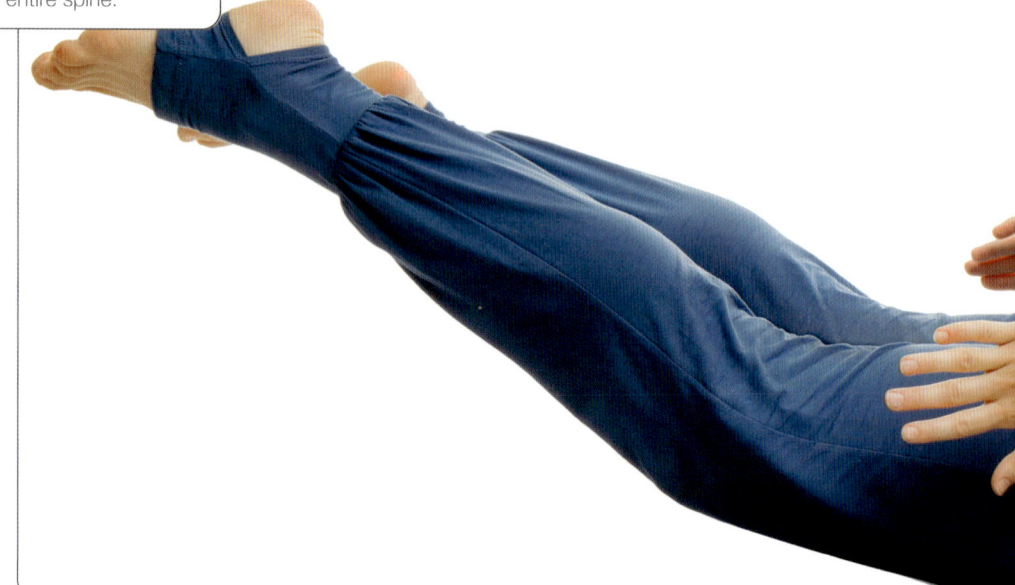

PRONUNCIATION & MEANING
- Salabhasana (sha-la-BAHS-anna)
- *salabha* = locust, grasshopper

BENEFITS
- Strengthens spine, buttocks, arms, and legs
- Stretches hip flexors, chest, and abdominals
- Stimulates digestion

CONTRA-INDICATIONS & CAUTIONS
- Back injury

LOCUST POSE • BACKBENDS

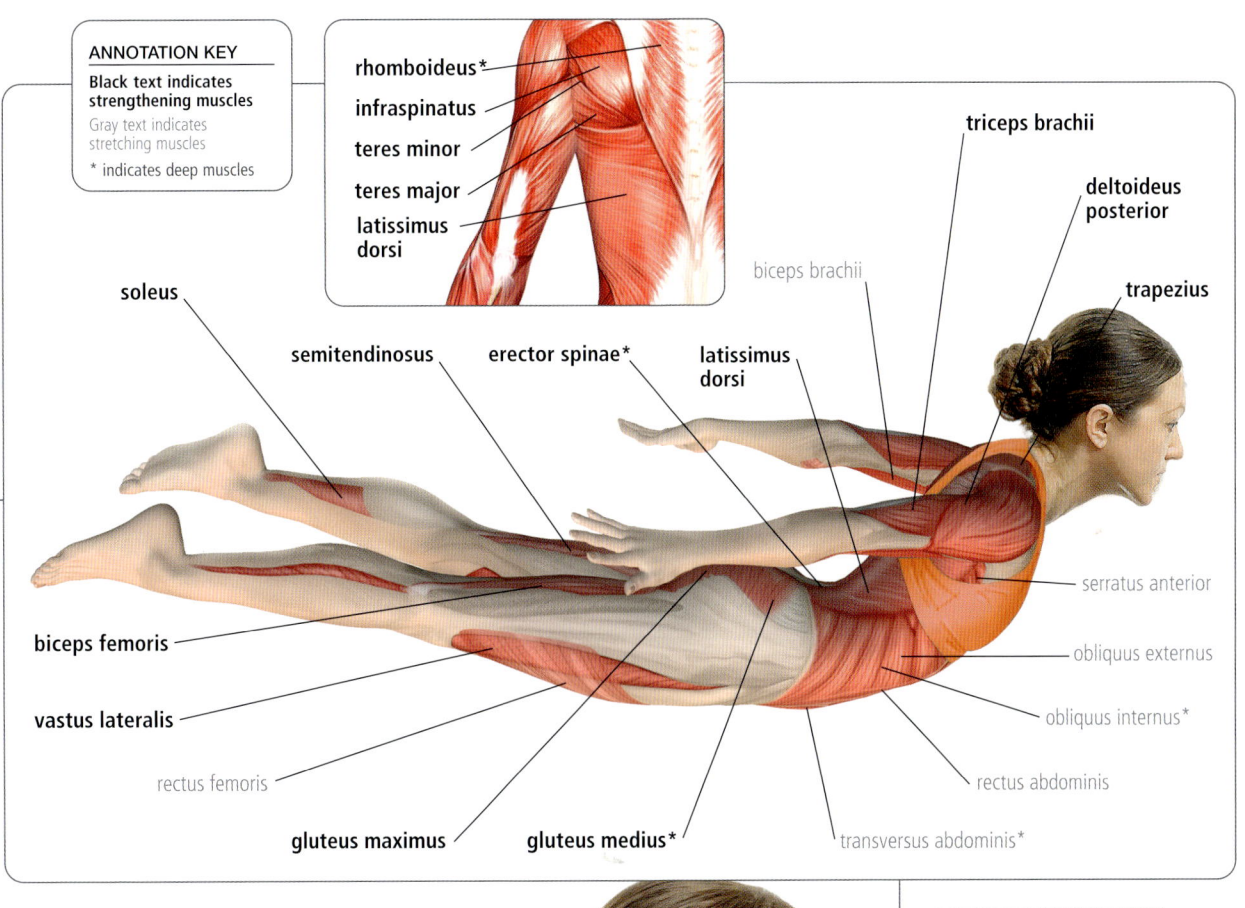

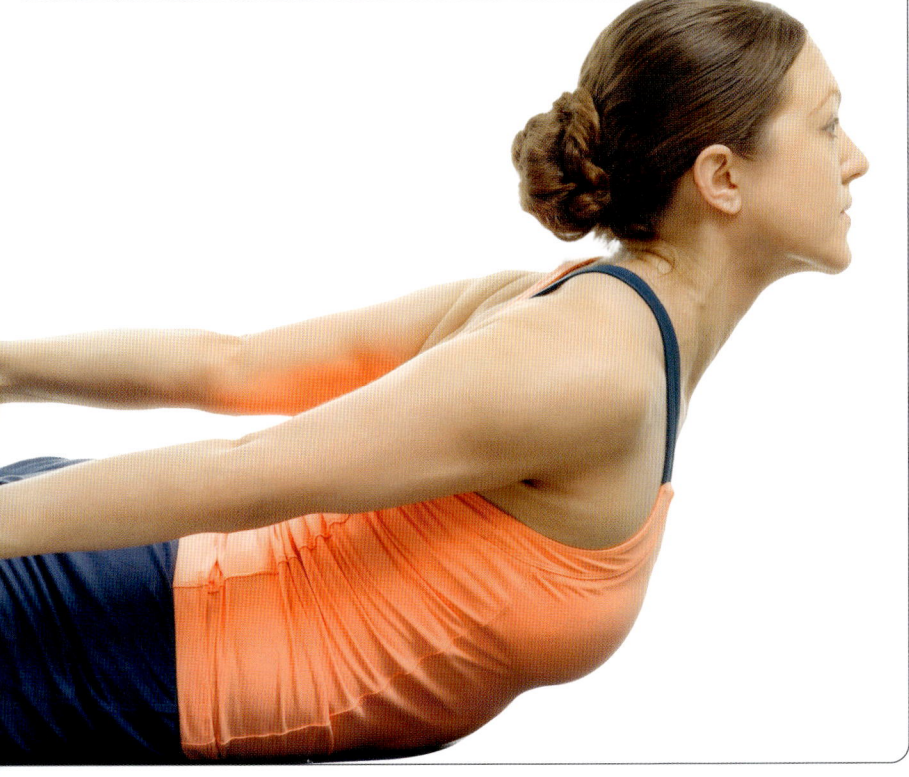

ANNOTATION KEY
Black text indicates strengthening muscles
Gray text indicates stretching muscles
* indicates deep muscles

- rhomboideus*
- infraspinatus
- teres minor
- teres major
- latissimus dorsi

- triceps brachii
- deltoideus posterior
- trapezius
- biceps brachii
- soleus
- semitendinosus
- erector spinae*
- latissimus dorsi
- serratus anterior
- biceps femoris
- vastus lateralis
- obliquus externus
- obliquus internus*
- rectus femoris
- rectus abdominis
- gluteus maximus
- gluteus medius*
- transversus abdominis*

BEST FOR
- rhomboideus
- infraspinatus
- teres major
- latissimus dorsi
- deltoideus
- erector spinae
- trapezius
- gluteus maximus
- gluteus medius

127

BACKBENDS

UPWARD-FACING BOW POSE
(URDHVA DHANURASANA)

❶ Lie supine on the floor. Bend your knees, and draw your heels as close to your buttocks as possible. Bend your elbows, and place your hands on the floor beside your head, with your fingertips pointing toward your shoulders.

❷ Exhale, and push down into your feet to lift your buttocks off the floor. Tighten your thighs, and keep your feet parallel. Push your hands into the floor to raise yourself onto the crown of your head.

❸ After a couple of breaths, exhale, and press into the floor with your hands and feet, lifting your hips up toward the ceiling. Straighten your arms, and allow your head to hang in between your shoulders. Push through your legs, straightening them as much as possible. Open your shoulders, and feel the extension through your entire spine.

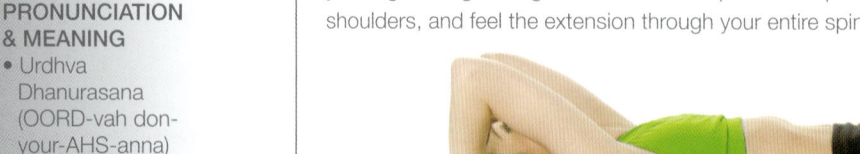

❹ Hold for 5 to 30 seconds. Exhale as you bend your arms, and slowly lower yourself to the floor. Repeat at least one more time.

PRONUNCIATION & MEANING
- Urdhva Dhanurasana (OORD-vah don-your-AHS-anna)
- *urdhva* = upward; *dhanu* = bow
- Also called Wheel Pose

BENEFITS
- Strengthens thighs and buttocks
- Stretches chest and spine
- Stimulates digestion
- Stimulates thyroid
- Reduces stress

CONTRA-INDICATIONS & CAUTIONS
- Back injury
- Carpal tunnel syndrome
- High or low blood pressure
- Headache

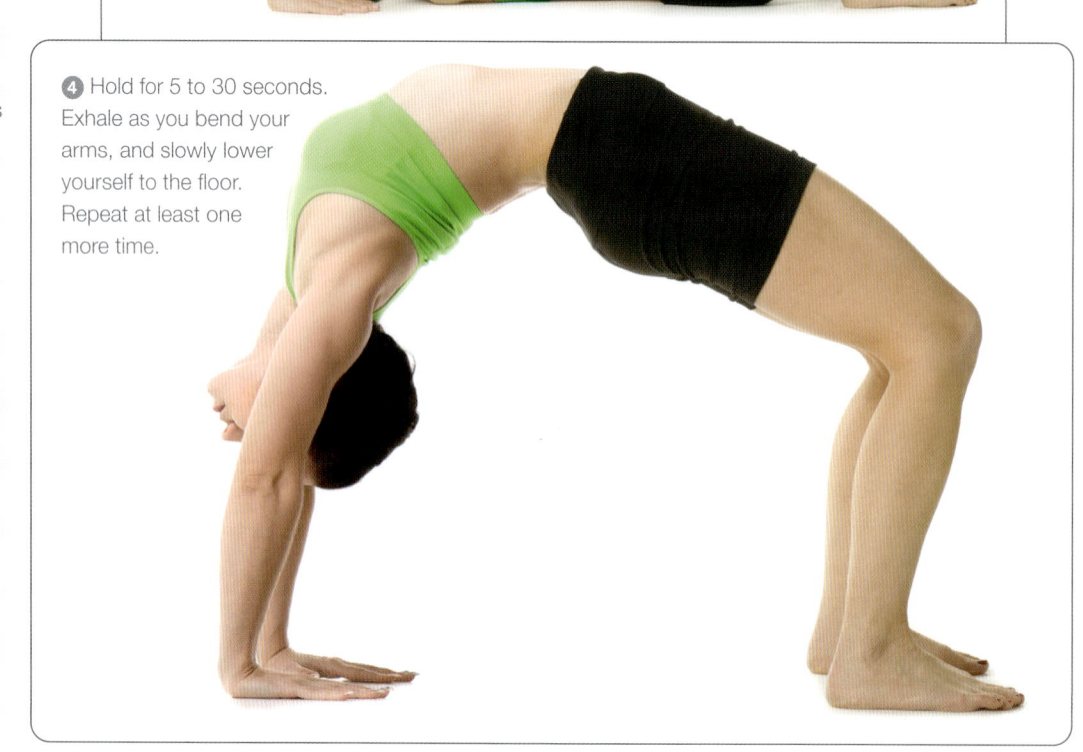

UPWARD-FACING BOW POSE • BACKBENDS

DO IT RIGHT
- Lift up, and extend through your shoulders, spine, and quadriceps, being careful not to put all the extension on your lower back.
- Keep your knees close together during the duration of the posture, making sure that they don't separate more than the width of your hips.

AVOID
- Turning your feet out.
- Splaying your elbows out to the sides to push up into the pose.

BEST FOR
- deltoideus medialis
- serratus anterior
- infraspinatus
- rhomboideus
- flexor carpi radialis
- latissimus dorsi
- trapezius
- erector spinae
- gluteus maximus
- vastus lateralis
- teres major
- teres minor

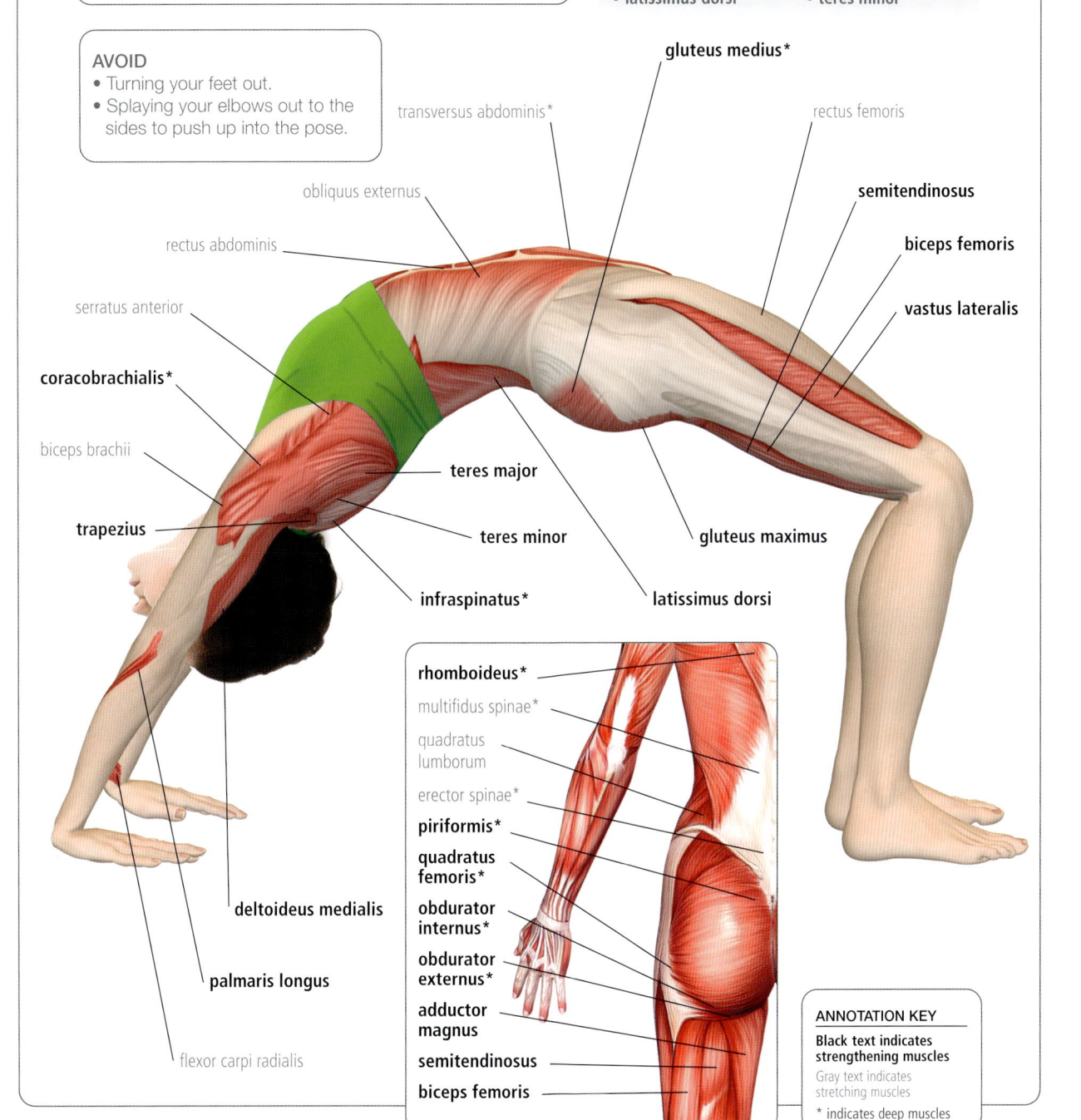

Labels on main figure:
- gluteus medius*
- rectus femoris
- transversus abdominis*
- semitendinosus
- biceps femoris
- obliquus externus
- vastus lateralis
- rectus abdominis
- serratus anterior
- coracobrachialis*
- biceps brachii
- teres major
- trapezius
- teres minor
- gluteus maximus
- infraspinatus*
- latissimus dorsi
- deltoideus medialis
- palmaris longus
- flexor carpi radialis

Labels on inset:
- rhomboideus*
- multifidus spinae*
- quadratus lumborum
- erector spinae*
- piriformis*
- quadratus femoris*
- obdurator internus*
- obdurator externus*
- adductor magnus
- semitendinosus
- biceps femoris

ANNOTATION KEY
Black text indicates strengthening muscles
Gray text indicates stretching muscles
* indicates deep muscles

129

SUPPORTED SHOULDERSTAND
(SALAMBA SARVANGASANA)

① Lie supine on the floor with your knees bent and arms by your sides.

② Tighten your abdominals, and lift your knees off the floor. Exhale, press your arms into the floor, and lift your knees higher so that your buttocks come off the floor.

③ Continue lifting your knees toward your face, and roll your back off the mat from your hips to your shoulders. With your upper arms firmly planted on the floor, bend your elbows, and place your hands on your lower back. Draw your elbows in closer to your sides.

④ Inhale, tuck your tailbone toward your pubis, and straighten your legs back toward your head. Your torso should be perpendicular to the floor.

⑤ With your next inhalation, extend your legs up toward the ceiling, opening your hips as you lift. Squeeze your buttocks, and press down with your elbows to create a straight, elongated line from your chest to your toes.

⑥ Hold for 30 seconds to 5 minutes before bending your knees and hips and returning to the floor.

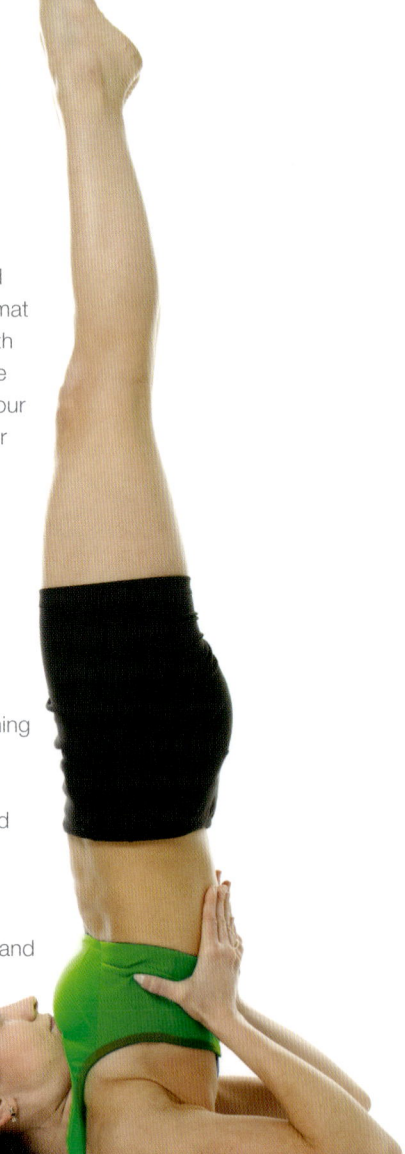

AVOID
- Bending at your hips once you are in the posture, because it puts added pressure on your neck and spine.
- Splaying your elbows out to the sides.

DO IT RIGHT
- Soften your throat, and relax your tongue.
- If you can't lift your pelvis into the inversion, practice a few feet away from a wall and walk your feet up the wall until you can place your hands on your back.
- Place folded blankets below your shoulders if the posture strains your neck.

PRONUNCIATION & MEANING
- Salamba Sarvangasana (sah-LOM-bah sar-van-GAHS-anna)
- *sa* = with; *alamba* = support; *sarva* = all; *anga* = limb

BENEFITS
- Relieves stress
- Stretches shoulders, neck, and upper spine
- Stimulates digestion

CONTRA-INDICATIONS & CAUTIONS
- High blood pressure
- Neck issues
- Headache or ear infection

ARM SUPPORTS & INVERSIONS

SUPPORTED SHOULDERSTAND • ARM SUPPORTS & INVERSIONS

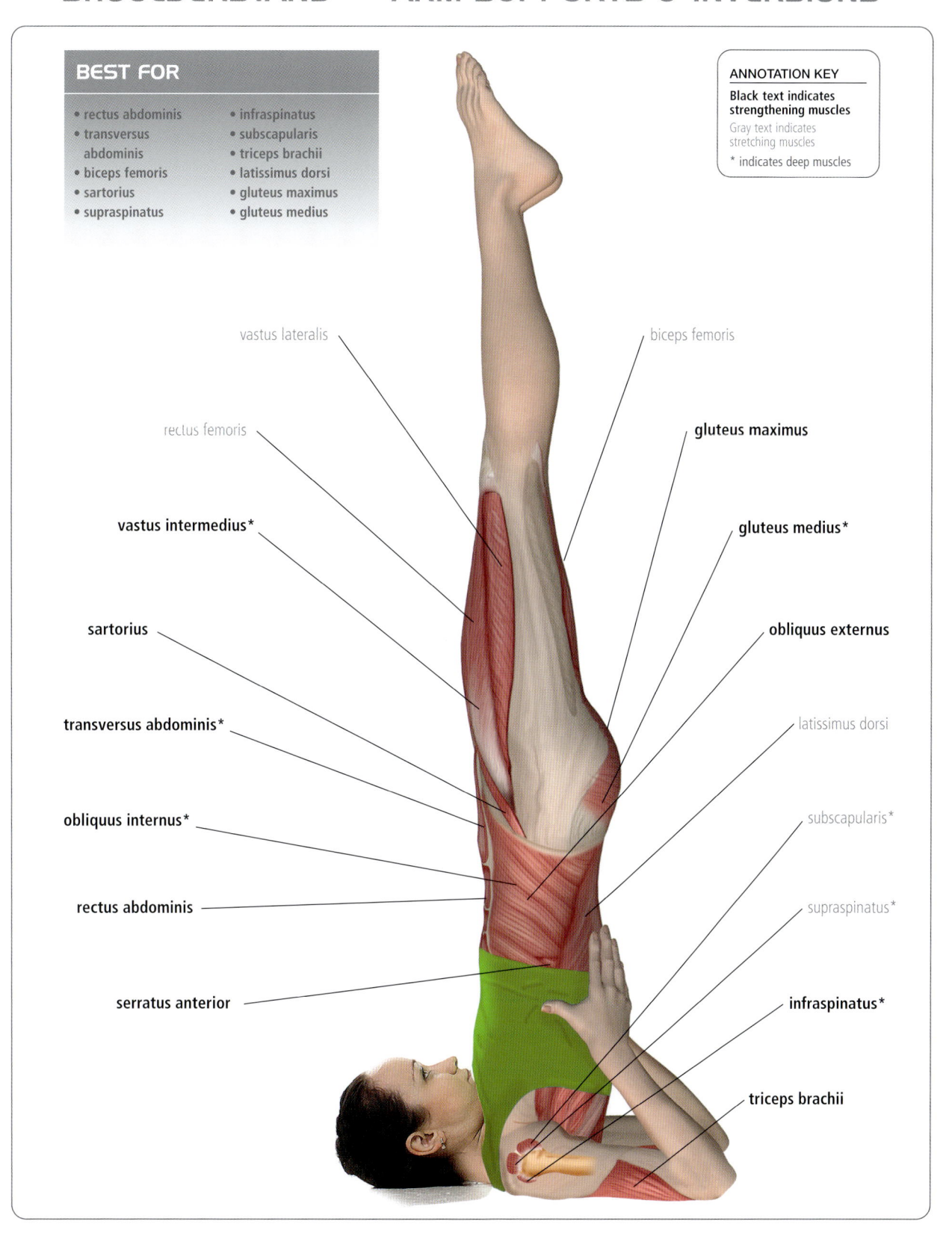

BEST FOR

- rectus abdominis
- transversus abdominis
- biceps femoris
- sartorius
- supraspinatus
- infraspinatus
- subscapularis
- triceps brachii
- latissimus dorsi
- gluteus maximus
- gluteus medius

ANNOTATION KEY
Black text indicates strengthening muscles
Gray text indicates stretching muscles
* indicates deep muscles

vastus lateralis

rectus femoris

vastus intermedius*

sartorius

transversus abdominis*

obliquus internus*

rectus abdominis

serratus anterior

biceps femoris

gluteus maximus

gluteus medius*

obliquus externus

latissimus dorsi

subscapularis*

supraspinatus*

infraspinatus*

triceps brachii

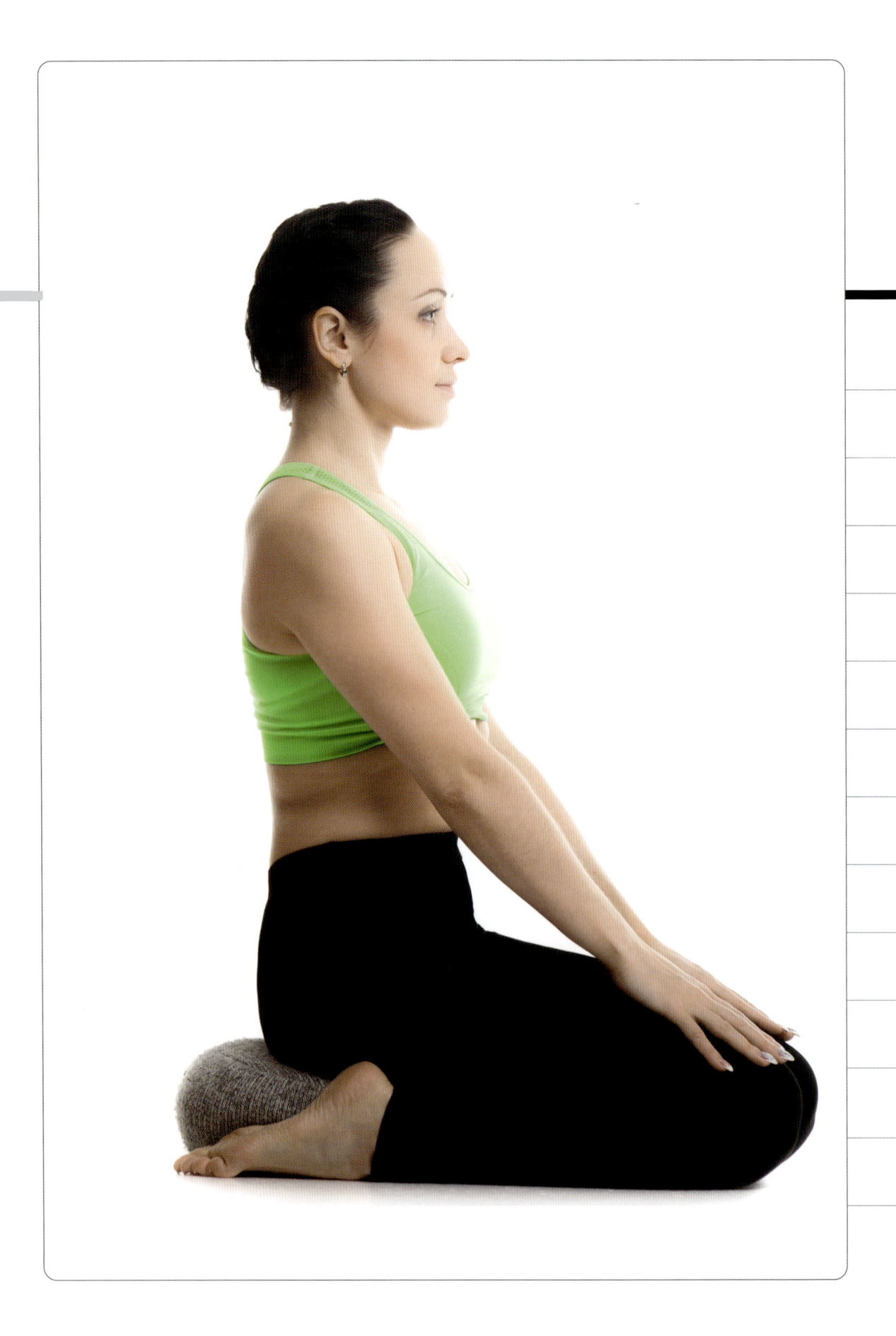

RESTORATIVE POSES

In yoga, the poses you engage in during the beginning and end of your session play pivotal roles in maximizing the benefits of the entire routine. Warm-up poses aim to activate your muscles, elevate your heart rate, and dissipate tension, which keeps you flexible and energized for your session. Conversely, cool-down poses help to soothe your muscles, decrease your heart rate, and offer relaxation after a strenuous session. Incorporating gentle stretches, particularly post-exercise, is crucial for warding off injuries. They also help you set the groundwork for or recover from other specific poses: Easy Pose and Staff Pose, for instance, are the foundation of most seated poses, while Knees-to-Chest can help you recover from backbends.

RESTORATIVE POSES

CHILD'S POSE
(BALASANA)

❶ Kneel on your hands and knees, hands planted shoulder-width apart.

❷ Bring your big toes together, and place your knees about hip-width apart.

❸ Shift your hips back toward your heels as you extend your torso forward, lowering your stomach onto your thighs. Let your shoulders round forward, allowing your forehead to rest gently on the floor.

❹ Slide your arms back along your thighs, with the palms of your hands facing upward. Breathe into the back of your body. Hold for the recommended breaths

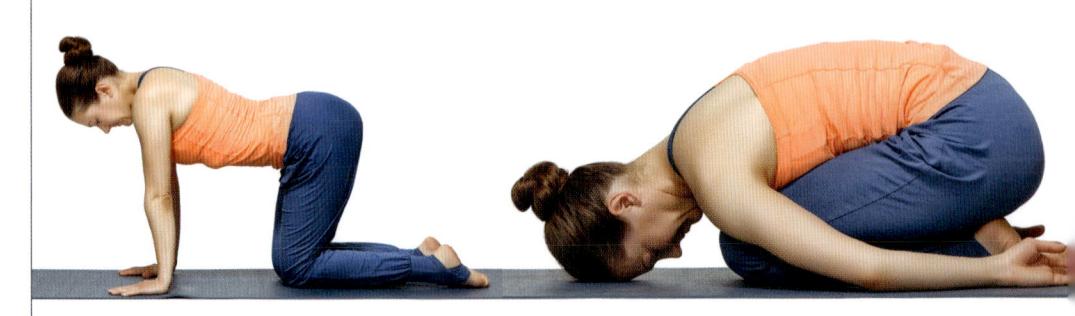

AVOID
- bringing your knees too far apart.

DO IT RIGHT
- Relax any tension you may be retaining in your jaw and face muscles.
- Place your forehead on a folded towel or low cushion if desired.
- Expand the space between your shoulder blades as you breathe.

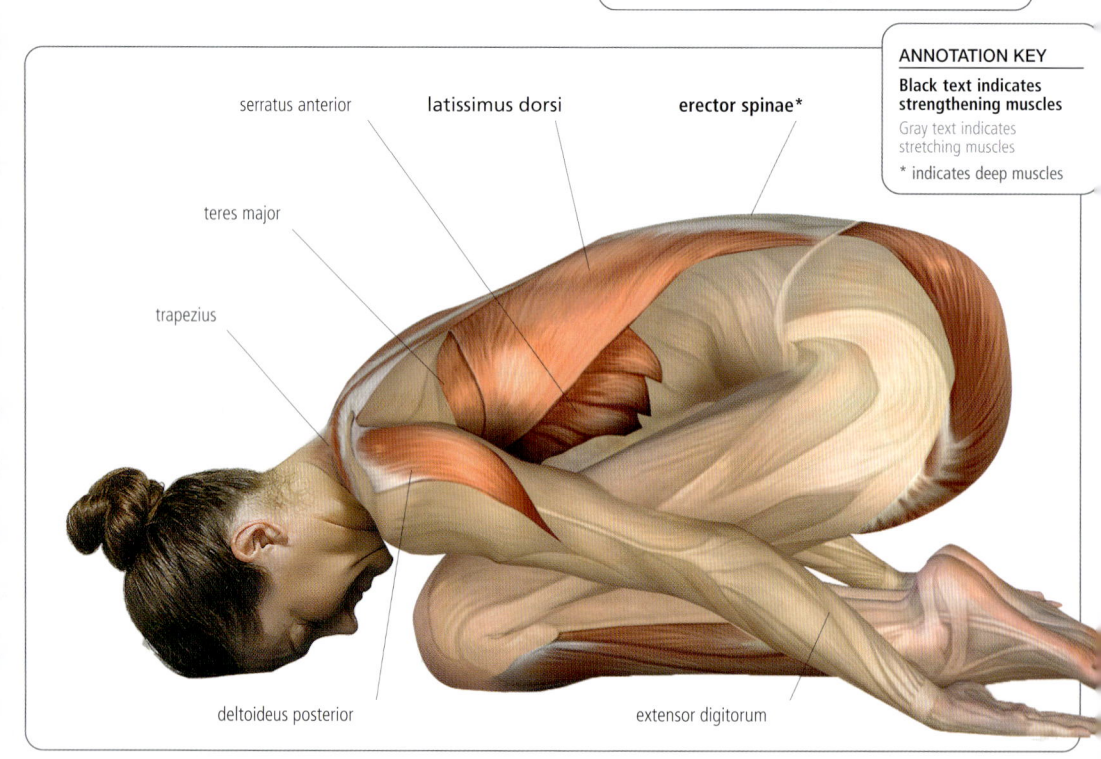

PRONUNCIATION & MEANING
- Balasana (bah-LAHS-anna)
- *bala* = child

BENEFITS
- Relaxes anterior muscles
- Passively stretches posterior muscles
- Reduces stress and anxiety
- Relieves back pain

CONTRA-INDICATIONS & CAUTIONS
- Diarrhea
- Knee injury
- Pregnancy

ANNOTATION KEY
Black text indicates strengthening muscles
Gray text indicates stretching muscles
* indicates deep muscles

serratus anterior
latissimus dorsi
erector spinae*
teres major
trapezius
deltoideus posterior
extensor digitorum

134

DOWNWARD-FACING DOG
(ADHO MUKHA SVANASANA)

RESTORATIVE POSES

❶ Kneel on your hands and knees with your knees directly below your hips. Stretch your hands out slightly in front of your shoulders with your fingertips facing forward. They should be placed one shoulder-width apart.

DO IT RIGHT
- If your hamstrings and shoulders are especially tight, practice the pose with your knees slightly bent and your heels lifted from the floor.
- Contract your thighs to lengthen your spine further, and keep pressure off your shoulders.

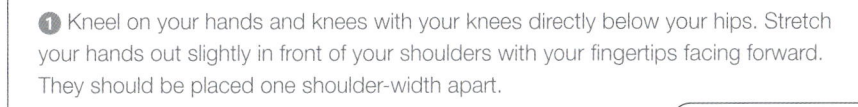

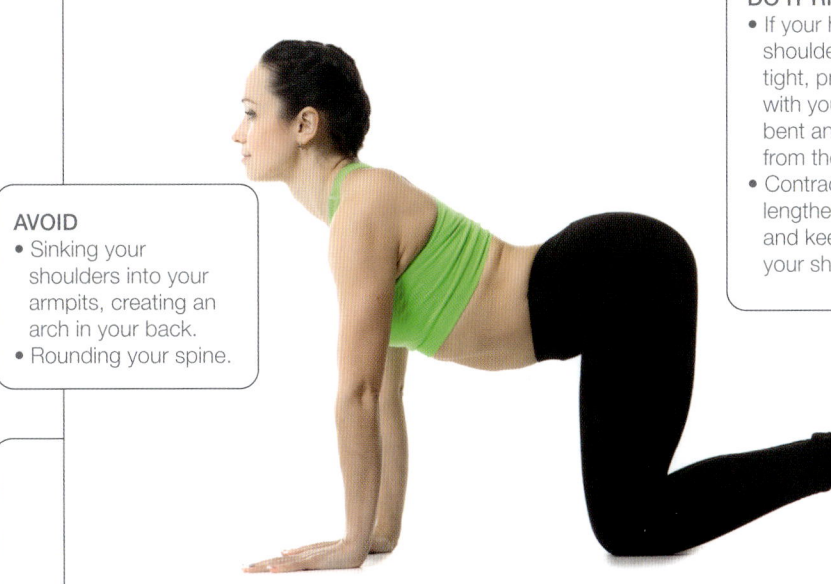

AVOID
- Sinking your shoulders into your armpits, creating an arch in your back.
- Rounding your spine.

❷ Exhale and press against the floor, keeping your elbows straight. Lift your sit bones up toward the ceiling and your knees away from the floor. Lengthen your hips away from your ribs to elongate your spine.

❸ Press your heels toward the floor, and contract your thighs. Try to straighten your knees. Turn your thighs slightly inward, and broaden your chest and shoulders. Position your head in between your arms.

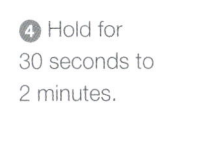

❹ Hold for 30 seconds to 2 minutes.

PRONUNCIATION & MEANING
- Adho Mukha Svanasana (AH-doh MOO-kah shvah-NAHS-anna)
- *adho* = downward; *mukha* = face; *shvana* = dog

LEVEL
- Beginner

BENEFITS
- Stretches shoulders, hamstrings, and calves
- Strengthens arms and legs
- Relives stress and headaches

CONTRA-INDICATIONS & CAUTIONS
- Carpal tunnel syndrome

135

KNEES-TO-CHEST POSE
(APANASANA)

RESTORATIVE POSES

① Lie on your back with your legs extended. On an exhalation, bend both knees and raise them toward your chest. Grasp your shins with both hands.

② Wrap your arms around your knees, placing each hand on your opposite elbow. Lengthen the back of your neck away from your shoulders. With each exhalation, gently pull your knees closer toward your chest, and flatten your back and shoulders on the floor.

③ Hold for 30 seconds to 1 minute.

PRONUNCIATION & MEANING
- Apanasana (ap-AN-ahs-anna)
- *apana* = waste-eliminating downward breath

BENEFITS
- Stretches lower back and hips
- Stimulates digestion

CONTRA-INDICATIONS & CAUTIONS
- Knee injury
- Pregnancy

AVOID
- Tensing your back or leg muscles.
- straining your neck; if you have difficulty placing your head on the mat, try resting it on a folded blanket.

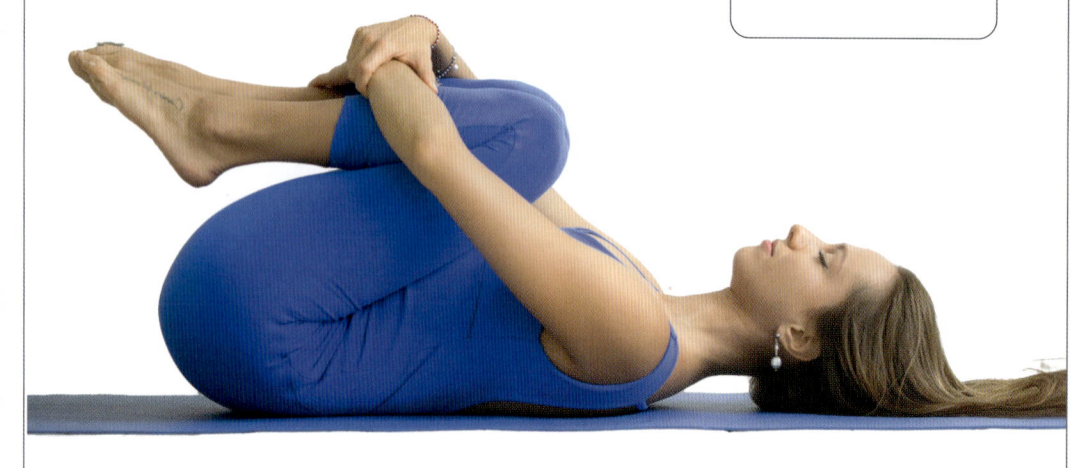

KNEES-TO-CHEST POSE • RESTORATIVE POSES

BEST FOR
- gluteus medius
- piriformis
- tractus iliotibialis
- quadratus femoris
- obturator externus
- adductor magnus
- biceps femoris
- semimembranosus
- gastrocnemius

DO IT RIGHT
- If you can't grasp your elbows while hugging your knees, place your hands directly on your knees.
- Draw your stomach inward.
- Press down into the mat with your back and shoulders.
- Lengthen the back of your neck.

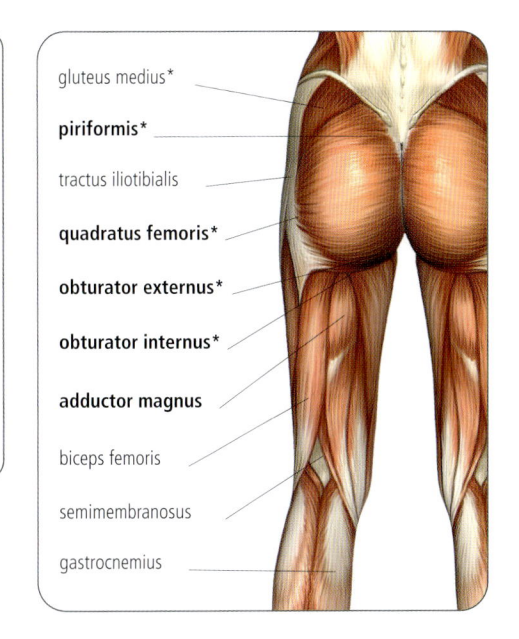

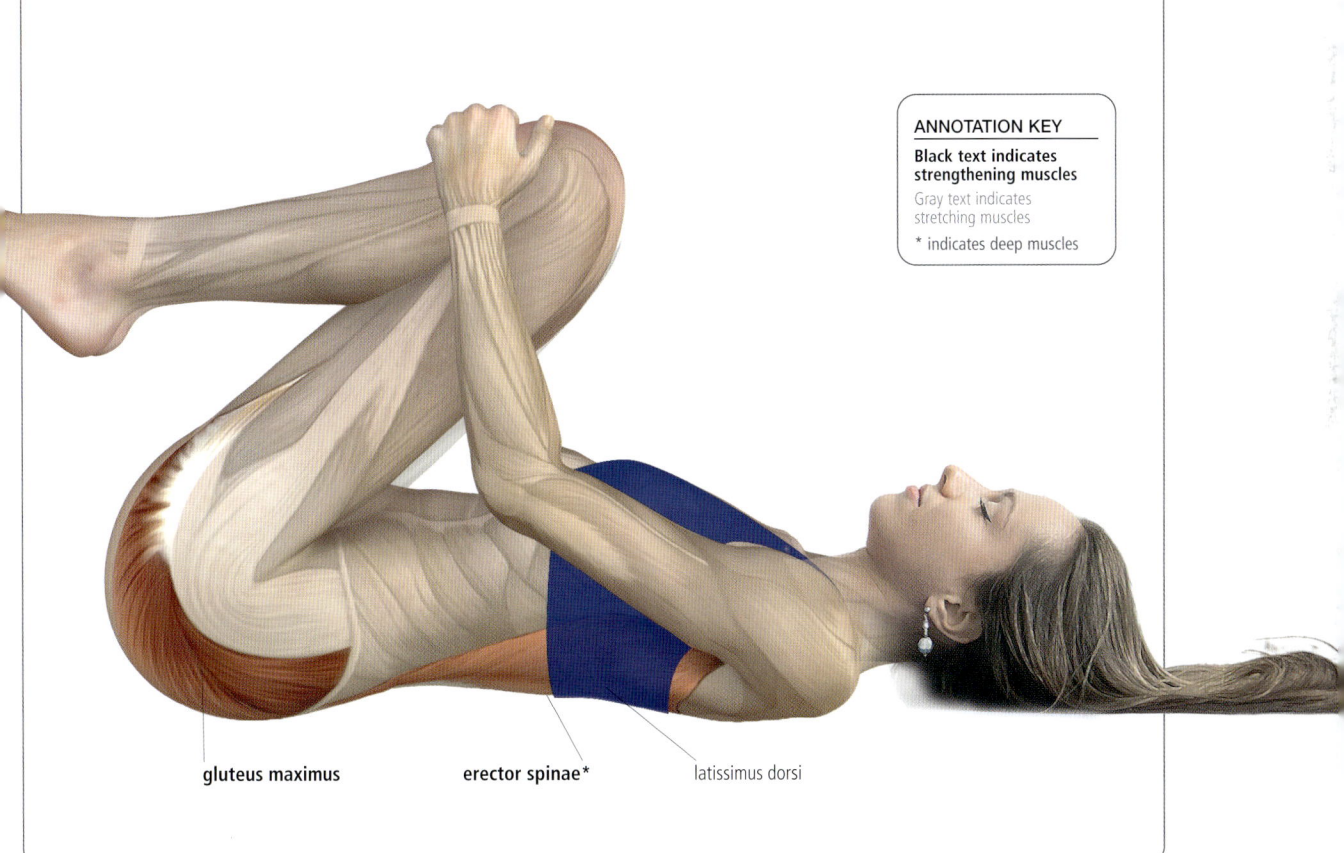

gluteus medius*
piriformis*
tractus iliotibialis
quadratus femoris*
obturator externus*
obturator internus*
adductor magnus
biceps femoris
semimembranosus
gastrocnemius

ANNOTATION KEY
Black text indicates strengthening muscles
Gray text indicates stretching muscles
* indicates deep muscles

gluteus maximus   erector spinae*   latissimus dorsi

137

RESTORATIVE POSES

CORPSE POSE
(SAVASANA)

① Sit on the floor on your buttocks with your knees bent. Lift your hips, and place your tailbone slightly closer to your heels. Elongate your lower back away from your tailbone before allowing your back to relax to the floor.

② Straighten your legs one at a time. Allow your legs to fall open, separated the same distance from the center of your body. The feet should be turned out equally.

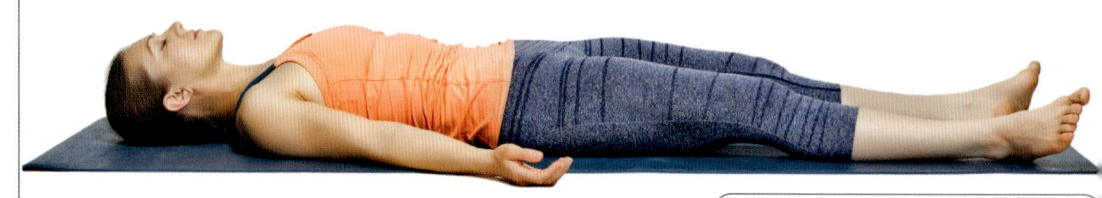

AVOID
- Moving once your body is aligned.
- Tensing your muscles.

PRONUNCIATION & MEANING
- Savasana (shah-VAHS-anna)
- *sava* = corpse

BENEFITS
- Calms the brain
- Relieves stress
- Relaxes the body

CONTRA-INDICATIONS & CAUTIONS
- Back injury

③ Relax your arms on the floor by your sides, leaving a space between your torso and your arms. Spread your shoulder blades and your collarbones, and turn your arms out so that your palms face up.

④ Lengthen your neck away from your shoulders, and try to release it comfortably toward the floor. Close your eyes. Breathe smoothly. Focus on your body alignment and your breath.

⑤ Relax every part of your body, starting with your toes and ending with your head. Feel each part sinking into the floor. Relax the muscles in your face and calm your brain.

⑥ Hold for 5 to 10 minutes. Gently come out of the pose by bending your knees to your chest and rolling over to one side. Bring your head up last.

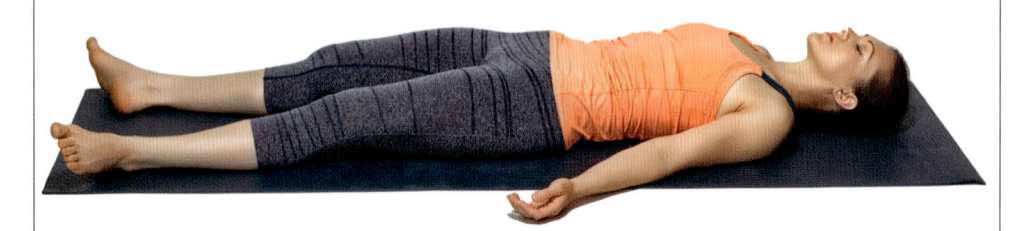

[alternate view]

DO IT RIGHT
- End your yoga practice with Corpse Pose.
- Pay attention to the alignment of your head, making sure that it is pulled away from your shoulders and does not tilt to one side.
- Practice with your knees bent and feet flat on the floor.

HERO POSE
(VIRASANA)

① Kneel on your hands and knees on the floor. Your thighs should be perpendicular to the floor, and your feet should be angled slightly wider than your hips.

② Bring your knees together until they touch, pushing the tops of your feet into the floor. Lean forward slightly with your torso, exhaling, and begin to sit back onto your buttocks.

③ Sit on the floor with your buttocks in between your heels.

④ Lift your chest, and press your shoulders back and down, lengthening your tailbone into the floor so that you are resting on your sit bones. Place your hands on the tops of your thighs. Pull your abdominals in toward your spine.

⑤ Hold for 30 seconds to 1 minute.

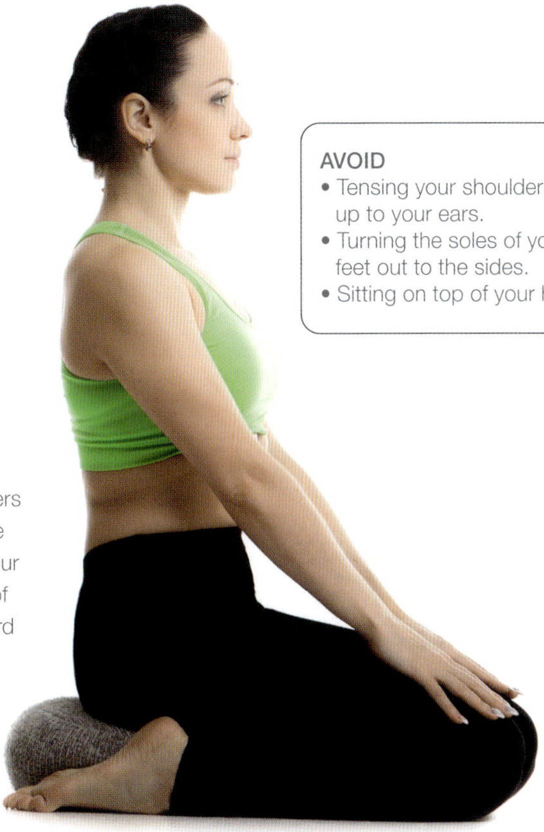

AVOID
- Tensing your shoulders up to your ears.
- Turning the soles of your feet out to the sides.
- Sitting on top of your heels.

DO IT RIGHT
- If you experience pain in your knees, place a folded blanket beneath you to elevate your hips. Point your big toes slightly inward so that the tops of your feet lie flat on the floor.

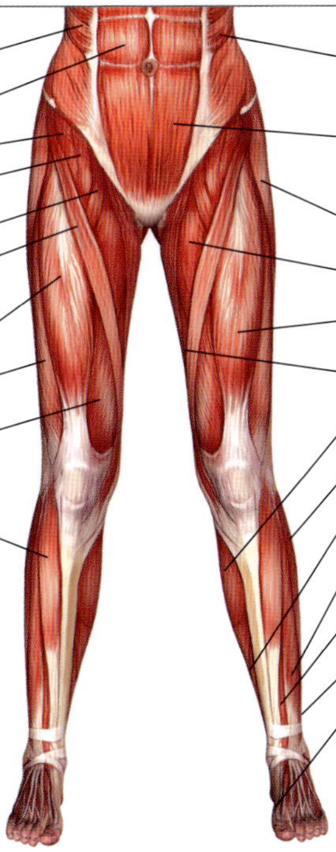

ANNOTATION KEY
Black text indicates strengthening muscles
Gray text indicates stretching muscles
* indicates deep muscles

BEST FOR
- rectus femoris
- vastus intermedius
- tensor fasciae latae
- sartorius
- vastus medialis
- vastus lateralis
- tibialis anterior
- extensor hallucis
- peroneus

Muscle labels:
- **obliquus internus**
- **rectus abdominis**
- **iliopsoas***
- **iliacus***
- **pectineus***
- sartorius
- vastus intermedius*
- vastus lateralis
- vastus medialis
- tibialis anterior
- **obliquus externus**
- **transversus abdominis***
- tensor fasciae latae
- **adductor longus**
- rectus femoris
- gracilis*
- soleus
- gastrocnemius
- flexor digitorum
- extensor digitorum
- extensor hallucis
- peroneus
- adductor hallucis

RESTORATIVE POSES

PRONUNCIATION & MEANING
- Virasana (veer-AHS-anna)
- vira = man, hero, chief

BENEFITS
- Loosens thighs, knees, and ankles
- Counterbalances hip-opening postures such as the Lotus Pose (Padmasana, see pages 108–109)
- Calms the brain for meditation
- Alleviates high blood pressure

CONTRA-INDICATIONS & CAUTIONS
- Knee injury
- Ankle injury

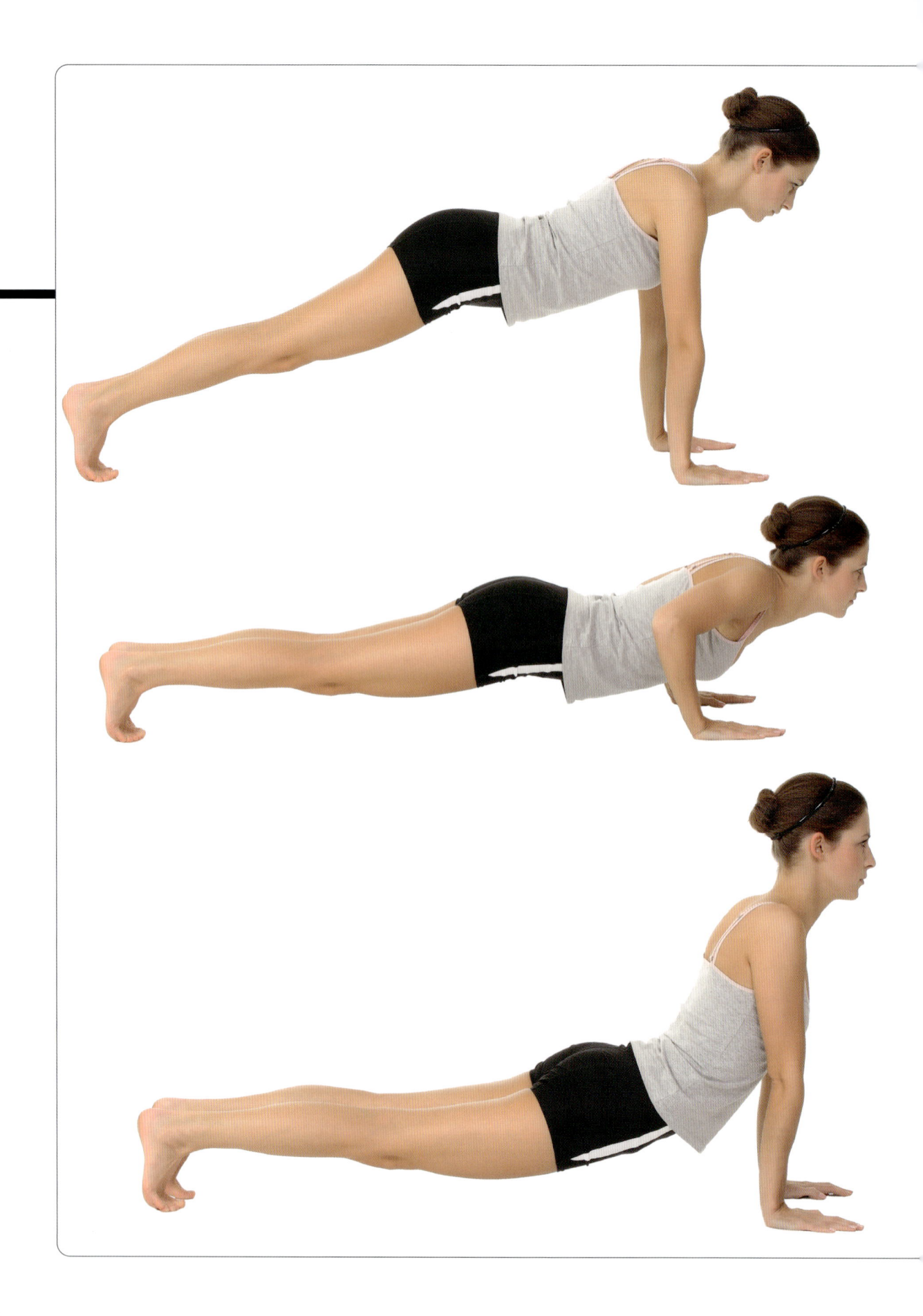

YOGA FLOWS

From the Sun Salutation that starts a day with a warming and energizing series of yoga asanas to a calming set of poses like the Spinal Flow to end it, yoga flows are poses that flow into each other—ideally in a smooth movement. For beginners, learning the individual poses is the first step, but even in a class, they will learn to move from one into the next. The pace is also a factor—the recommended number of breaths to hold a pose can be increased to create a more cardio-based session, while breaths can be increased to for a more strengthening experience. Whatever your pace, flowing from one pose to the next, almost as if in a dance, allows you to maximize the strength and flexibility that you will gain throughout your entire body.

PUTTING IT ALL TOGETHER

For beginning practitioners, one of the most challenges aspects of yoga is not learning the many pose, but instead putting them together in graceful flows that move smoothly from one pose to the next.

Familiarizing yourself with various yoga asanas is only the first step in your yoga practice. The next step is learning how to incorporate these asanas into sequences. Most flows begin with gentler poses, and then build up to those that are more challenging, before ending with a cool-down asana. The traditional way to start your day is with an invigorating Surya Namasjara—better known as a Sun Salutation. For other yoga practice there are endless combinations of asanas, from those that calm your spirit to those that strengthen your body. The sequences featured in this chapter are a guide to get you started at combining poses, but with each individual one, focus on attaining the proper body position before moving on to the next. Don't feel as if you must slavishly follow any one flow; you can combine other poses to add variety and create a yoga practice that best suits your body's needs and capabilities.

COMBINING POSES

Certain poses flow particularly well together. When combining poses, aim to move seamlessly from one to the next, with no rest between them. Combination Poses can also be modifications and variations of the original move, such as moving from a Standing Half Forward Bend to Head-to-Knee Forward Bend. Here is a short list of some beginner poses that allow you to transition from one to the other in a natural motion.

- Prayer Pose to Garland Pose
- Chair Pose to Standing Forward Bend
- Downward-facing Dog to High Lunge
- Plank Pose to Four-Limbed Staff Pose
- Plank Pose to Side Plank Pose
- Four-Limbed Staff Pose to Cobra Pose
- Cat Pose to Cow Pose
- Warrior I to Warrior II
- Extended Side Angle Pose to Triangle Pose

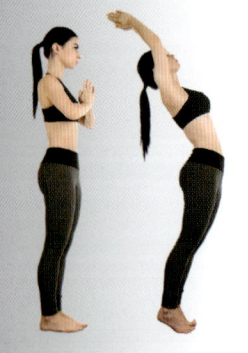

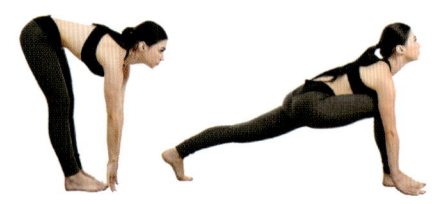

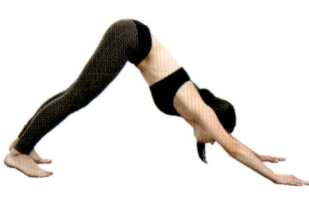

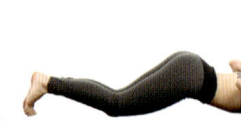

PUTTING IT ALL TOGETHER • YOGA FLOWS

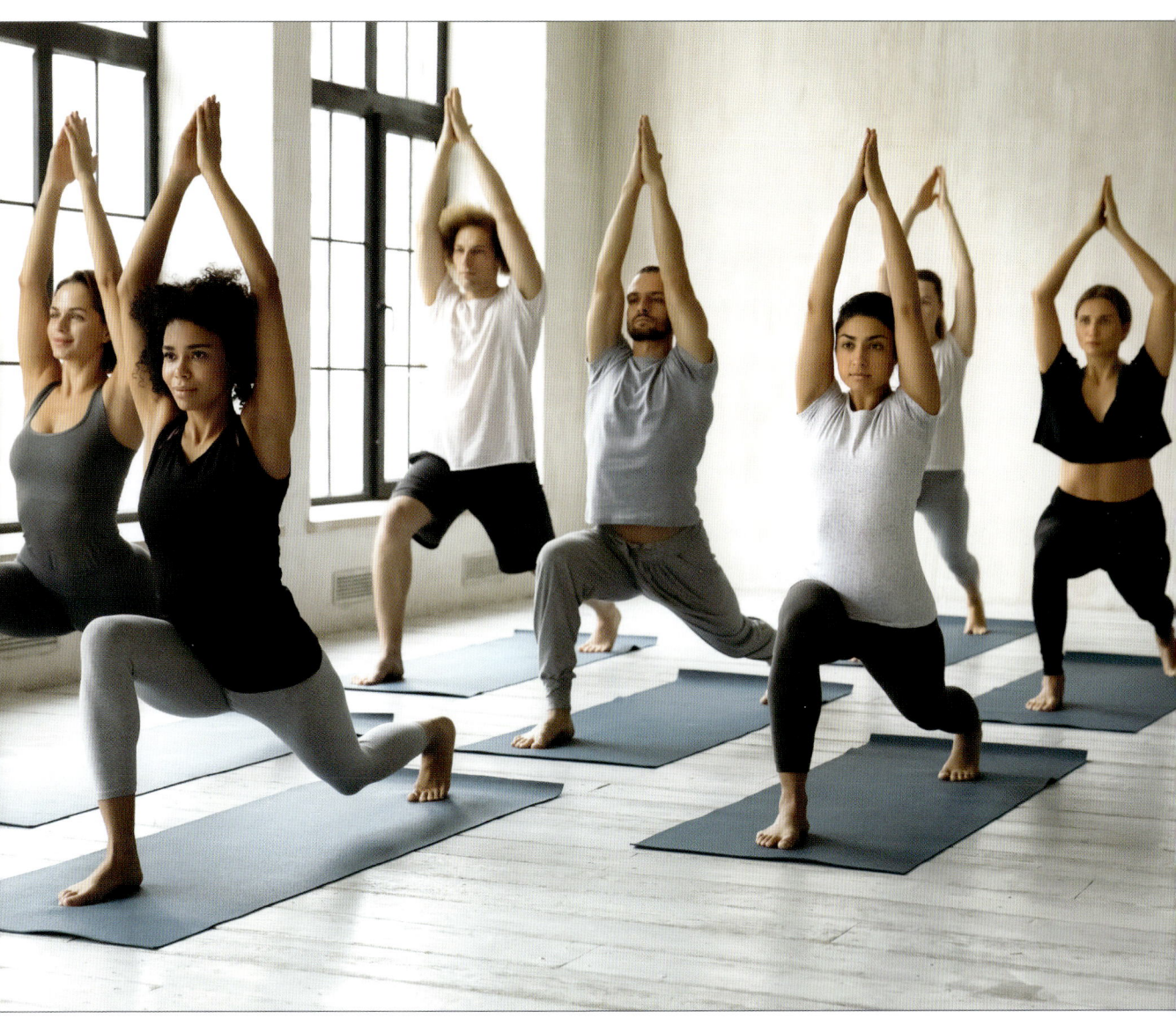

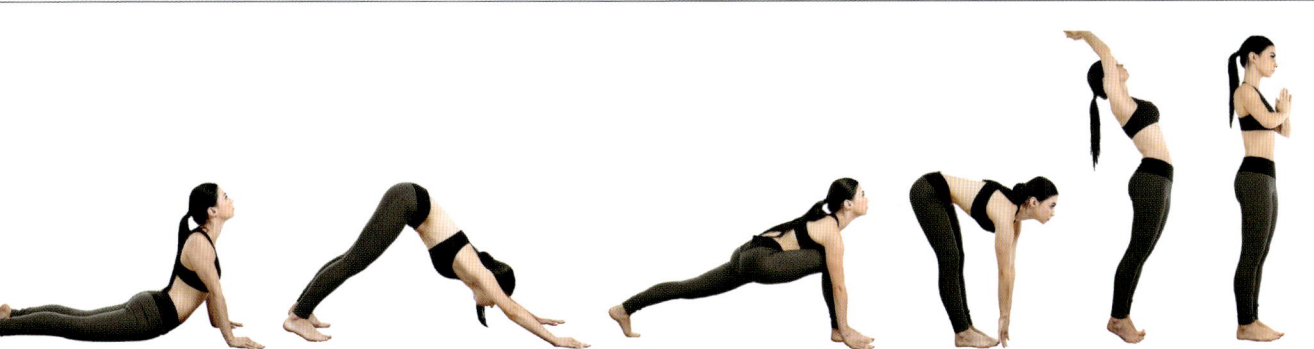

YOGA FLOWS

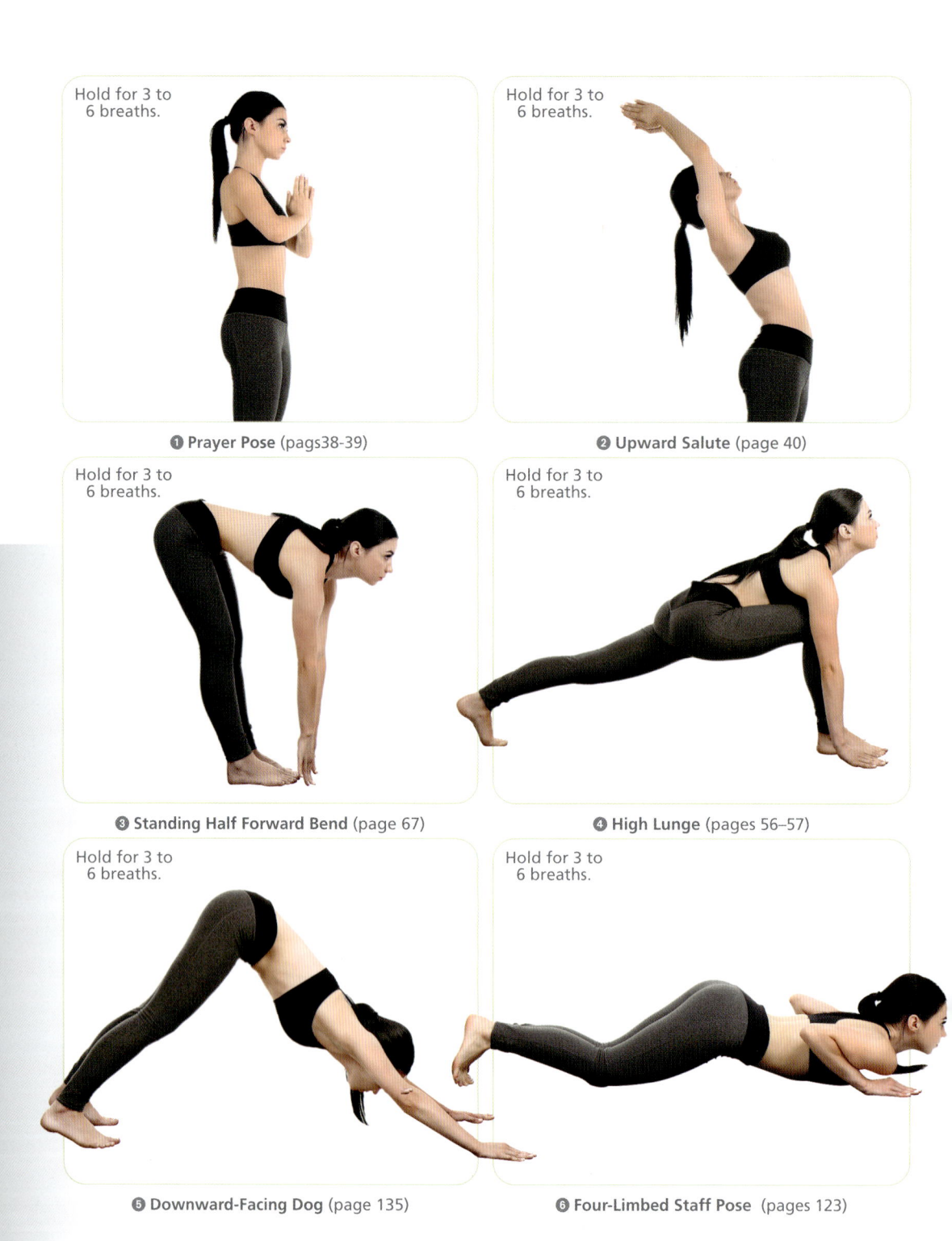

SUN SALUTATION

Hold for 3 to 6 breaths.

❶ Prayer Pose (pags38-39)

Hold for 3 to 6 breaths.

❷ Upward Salute (page 40)

Hold for 3 to 6 breaths.

❸ Standing Half Forward Bend (page 67)

Hold for 3 to 6 breaths.

❹ High Lunge (pages 56–57)

Hold for 3 to 6 breaths.

❺ Downward-Facing Dog (page 135)

Hold for 3 to 6 breaths.

❻ Four-Limbed Staff Pose (pages 123)

144

SUN SALUTATION • YOGA FLOWS

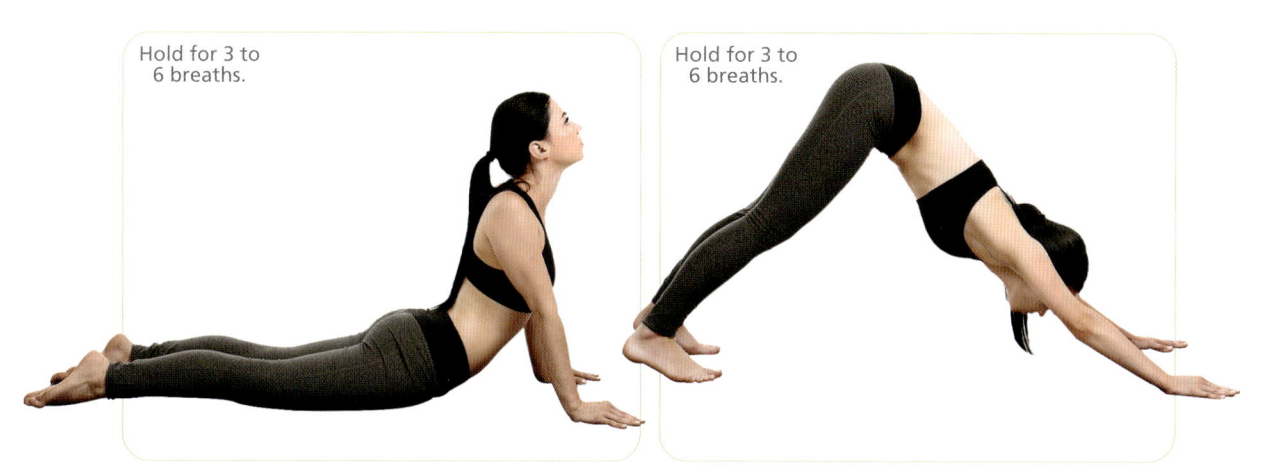

Hold for 3 to 6 breaths.

7 Cobra Pose (pages 80-81)

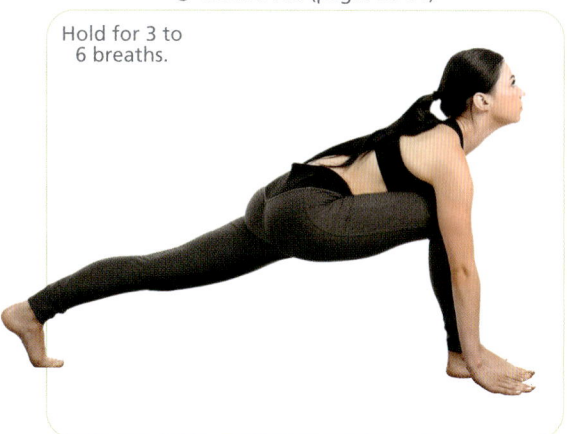

Hold for 3 to 6 breaths.

8 Downward-Facing Dog (page 135)

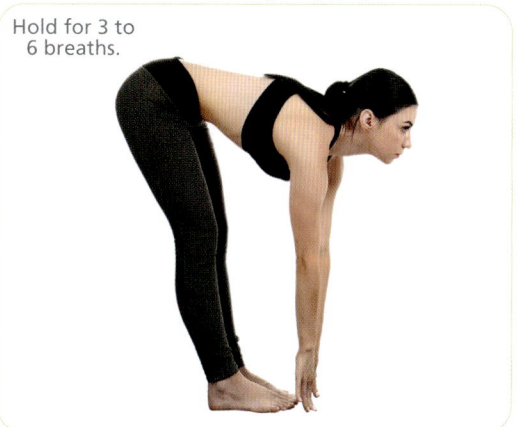

Hold for 3 to 6 breaths.

9 High Lunge (pages 56–57)

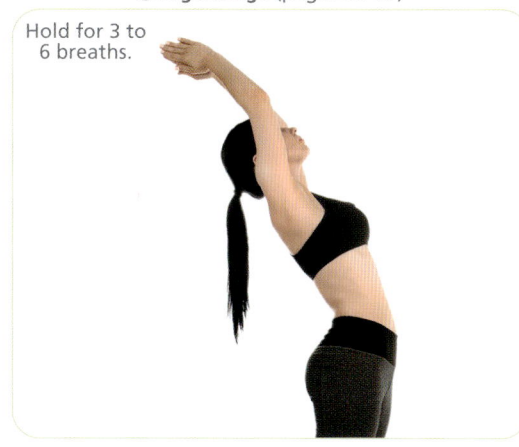

Hold for 3 to 6 breaths.

10 Standing Half Forward Bend (page 67)

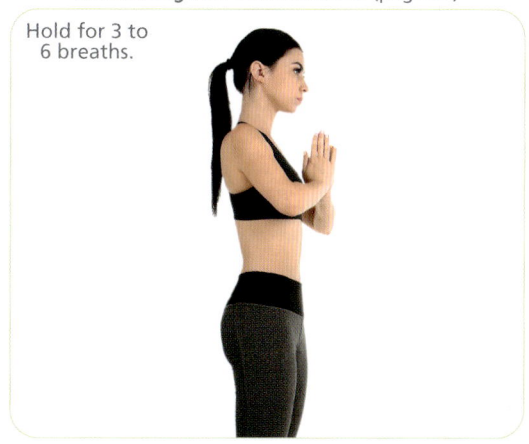

Hold for 3 to 6 breaths.

11 Upward Salute (page 40)

Hold for 3 to 6 breaths.

1 Prayer Pose (pags38-39)

145

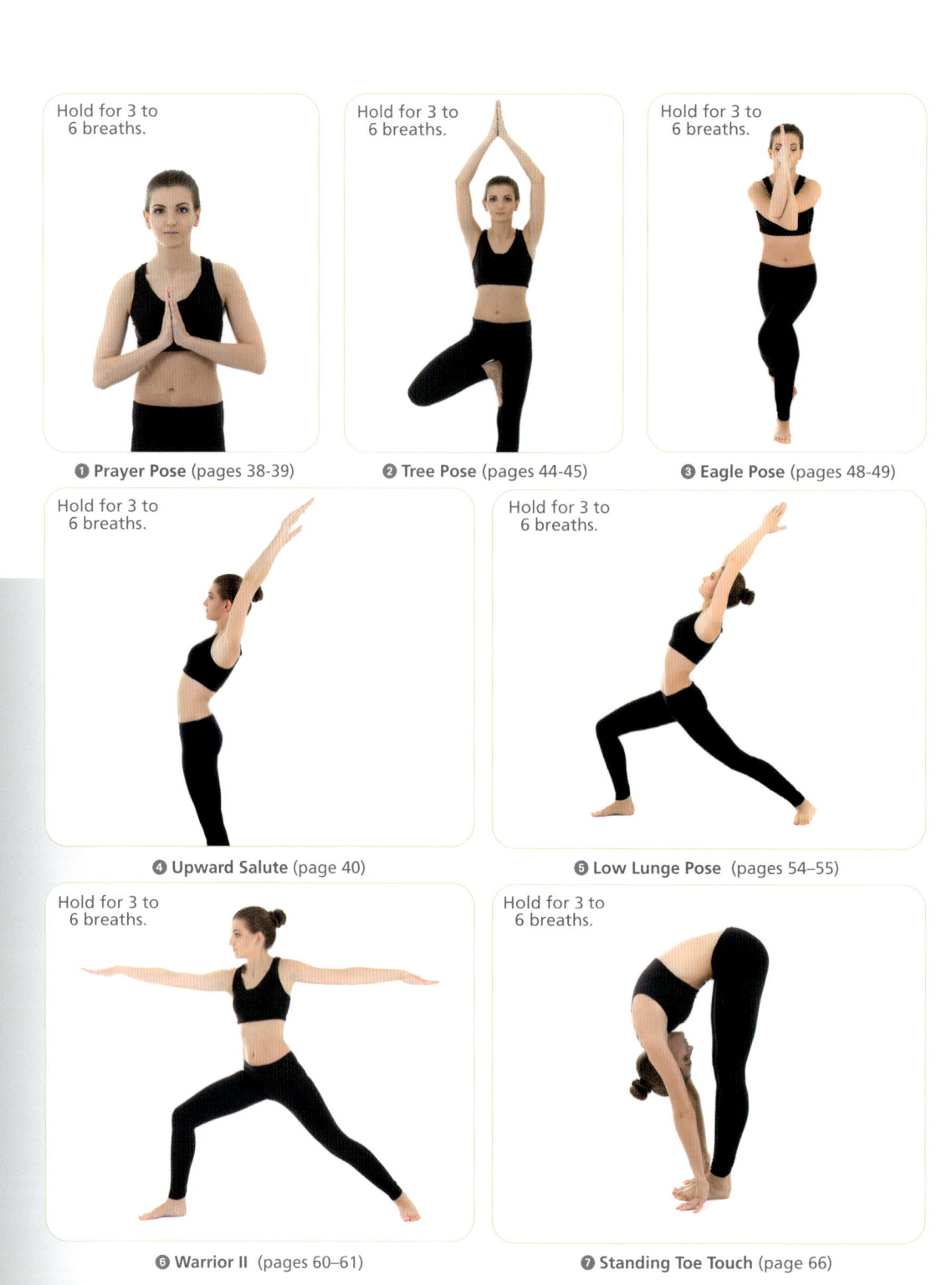

NOVICE FLOW

YOGA FLOWS

Hold for 3 to 6 breaths.

❶ **Prayer Pose** (pages 38-39)

Hold for 3 to 6 breaths.

❷ **Tree Pose** (pages 44-45)

Hold for 3 to 6 breaths.

❸ **Eagle Pose** (pages 48-49)

Hold for 3 to 6 breaths.

❹ **Upward Salute** (page 40)

Hold for 3 to 6 breaths.

❺ **Low Lunge Pose** (pages 54–55)

Hold for 3 to 6 breaths.

❻ **Warrior II** (pages 60–61)

Hold for 3 to 6 breaths.

❼ **Standing Toe Touch** (page 66)

NOVICE FLOW • YOGA FLOWS

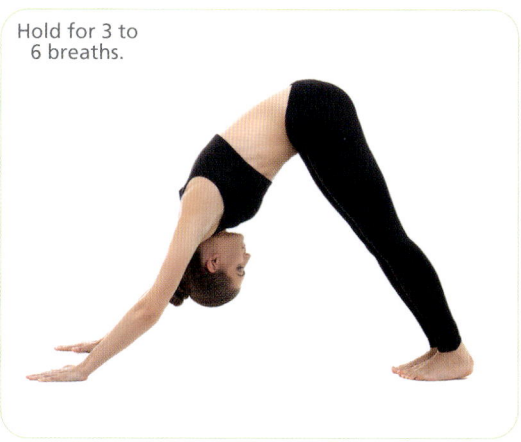

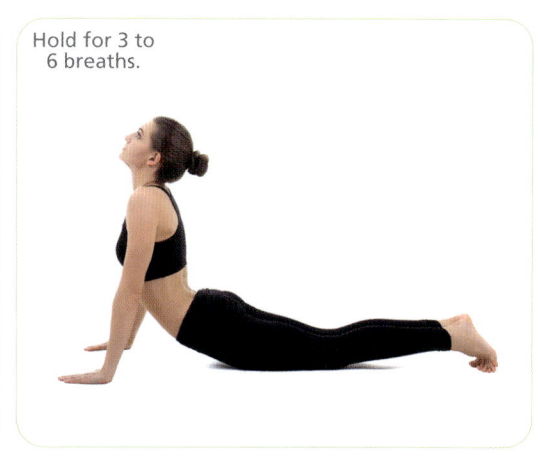

Hold for 3 to 6 breaths.

❽ **Downward-Facing Dog** (page 135)

Hold for 3 to 6 breaths.

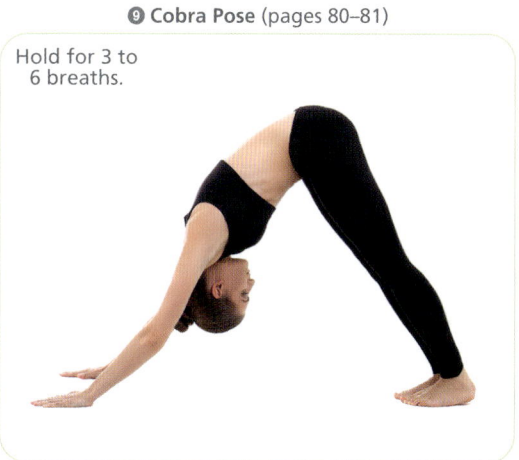

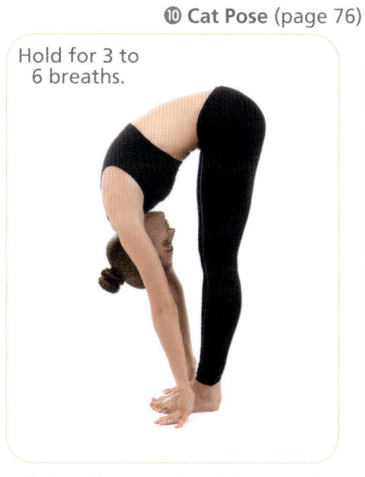

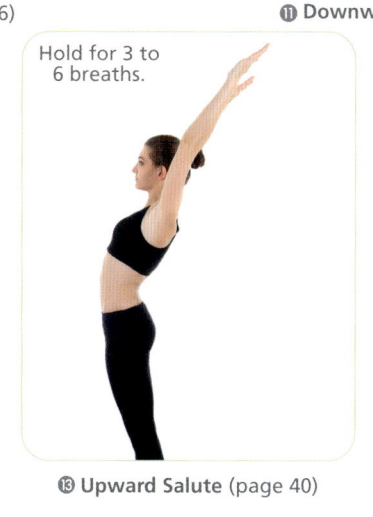

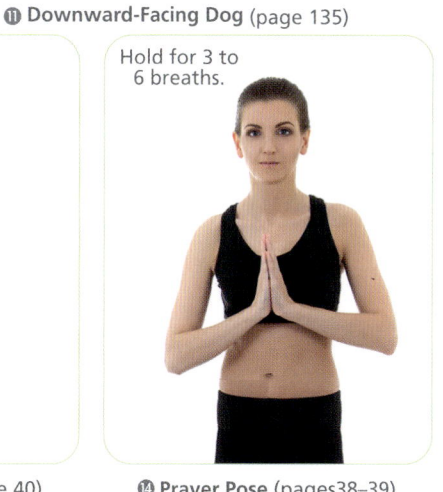

❾ **Cobra Pose** (pages 80–81)

Hold for 3 to 6 breaths.

❿ **Cat Pose** (page 76)

Hold for 3 to 6 breaths.

⓫ **Downward-Facing Dog** (page 135)

Hold for 3 to 6 breaths.

⓬ **Standing Toe Touch** (page 66)

Hold for 3 to 6 breaths.

⓭ **Upward Salute** (page 40)

Hold for 3 to 6 breaths.

⓮ **Prayer Pose** (pages 38–39)

EXTENDED NOVICE FLOW

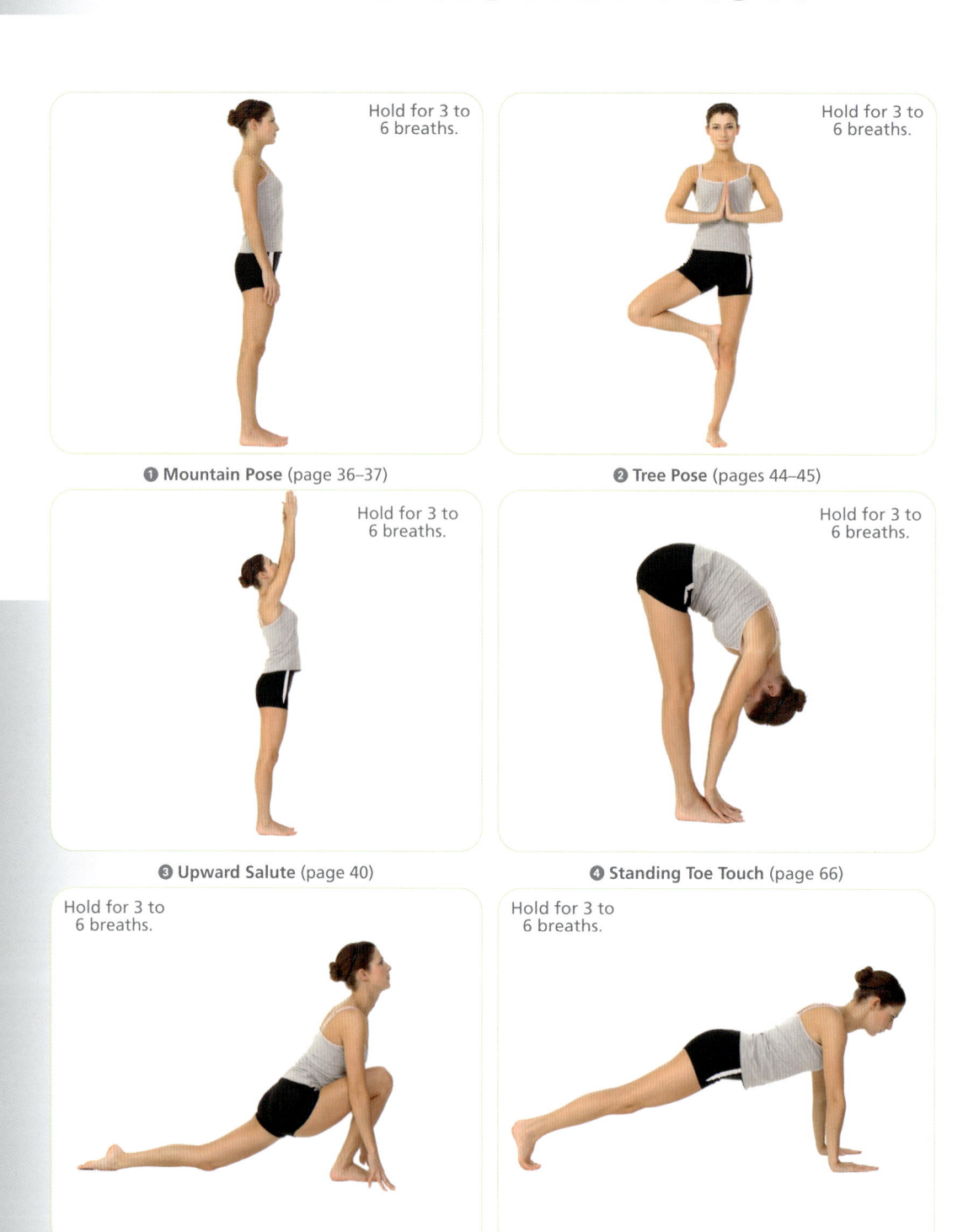

YOGA FLOWS

Hold for 3 to 6 breaths.

❶ **Mountain Pose** (page 36–37)

Hold for 3 to 6 breaths.

❷ **Tree Pose** (pages 44–45)

Hold for 3 to 6 breaths.

❸ **Upward Salute** (page 40)

Hold for 3 to 6 breaths.

❹ **Standing Toe Touch** (page 66)

Hold for 3 to 6 breaths.

❺ **High Lunge** (pages 56–57)

Hold for 3 to 6 breaths.

❻ **Plank Pose** (page 122)

148

EXTENDED NOVICE FLOW • YOGA FLOWS

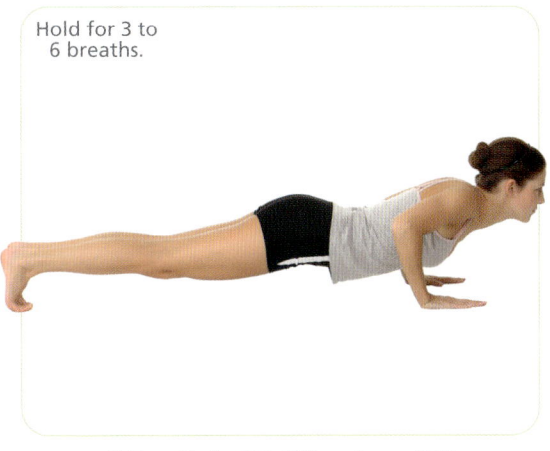

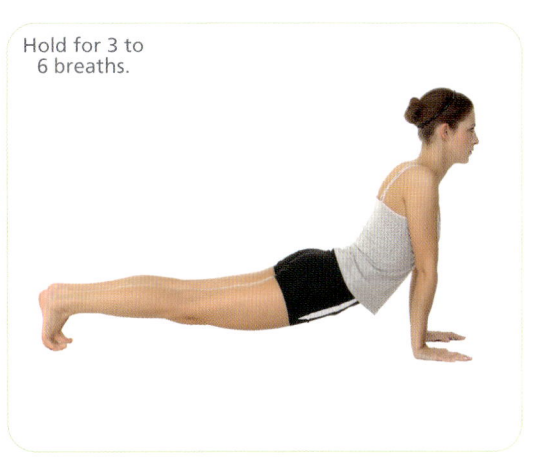

Hold for 3 to 6 breaths.

⑦ Four-Limbed Staff Pose (page 123)

Hold for 3 to 6 breaths.

⑧ Cobra Pose (pages 80–81)

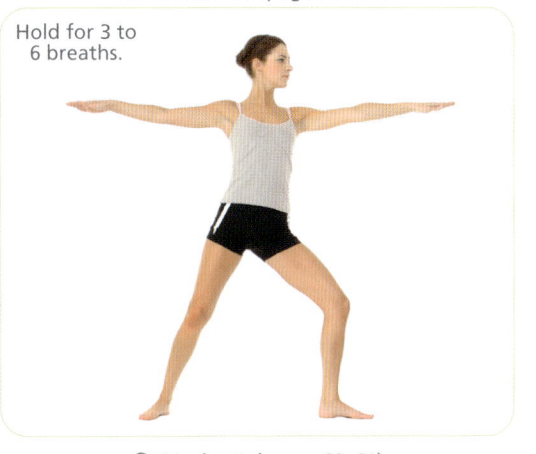

Hold for 3 to 6 breaths.

⑨ Downward-Facing Dog (page 135)

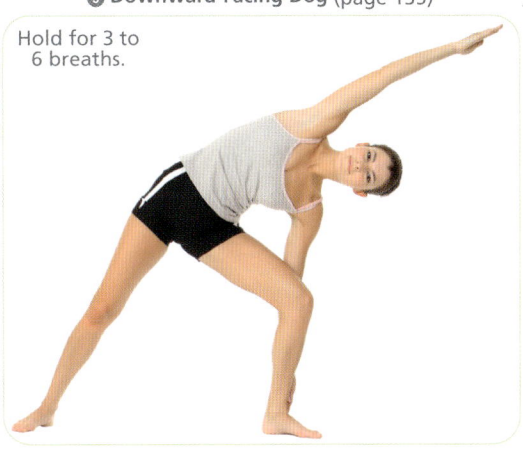

Hold for 3 to 6 breaths.

⑩ Warrior II (pages 60–61)

Hold for 3 to 6 breaths.

⑪ Extended Side Angle Pose (pages 52–53)

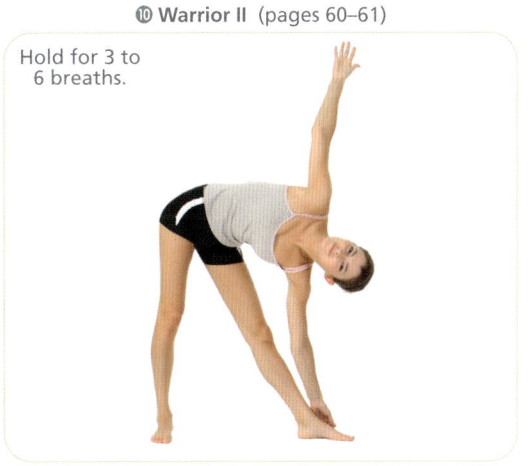

Hold for 3 to 6 breaths.

⑫ Triangle Pose (pages 50–51)

149

EXTENDED NOVICE FLOW CONTD.

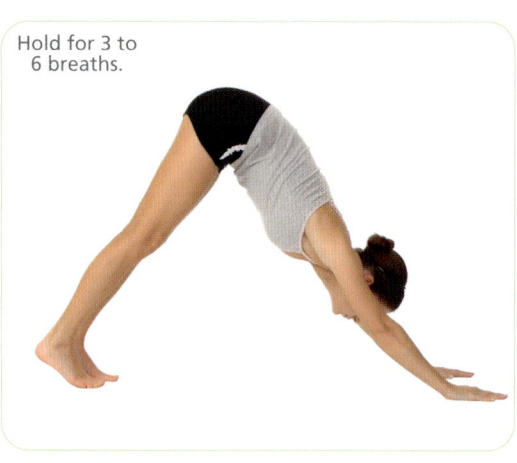

YOGA FLOWS

Hold for 3 to 6 breaths.

⑬ **Downward-Facing Dog** (pages 135)

Hold for 3 to 6 breaths.

⑭ **Cobra Pose** (pages 80–81)

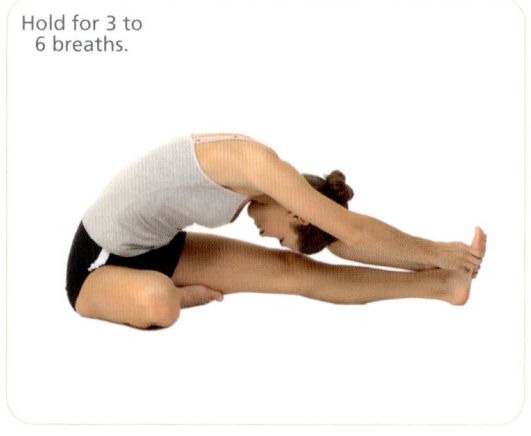

Hold for 3 to 6 breaths.

⑮ **Garland Pose** (pages 46–47)

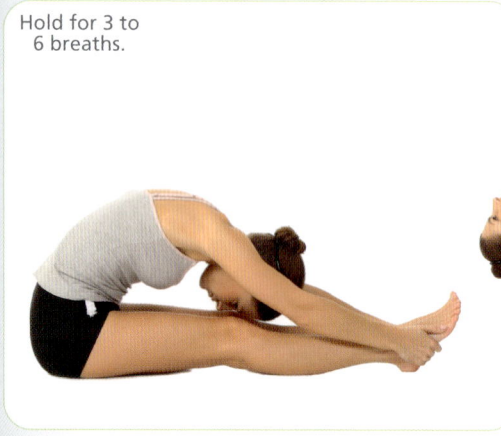

Hold for 3 to 6 breaths.

⑯ **Head-to-Knee Forward Bend** (pages 68-69)

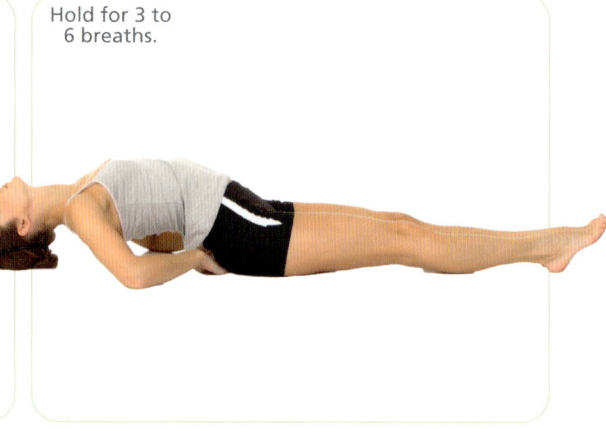

Hold for 3 to 6 breaths.

⑰ **Seated Forward Bend** (pags 70–71)

Hold for 3 to 6 breaths.

⑱ **Fish Pose** (pages 90–91)

EXTENDED NOVICE FLOW • YOGA FLOWS

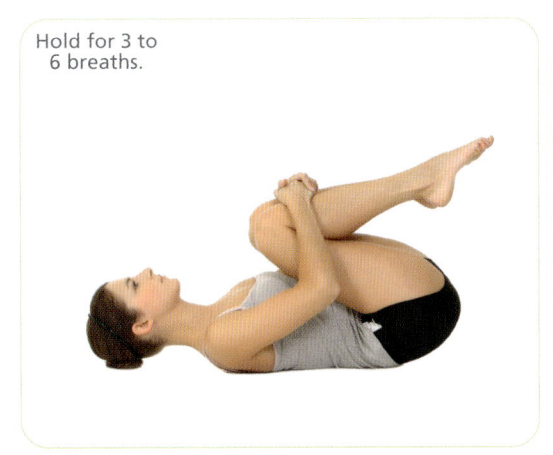

Hold for 3 to 6 breaths.

⑲ **Knees-to-Chest Pose** (page 136-37)

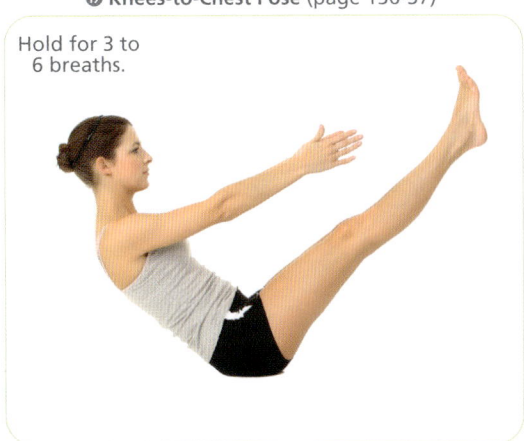

Hold for 3 to 6 breaths.

⑳ **Seated Forward Bend** (page 70–71)

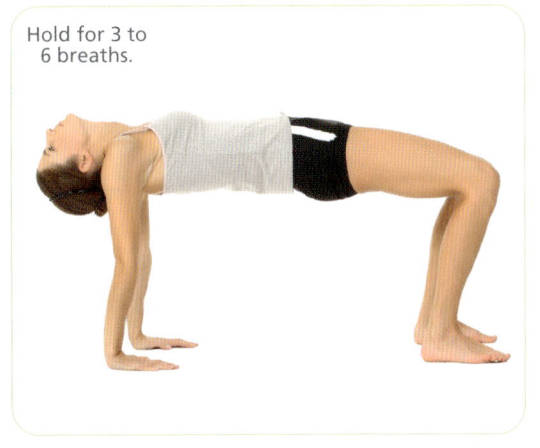

Hold for 3 to 6 breaths.

㉑ **Boat Pose** (pages 108–109)

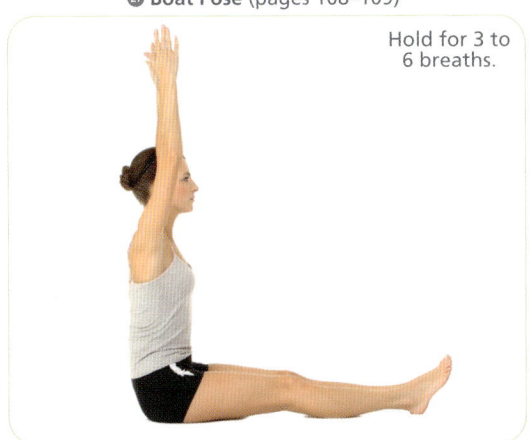

Hold for 3 to 6 breaths.

㉒ **Upward-Facing Bow Pose** (pages 128–129)

Hold for 3 to 6 breaths.

㉓ **Staff Pose** (pages 98–99)

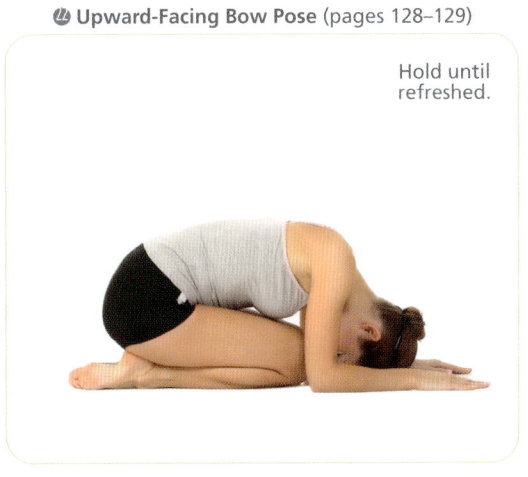

Hold until refreshed.

● **Child's Pose** (page 134)

SPINAL FLOW

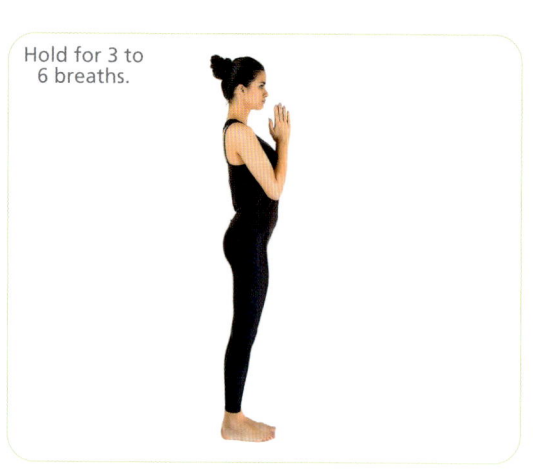

YOGA FLOWS

Hold for 3 to 6 breaths.

❶ **Prayer Pose** (page 38–9)

Hold for 3 to 6 breaths.

❷ **Upward Salute** (page 40)

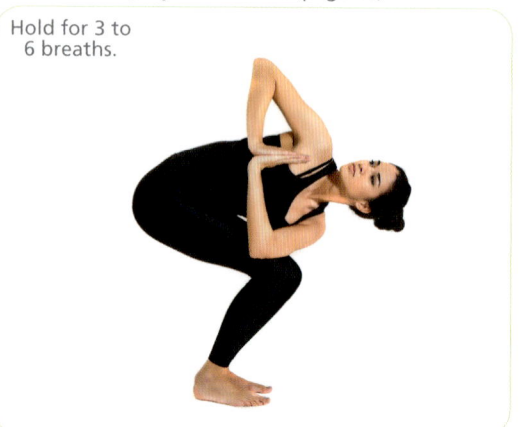

Hold for 3 to 6 breaths.

❸ **High Lunge** (pages 56–57)

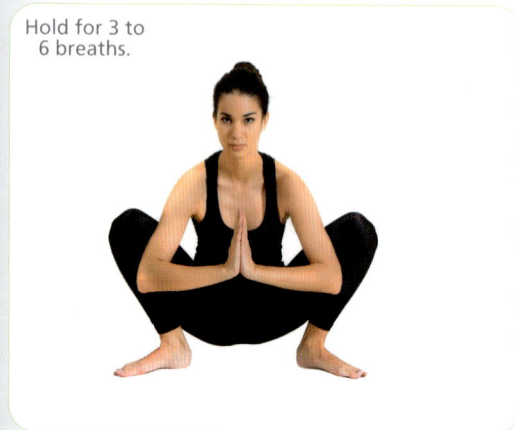

Hold for 3 to 6 breaths.

❹ **Twisting Chair Pose** (page 42-3)

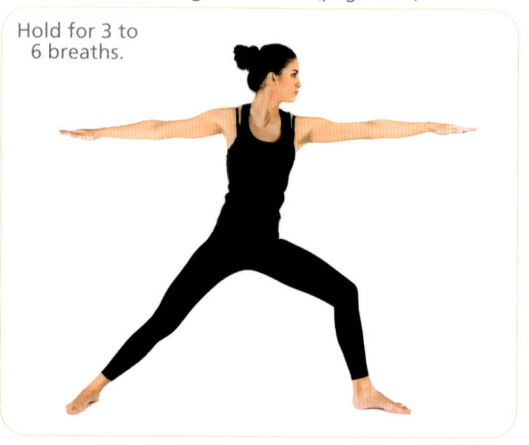

Hold for 3 to 6 breaths.

❿ **Garland Pose** (pages 46–47)

Hold for 3 to 6 breaths.

❺ **Warrior II** (pages 60–61)

152

SPINAL FLOW • YOGA FLOWS

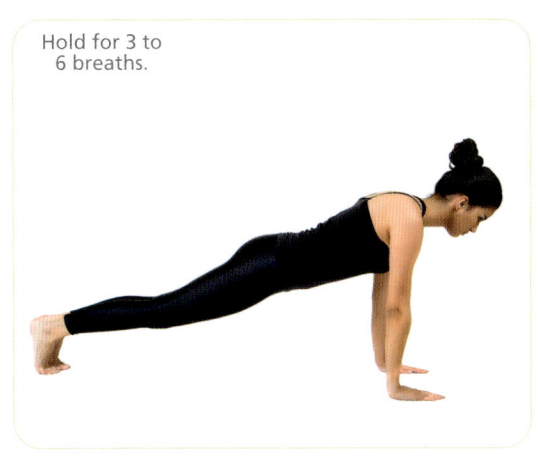

Hold for 3 to 6 breaths.

⑦ Plank Pose (page 122)

Hold for 3 to 6 breaths.

⑧ High Lunge (pages 56–57)

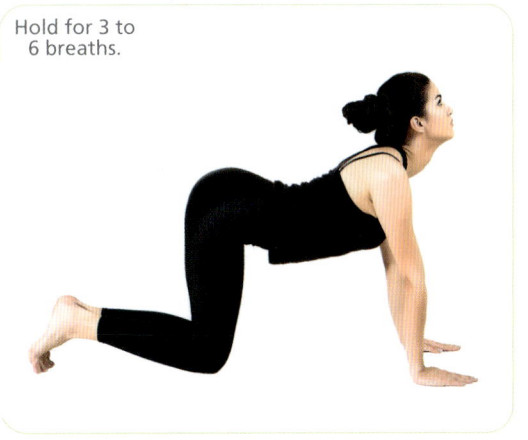

Hold for 3 to 6 breaths.

⑨ Downward-Facing Dog (page 135)

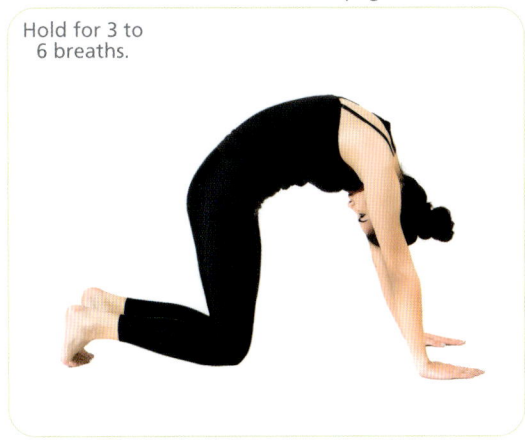

Hold for 3 to 6 breaths.

⑩ Cat Pose (page 76)

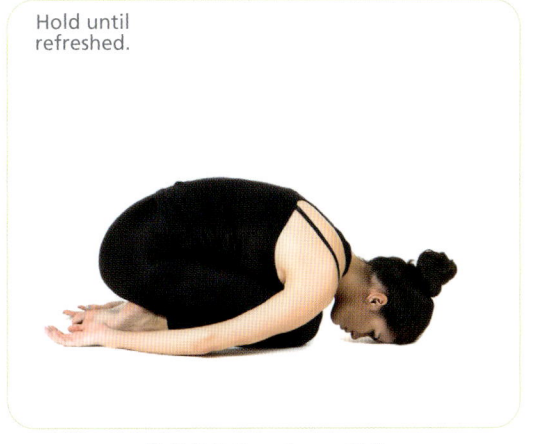

Hold for 3 to 6 breaths.

⑪ Cow Pose (page 77)

Hold until refreshed.

⑫ Child's Pose (page 134)

BALANCED FLOW

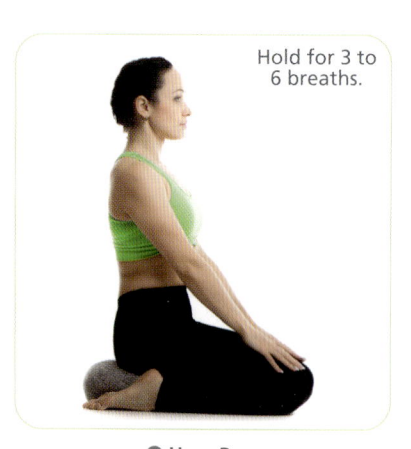

YOGA FLOWS

Hold for 3 to 6 breaths.

① Hero Pose
(page 139)

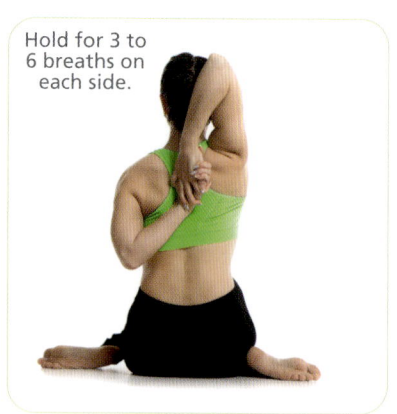

Hold for 3 to 6 breaths on each side.

② Cow-Face Pose
(pages 104-105)

Hold for 3 to 6 breaths.

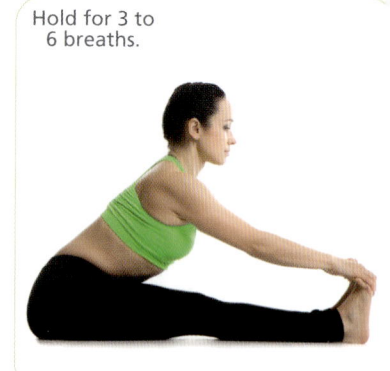

③ Seated Forward Bend
(pages 70-71)

Hold for 3 to 6 breaths on each side.

④ Marichi's Pose
(pages 112-113)

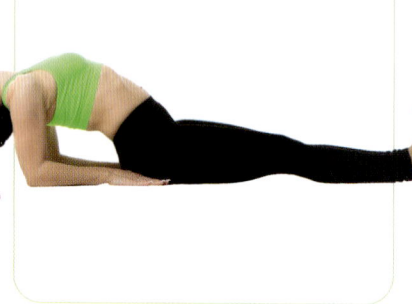

Hold for 3 to 6 breaths.

⑤ Fish Pose
(pages 90+91)

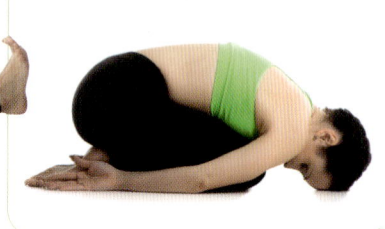

Hold until refreshed.

⑥ Child's Pose
(page 134)

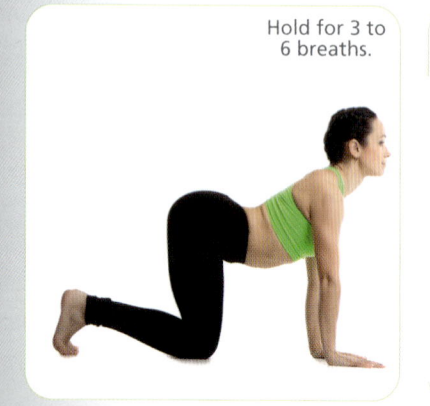

Hold for 3 to 6 breaths.

⑦ Cat Pose
(page 76)

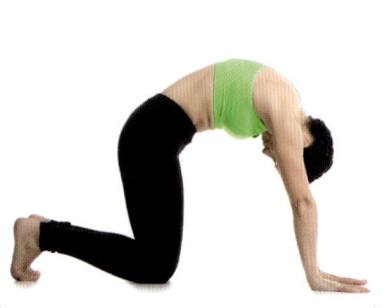

Hold for 3 to 6 breaths.

⑧ Cow Pose
(page 77)

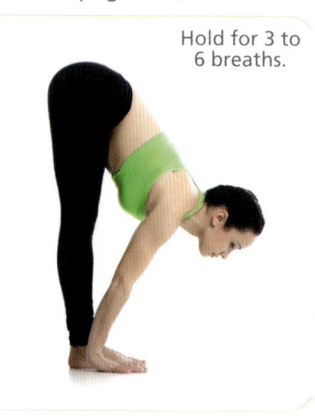

Hold for 3 to 6 breaths.

⑨ Standing Half Forward Bend
(page 67)

BALANCED FLOW • YOGA FLOWS

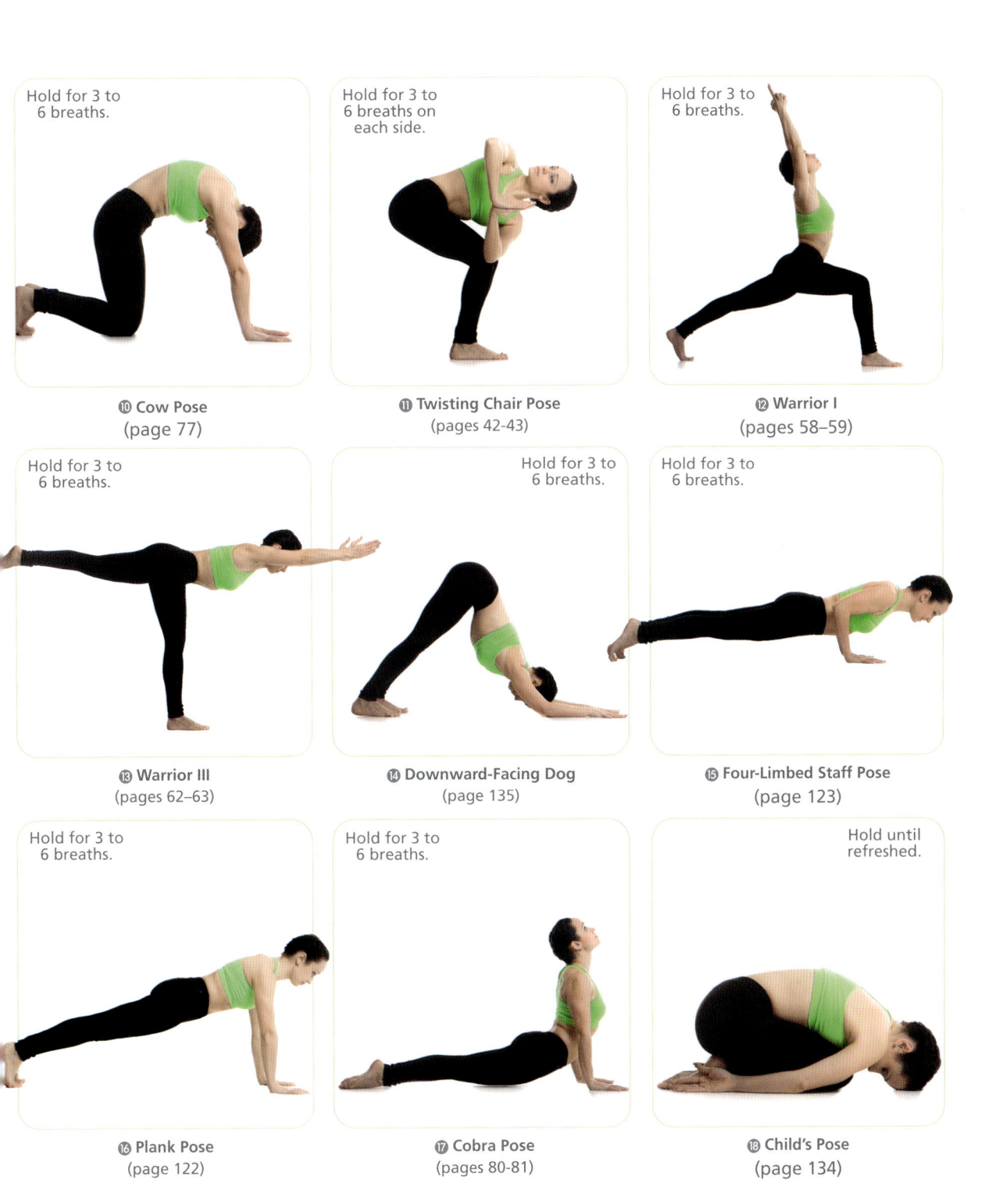

Hold for 3 to 6 breaths.

⑩ Cow Pose
(page 77)

Hold for 3 to 6 breaths on each side.

⑪ Twisting Chair Pose
(pages 42–43)

Hold for 3 to 6 breaths.

⑫ Warrior I
(pages 58–59)

Hold for 3 to 6 breaths.

⑬ Warrior III
(pages 62–63)

Hold for 3 to 6 breaths.

⑭ Downward-Facing Dog
(page 135)

Hold for 3 to 6 breaths.

⑮ Four-Limbed Staff Pose
(page 123)

Hold for 3 to 6 breaths.

⑯ Plank Pose
(page 122)

Hold for 3 to 6 breaths.

⑰ Cobra Pose
(pages 80–81)

Hold until refreshed.

⑱ Child's Pose
(page 134)

155

MUSCLE GLOSSARY

The following glossary explains the Latin terminology used to describe the body's musculature. Certain words are derived from Greek; these have been indicated in each instance.

Neck

levator scapulae: *levare*, "to raise," and *scapulae*, "shoulder [blades]"

scalenes: Greek *skalénós*, "unequal"

splenius: Greek *splénion*, "plaster, patch"

sternocleidomastoideus: Greek *stérnon*, "chest," Greek *kleís*, "key," and Greek *mastoeidés*, "breast-like"

Back

erector spinae: *erectus*, "straight," and *spina*, "thorn"

latissimus dorsi: *latus*, "wide," and *dorsum*, "back"

multifidus spinae: *multus*, "much," *findere*, "to split," and *spina*, "thorn"

quadratus lumborum: *quadratus*, "square" or "rectangular," and *lumbus*, "loin"

rhomboideus: Greek *rhembesthai*, "to spin"

trapezius: Greek *trapezion*, "small table"

Chest

coracobrachialis: Greek *korakoeidés*, "raven-like," and *brachium*, "arm"

pectoralis [major and minor]: *pectus*, "breast"

Shoulders

deltoideus [anterior, posterior, and medialis]: Greek *deltoeidés*, "delta-shaped"

infraspinatus: *infra*, "under," and *spina*, "thorn"

subscapularis: *sub*, "below," and *scapulae*, "shoulder [blades]"

supraspinatus: *supra*, "above," and *spina*, "thorn"

teres [major and minor]: *teres*, "rounded"

Core

obliquus externus: *obliquus*, "slanting," and *externus*, "outward"

obliquus internus: *obliquus*, "slanting," and *internus*, "within"

rectus abdominis: *rego*, "straight, upright," and *abdomen*, "belly"

serratus anterior: *serra*, "saw," and *ante*, "before"

transversus abdominis: *transversus*, "athwart," and *abdomen*, "belly"

Hips

gemellus inferior: *geminus*, "twin" and *inferus*, "under"

gemellus superior: *geminus*, "twin" and *super*, "above"

gluteus maximus: Greek *gloutós*, "rump," with Latin *maximus*, "largest"

gluteus medius: Greek *gloutós*, "rump," with Latin *medialis*, "middle"

iliacus: *ilia*, "groin"

MUSCLE GLOSSARY • APPENDICES

iliopsoas: *ilia*, "groin," and Greek *psoa*, "groin muscle"

iliotibial band: *ilia*, "groin," and *tibia*, "reed pipe"

obturator externus: *obturare*, "to block," and *externus*, "outward"

obturator internus: *obturare*, "to block," and *internus*, "within"

pectineus: *pectin*, "comb"

piriformis: *pirum*, "pear," and *forma*, "shape"

quadratus femoris: *quadratus*, "square" or "rectangular," and *femur*, "thigh"

Upper Arm

biceps brachii: *biceps*, "two-headed," and *brachium*, "arm"

brachialis: *brachium*, "arm"

triceps brachii: *triceps*, "three-headed," and *brachium*, "arm"

Lower Arm

brachioradialis: *brachium*, "arm," and *radius*, "spoke"

extensor carpi radialis: *extendere*, "to bend"; Greek *karpós*, "wrist"; and *radius*, "spoke"

extensor digitorum: *extendere*, "to bend," and *digitus*, "finger, toe"

flexor carpi radialis: *lectere*, "to bend"; Greek *karpós*, "wrist"; and *radius*, "spoke"

flexor digitorum: *flectere*, "to bend," and *digitus*, "finger" or "toe"

Upper Leg

adductor longus: *adducere*, "to contract," and *longus*, "long"

adductor magnus: *adducere*, "to contract," and *magnus*, "major"

biceps femoris: *biceps*, "two-headed," and *femur*, "thigh"

gracilis: *gracilis*, "slim, slender"

rectus femoris: *rego*, "straight" or "upright," and *femur*, "thigh"

sartorius: *sarcio*, "to patch" or "to repair"

semimembranosus: *semi*, "half," and *membrum*, "limb"

semitendinosus: *semi*, "half," and *tendo*, "tendon"

tensor fasciae latae: *tenere*, "to stretch"; *fasciae*, "band"; and *latae* "laid down"

vastus intermedius: *vastus*, "immense, huge," and *intermedius*, "between"

vastus lateralis: *vastus*, "immense, huge," and *lateralis*, "of the side"

vastus medialis: *vastus*, "immense, huge," and *medialis*, "middle"

Lower Leg

extensor hallucis: *extendere*, "to bend," and *hallex*, "big toe"

flexor hallucis: *flectere*, "to bend," and *hallex*, "big toe"

gastrocnemius: Greek *gastroknémía*, "calf [of the leg]"

peroneus: *peronei*, "of the fibula"

soleus: *solea*, "sandal"

tibialis anterior: *tibia*, "reed pipe," and *ante*, "before"

tibialis posterior: *tibia*, "reed pipe," and *posterus*, "coming after"

INDEX OF POSE NAMES

APPENDICES

Awkward Pose	141	High Lunge	56-57
Bharadvaja's Twist	110-11	Knees-to-Chest Pose	136-7
Boat Pose	108-9	Locust Pose	126-7
Bound angle pose	100	Low Lunge Pose	54-55
Bound angle pose	101	Marichi's pose	112-3
Bow Pose	82-83	Mountain Pose	36-37
Bridge Pose	84-85	Plank Pose	122
Camel Pose	86-87	Prayer Pose	38-39
Cat Pose to Cow Pose	76-77	Reclining twist	116-7
Child's Pose	134-5	Reverse Tabletop Pose	88-89
Cobra Pose	80-81	Seated Forward Bend	70-71
Corpse Pose	138	Side Plank Pose	124-5
Cow-Face Pose	104-5	Staff Pose	98-99
Downward-Facing Dog	135	Standing Half Forward Bend	67
Eagle Pose	48-49	Standing Toe Touch	66
Easy Pose	96-97	Supported Shoulderstand	130-31
Extended Puppy Pose	74-75	Tree Pose	44-45
Extended Side Angle Pose	52-53	Triangle Pose	50-51
Fire log pose	102-3	Twisting chair pose	42-43
Fish Pose	90-91	Upward-Facing Bow Pose	128-9
Four-Limbed Staff Pose	123	Upward-Facing Dog Pose	78-79
Full lotus pose	107	Upward Plank Pose	120-21
Garland Pose	46-47	Upward Salute	40
Half-Frog Pose	92-93	Warrior Pose I	58-59
Half lord of the fishes	114-5	Warrior Pose II	60-61
Half lotus pose	106	Warrior Pose III	62-63
Head-to-Knee Forward Bend	68-69	Wide-Legged Forward Bend	72-73
Hero pose	139		

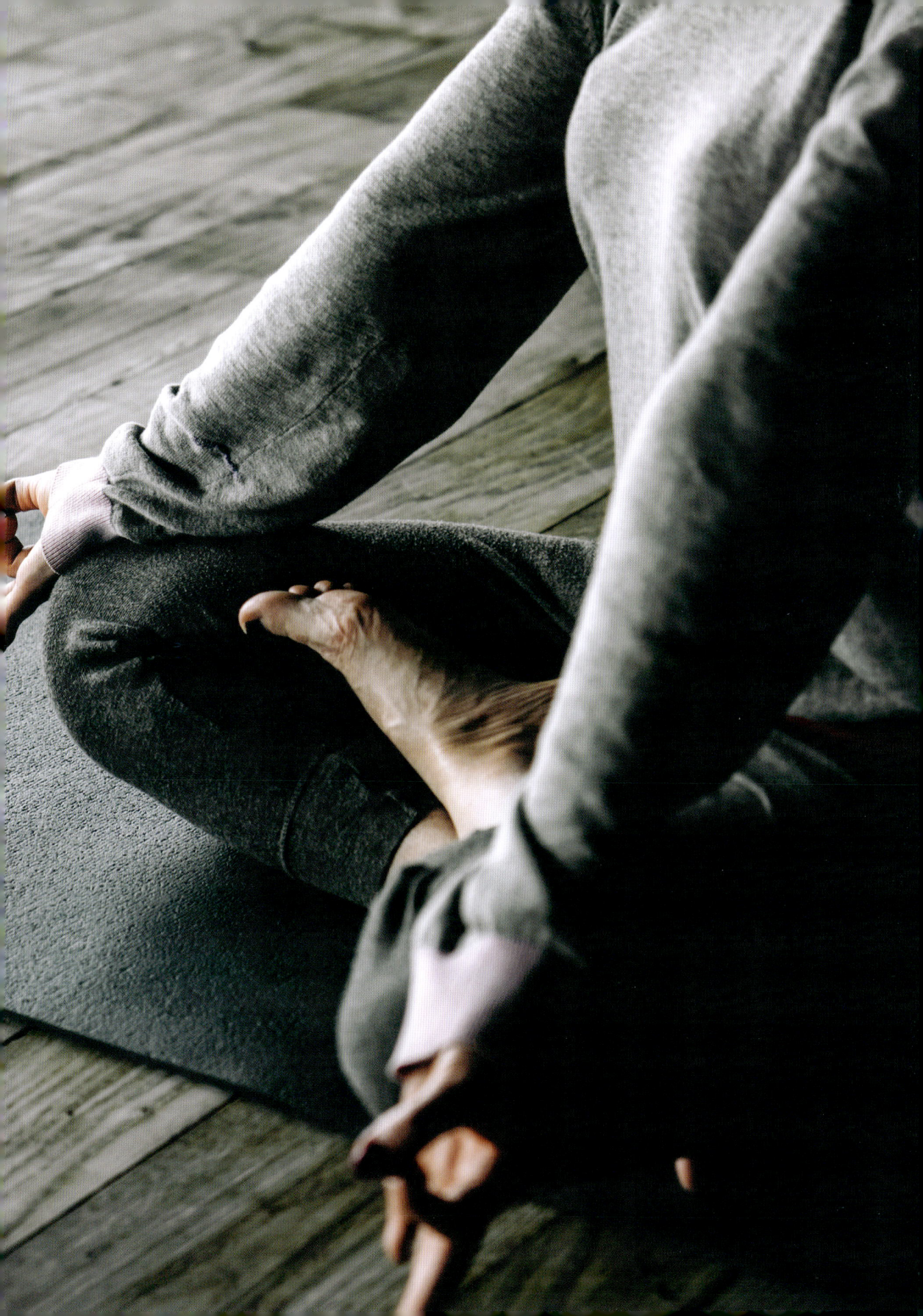

PHOTO CREDITS

APPENDICES

All images are from Shutterstock.com and Moseleyroad inc.

For detailed credits, please contact info@moseleyroad.com

All image manipulation by Adam Moore.